Kempe's Operative Neurosurgery

VOLUME TWO

POSTERIOR FOSSA, SPINAL AND PERIPHERAL NERVE

SECOND EDITION

Springer
New York
Berlin
Heidelberg
Hong Kong
London
Milan
Paris
Tokyo

Kempe's Operative Neurosurgery

VOLUME TWO

POSTERIOR FOSSA, SPINAL AND PERIPHERAL NERVE

SECOND EDITION

With 284 figures

Michael Salcman, MD
Chief, Division of Neurosurgery
Sinai Hospital
Baltimore, Maryland

Roberto C. Heros, MD
Professor, Co-chairman and Program Director
Department of Neurological Surgery
University of Miami School of Medicine
Miami, Florida

Edward R. Laws, Jr., MD
Professor of Neurosurgery
Professor of Medicine
Department of Neurological Surgery
University of Virginia Health Sciences Center
Charlottesville, Virginia

Volker K. H. Sonntag, MD
Clinical Professor of Neurosurgery
University of Arizona
Director of Resident Neurosurgery Program
Barrow Neurological Institute
Phoenix, Arizona

Springer

The Editors would like to thank the following illustrators for their invaluable contribution to both volumes of *Kempe's Operative Neurosurgery*: Birck Cox, Nicole Mock, Wiesia Langenfeld, Beth La Row, Anne Rains, Ann Saydlowski, and Paul Schiffmacher. This project was brought to completion by Elise Paxson, Senior Development Editor at Current Medicine. We are also very grateful to the senior staff at Springer-Verlag in New York.

The Library of Congress has catalogued the first volume as follows:

Library of Congress Cataloging-in-Publication Data

Kempe's operative neurosurgery. --2nd ed.
p. ; cm.
Includes bibliographical references and index.
ISBN 0-387-98537-9 (hard cover : alk. paper)
1. Nervous system--Surgery--Atlases. I. Title: Operative Neurosurgery. II. Salcman, Michael. III. Kempe, Ludwig G. Operative neurosurgery.
[DNLM: 1. Nervous System Diseases--surgery--Atlases. 2. Neurosurgical Procedures--Atlases. WL 17 K32 2000]
RD593 .K4 2000
617.4'8--dc21

99-045301

Kempe's Operative Neurosurgery, Volume Two, ISBN 0-387-98536-0 Printed on acid-free paper.

Printed in the United States of America.

9 8 7 6 5 4 3 2 1 SPIN 10678960

www.springer-ny.com

Springer-Verlag New York Berlin Heidelberg
A member of BertelsmannSpringer Science+Business Media GmbH

Preface

This second volume of the revised edition of *Kempe's Operative Neurosurgery* continues to follow the organization of its original model. The topics are presented in a "top down" anatomical sequence from the posterior fossa to the lumbar spine and peripheral nerves. Significant additions include a chapter on carotid endarterectomy and several new sections on spinal instrumentation. We have attempted to keep the text brief and to the point; further details can be found in the very few references that are cited. The inevitable omissions and inadvertent errors in a work of this scope are entirely my responsibility. This second volume could not have been completed without the contributions of my co-editors, dear friends and passionate scholars all.

Michael Salcman, MD

Contents

CHAPTER

25

Suboccipital Craniectomy: Retromastoid Approach for Acoustic Schwannoma

The most common position for posterior fossa operations in adults is the lateral decubitus or "park bench" position; this approach has largely replaced the use of the sitting position for most procedures. After intubation and placement of a three-point head fixation device, the patient is turned on his side and the shoulder contralateral to the lesion supported by a roll in the axilla; the ipsilateral shoulder is rolled forward and pulled down with tape (Fig. 25-1). The dependent arm can be suspended by a sling in the crook of the Mayfield attachment. All pressure points are carefully padded. In lesions of the cerebellopontine angle, the head is kept in a relatively neutral position and the body is slightly elevated (reverse Trendelenberg). A straight retromastoid incision is used for most lesions centered on the internal acoustic meatus and for exploration of the cranial nerves (see Chapter 26). The incision is usually 8 to 10 cm long and is made one fingerbreadth medial to the mastoid process and digastric groove (Fig. 25-2). The incision extends from a line just above the top of the pinna of the ear to a point just below the mastoid tip. Care in splitting the muscle at the inferior end is important in avoiding an ectactic vertebral artery. For very large lesions, the superior end of the incision can be extended medially to a point 2 cm above the inion and curved toward the midline (inverted hockeystick) (Fig. 25-3). Once the linear retromastoid incision is cleared down to the bone, it can usually be held open by one or two curved cerebellar retractors.

The first bur hole should be placed near the center of the exposure to avoid the junction of the transverse and sigmoid sinuses in the superolateral corner. Although some surgeons turn a craniotomy flap, it is probably safer to perform a craniectomy. The suboccipital bone is thinned down with a large bur and then removed with rongeurs until a 5-cm-diameter exposure is achieved. The following structures form the boundaries of this exposure: the inferior edge of the transverse sinus superiorly, and the floor of the suboccipital fossa inferiorly (Fig. 25-4). In large lesions, the midline dura medially and the foramen magnum inferiorly should also be exposed. The dura is opened in a semilunar fashion and the edges sewn back to the muscle or placed in traction with hemostats (Fig. 25-5). The delicate surface of the cerebellum should be protected with a rubber dam cut to fit from a surgical glove and covered with a large moist cottonoid before a retractor blade is placed against it. If the cerebellum is "full," spinal fluid can be drained from a previously placed lumbar catheter, or the cisterna magna can be opened in the inferior portion of the field near cranial nerves IX, X, and XI. In dealing with extremely large tumors in the cerebellopontine angle, it is sometimes necessary to resect the thin rim of the cerebellar hemisphere as it caps the tumor so as to avoid postoperative hemorrhage and swelling. Once the cerebellum is relaxed, a narrow-tipped Sugita blade can be slipped over the lateral surface at the midpoint of the exposure and directed toward the flocculus (Fig. 25-6). After the initial approach, two small rectractors placed superiorly and inferiorly in the field sometimes provide better retraction with less bruising of the cerebellum. Prolonged retraction at any single site should be avoided.

So-called "acoustic schwannomas" usually arise from the superior vestibular nerve of the eighth cranial nerve complex within the internal auditory meatus (porus acousticus). Early symptoms include tinnitus and poor speech discrimination while using the telephone. Progressive hearing loss, facial nerve weakness, facial numbness, and unsteady gait are late signs. Modern audiometry and imaging studies, particularly magnetic resonance imaging, allow early diagnosis and, as a result, removal of small tumors. On rare occasions, tumors come to attention only after they have produced pressure on the pons, medulla, and cranial nerves, or have caused increased intracranial pressure. The removal of a medium-sized acoustic schwannoma will be used to further illustrate the principles of the retromastoid approach.

The anatomic relationships of this tumor are illustrated in Figures 25-5, 25-7, and 25-8. The facial nerve, more or less adherent to the tumor capsule, is pushed toward the ventral surface of the tumor. It then passes anteriorly toward the roots of the trigeminal nerve. The facial nerve enters the internal auditory meatus at its anterior extent either in the upper or lower quadrant. The main vascular supply to this tumor is from the posterior inferior and anterior inferior cerebellar arteries, as shown in Figures 25-7 and 25-8. Venous drainage is from the dorsal aspect of the tumor to the petrosal sinus.

The goal in the surgical treatment of this lesion is total removal of the tumor with preservation of the facial nerve. The goal is not always attainable. In small intracanalicular tumors, it is sometimes possible to preserve hearing. In very large tumors, the capsule may be so adherent to the pons and medulla that total removal would result in contusion or infarction of the brain stem. In some situations, a radical intracapsular excision or radiosurgery is preferable to an attempt at complete microsurgical removal. It is not always possible to preserve the seventh nerve. Even though it is carefully identified proximally, close to the brain stem, and distally, as it leaves through the porus acousticus, the facial nerve is most easily injured in the area in between. The nerve often is thin and spread out over the capsule of the tumor. The larger the tumor, the more difficult it will be to preserve the facial nerve.

After the initial steps of the retromastoid exposure have been completed, gentle retraction of the cerebellum places the arachnoid under tension so that it can easily be opened with microforceps and microscissors. Care must be taken not to stir up bleeding on the subjacent surface of the tumor. The arachnoid is frequently thickened in the vicinity of nerves IX, X, and XI at the inferior pole of the tumor (Fig. 25-9). In the upper portion of the field, cranial nerve V is often seen draped over the superior pole of the tumor. Some acoustic schwannomas have a cystic component, and there is often a cyst over the posteroinferior portion of the tumor. On aspirating the cyst, an amber, highly proteinatious fluid is obtained. With collapse of the cyst and opening of the arachnoid, the limits and size of the lesion can now be established. If, at this point, it is apparent that the tumor is so large that a great deal of retraction of the cerebellum is necessary to gain exposure, the thin rim of cerebellum that caps the tumor should be removed. Further exposure can be created by performing a small intracapsular removal (Fig. 25-10). The tumor capsule is entered in an avascular area. The tumor is gutted using a microbipolar forceps and suction or an ultrasonic aspirator. In intracapsular removal, two points must be kept in mind: 1) because the medial extension of the tumor has not been defined, extreme caution must be taken to avoid injury to the brain stem, and 2) because the facial nerve is usually anterior or ventral to the tumor, the capsule must not be violated in these areas. Intraoperative recordings from the facial muscles and electrical stimulation help identify the location of the VIIIth nerve in those rare situations in which it courses through the body of the tumor. It is critical to obtain complete hemostasis when early intracapsular removal has been performed prior to identification of nervous and vascular structures on either the mesial or lateral surface of the tumor.

In small- and medium-sized tumors, the anatomic dissection should precede partial removal of the lesion. The IXth, Xth, and XIth nerves are freed from the capsule of the tumor and covered with a protecting, wet cotton pledget or rubber dam (Fig. 25-10). In the dissection of the inferior capsule, large feeding branches from the posterior inferior cerebellar artery or directly from the vertebral artery must be clipped and divided. Monopolar coagulation should be avoided in this area. The tumor capsule is then gently elevated and the facial nerve is identified on its ventral aspect (Fig. 25-11). Electrical stimulation aids in identifying the nerve. It may be possible to isolate the facial nerve for only a few millimeters at this point because the nerve passes anteriorly toward the roots of the trigeminal nerve on its way toward the porus acousticus, and this portion of the course of the nerve is still obscured by the tumor.

Having identified the facial nerve proximally (Fig. 25-11), it must now be exposed distally at the internal auditory meatus. As the VIIth nerve is protected, the tumor is then divided at the meatus (Fig. 25-12). Attention is now directed to the anterosuperior extension. As the tumor is most gently retracted inferiorly, the veins draining from the tumor into the superior petrosal sinus can be identified. These vessels are clipped or coagulated with bipolar current and divided. Moving medially, arterial branches to the tumor from the anterior inferior cerebellar artery are visualized, clipped, and divided (Fig. 25-13). If the tumor extends upward through the tentorial incisura, it may even be supplied by branches from the superior cerebellar artery. The fifth nerve is almost always very easily dissected free of the tumor capsule, but it is at this point anteriorly that the facial nerve is most difficult to preserve. As the tumor is gradually retracted inferiorly, the facial nerve may be identified as many thinned-out single fascicles.

The angle of retraction is changed from inferior to lateral, and the crucial medial dissection is now carried out. As previously mentioned, at times it will be best for the patient if a small portion of the capsule that is adherent to the brain stem is left behind. After removing the remaining capsule, bleeding veins on the surface of the pons and medulla can be controlled by applying a wet cotton pledget and temporarily leaving that area.

Having removed the bulk of the tumor, attention is turned to the remaining nubbin in the porus acousticus (Figs. 25-13). Under magnification, the dura is incised at the posterior aspect of the porus and elevated (Fig. 25-14 and 25-15*A*). A high-speed drill, cooled by irrigation, can be used to remove the posterior wall of the porus and expose the remaining tumor (25-15*B*). A diamond bur should be used in the final stages of drilling (Fig. 25-16*A*). It is important to coat this bony margin with bone wax to avoid a postoperative cerebrospinal fluid fistulae. The intrameatal dura is incised (Fig. 25-16*B*); note the orientation of the nerves in the meatus (Fig. 25-16*C*). The tumor is teased out of the canal with small needles and microfreers while the facial nerve is supported on gel foam (Fig. 25-15*B*). The small artery accompanying the facial nerve is protected and preserved in the same manner. Any bleeding from within the canal can be controlled with bipolar coagulation.

The tumor bed is checked for meticulous hemostasis. All cotton pledgets and strips are freed using irrigation and removed. A water-tight dural closure is attained and the remainder of the wound closed in layers.

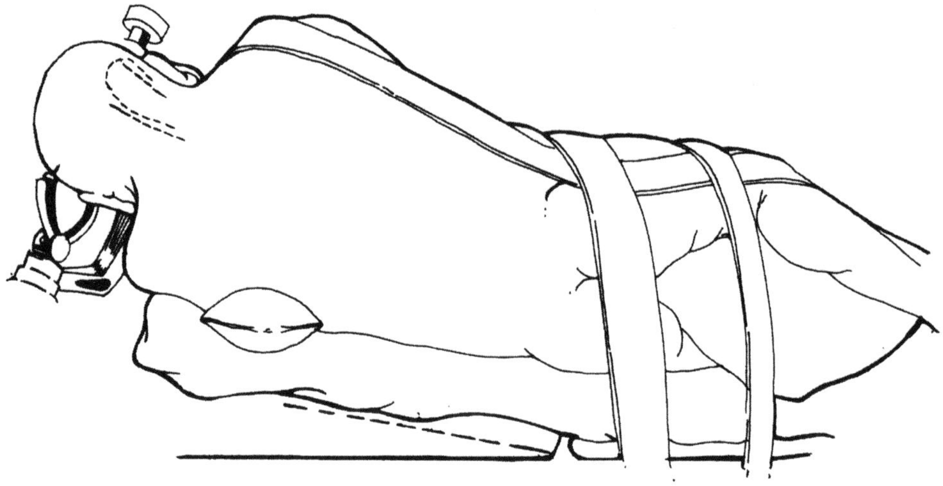

Figure 25-1. Lateral decubitus position. Patient is completely padded with head rotated down and forward. The ipsilateral shoulder is rolled away from the surgeon.

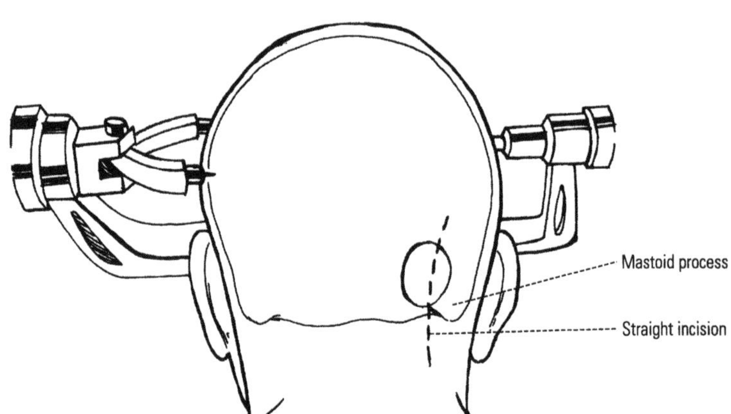

Figure 25-2. Retromastoid incision for most cerebellopontine angle lesions. The incision extends from just above the pinna of the ear to below the mastoid tip, one to two finger breadths medial to the mastoid process.

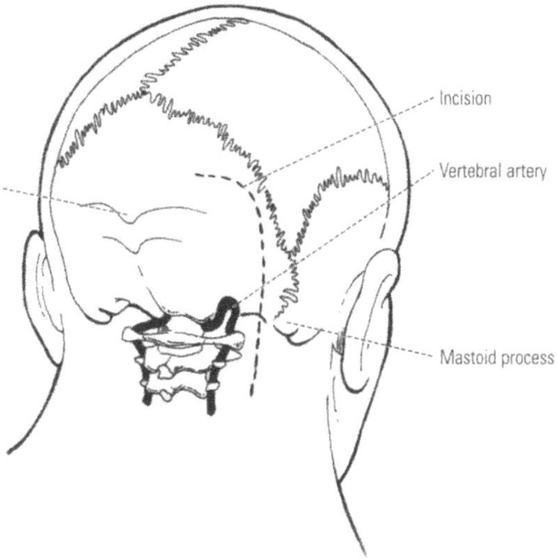

Figure 25-3. Retromastoid incision: inverted hockeystick for very large lesions. Top of incision curves medially 2 cm above inion and is extended below mastoid process. Note ectactic vertebral artery.

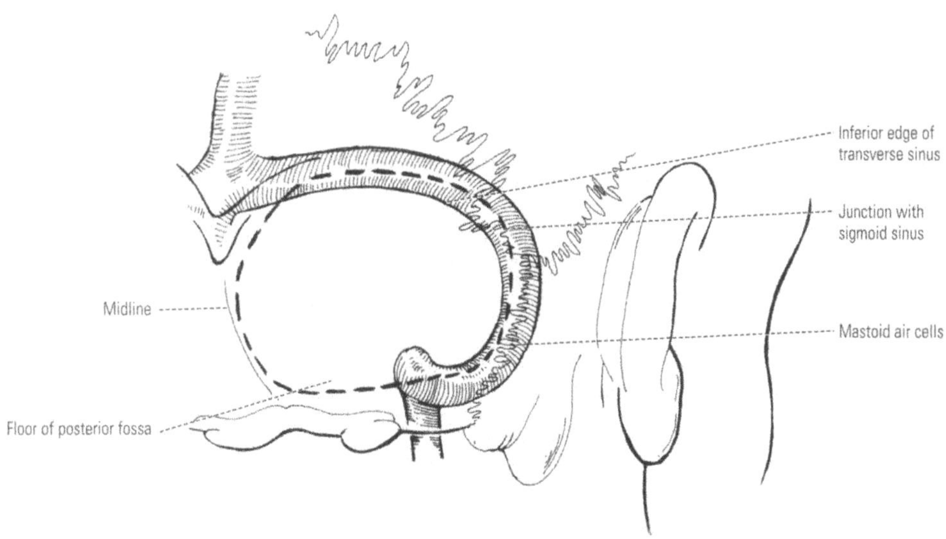

Figure 25-4. Anatomical boundaries of unilateral suboccipital craniectomy. Note transverse sinus above, junction with sigmoid sinus superolateral, mastoid air cells lateral, suboccipital floor below and midline. Only the lateral half is needed for most cerebellopontine lesions.

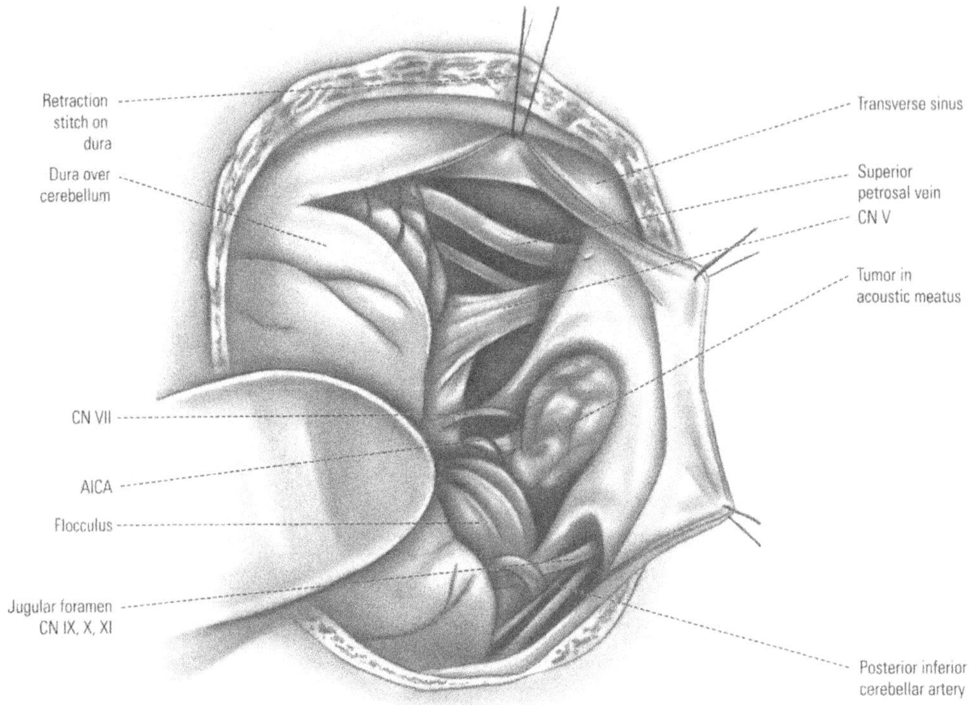

Figure 25-5. Retromastoid dural incision and intradural landmarks. Note semilunar incision and dura folded over cerebellar hemisphere. Note structures exposed in cerebellopontine angle and inferior posterior fossa. Note small tumor in acoustic meatus.

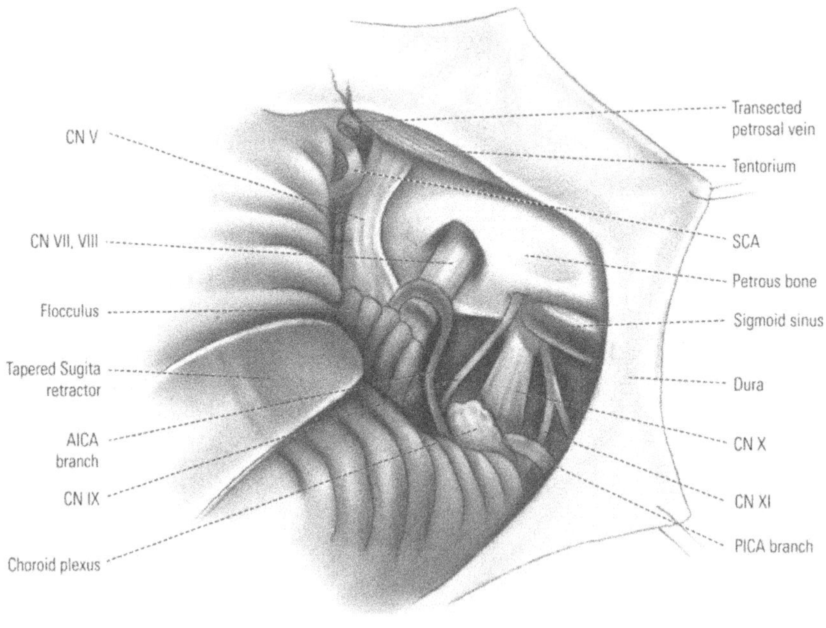

Figure 25-6. Initial approach to cerebellopontine angle. Note retractor is perpendicular to cerebellum at midpoint of exposure. Look for flocculus of cerebellum and choroid plexus as guide to location of VII and VIII complex. Note: only normal anatomy is demonstrated. PICA—posterior inferior cerebellar artery; SCA—superior cerebellar artery.

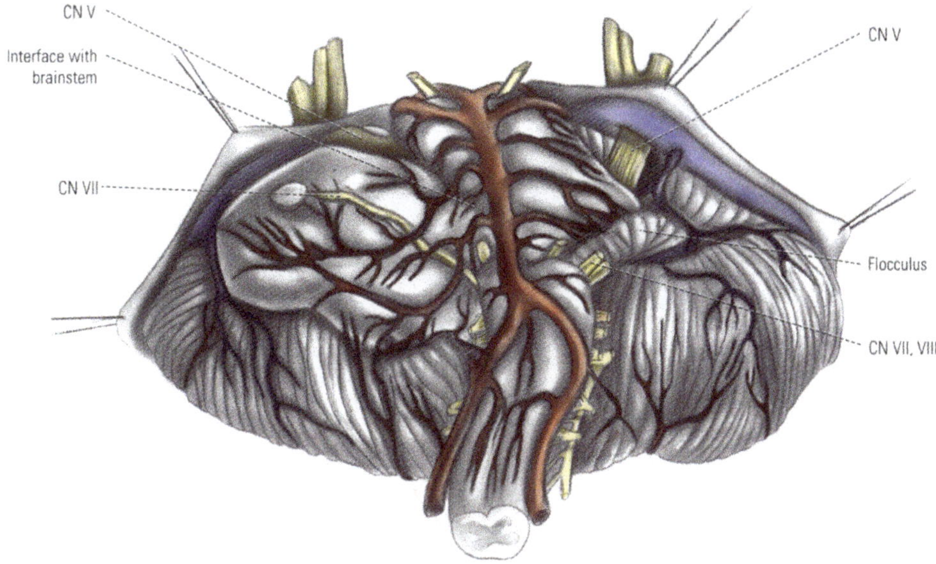

Figure 25-7. Anatomical relations of large tumor seen from its ventral surface. Note anteroventral displacement of cranial nerve VII, medial involvement of brain stem.

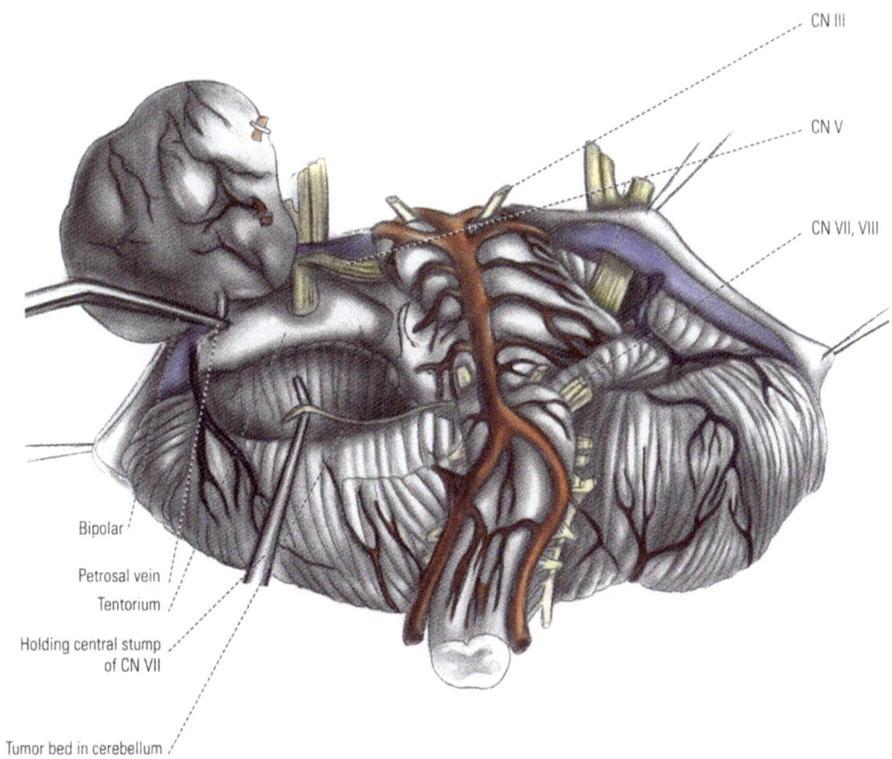

Figure 25-8. Anatomical relations of tumor bed seen from ventral surface.

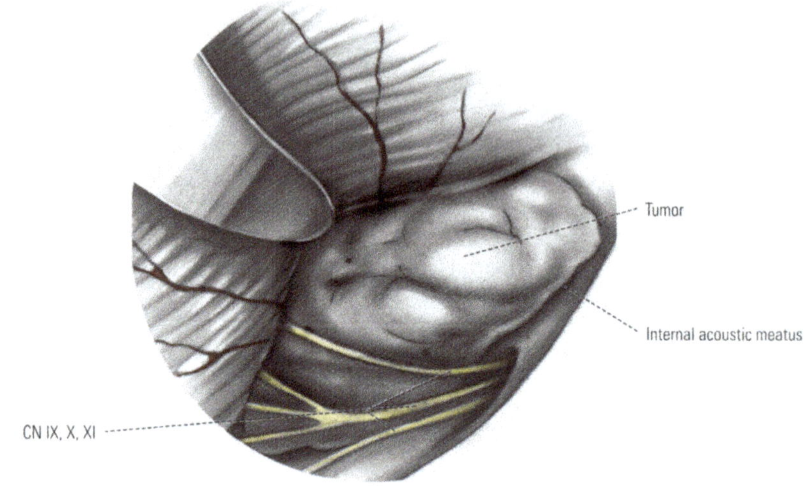

Figure 25-9. Exposure of cerebellopontine angle. The lower pole and lateral extent of tumor are visible.

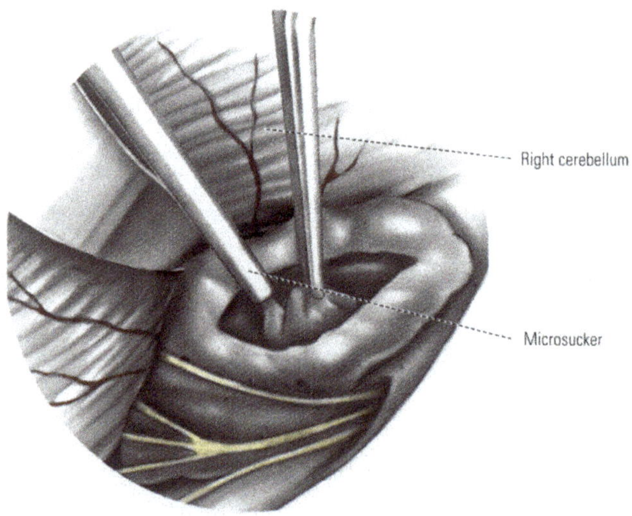

Figure 25-10. Incision of tumor capsule permits intracapsular removal.

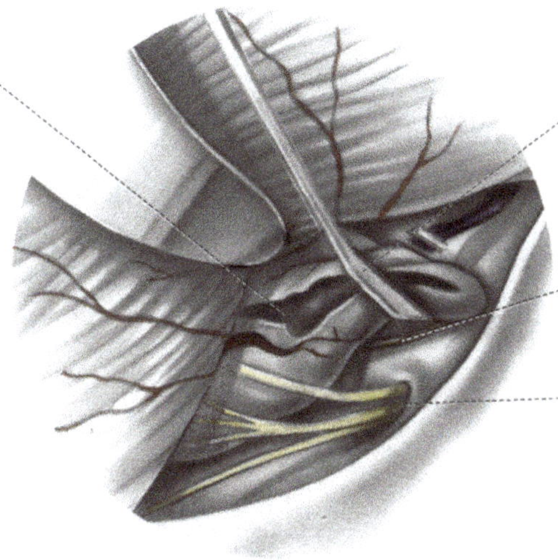

Figure 25-11. Elevation of inferior pole of tumor. After a small intracapsular removal, the tumor is elevated off the IX, X, and XIth cranial nerves. The VIIth nerve is seen ventrally and anteriorly entering the acoustic meatus.

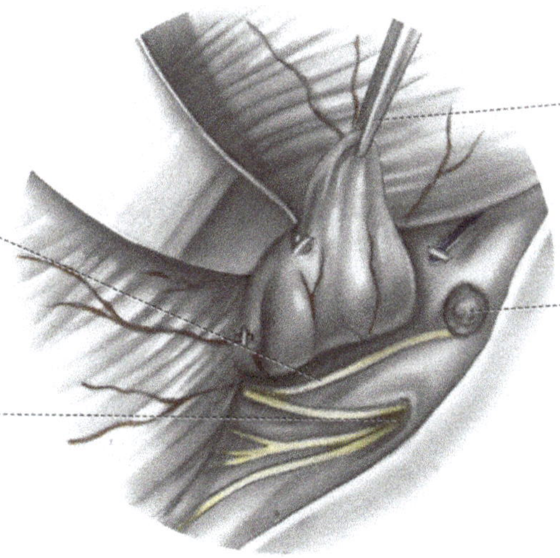

Figure 25-12. Lateral dissection of tumor. After the VIIth nerve is identified, the tumor is transected at the meatus and retracted superiorly.

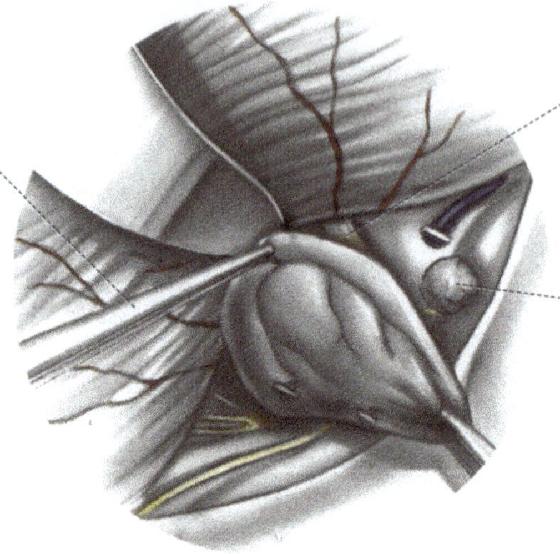

Figure 25-13. Superomesial dissection of tumor. Note exposure of Vth nerve superiorly and gentle downward retraction of tumor mass. Only vessels entering the capsule directly are taken, especially on brainstem side of tumor.

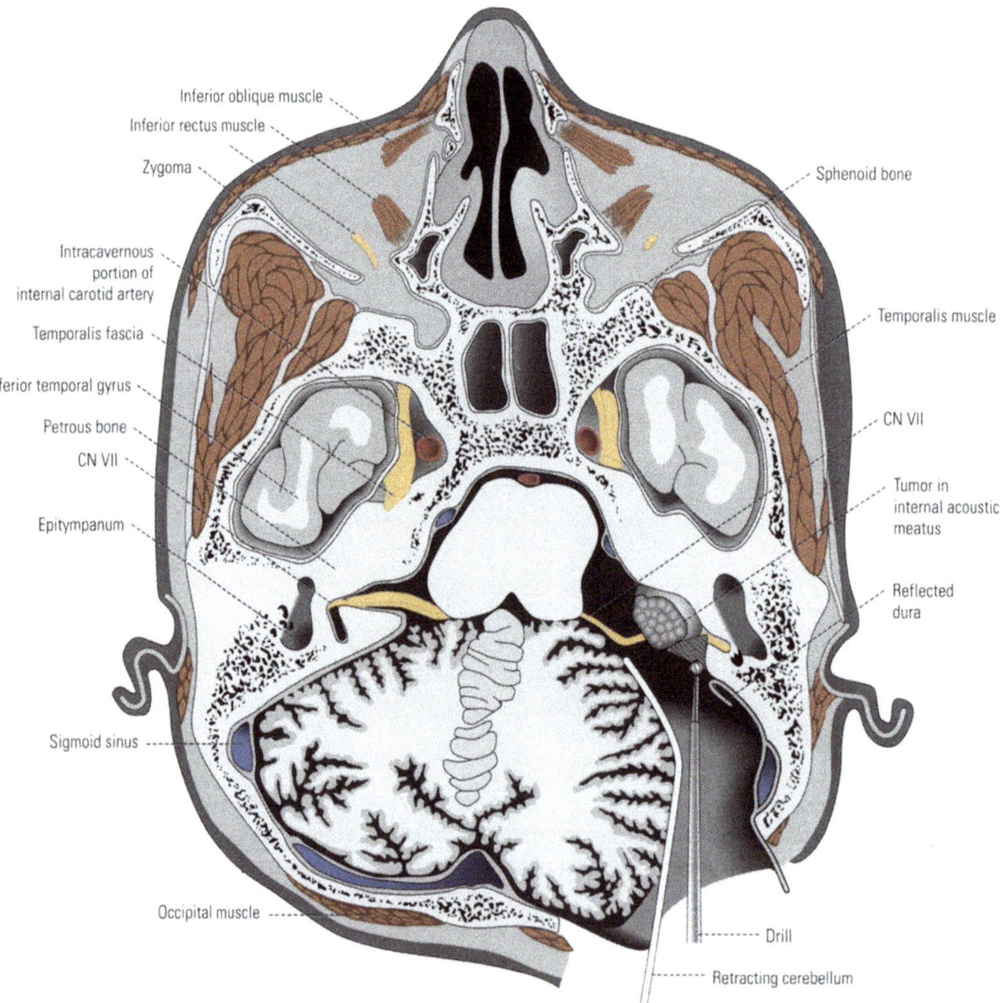

Figure 25-14. General orientation for meatal dissection.

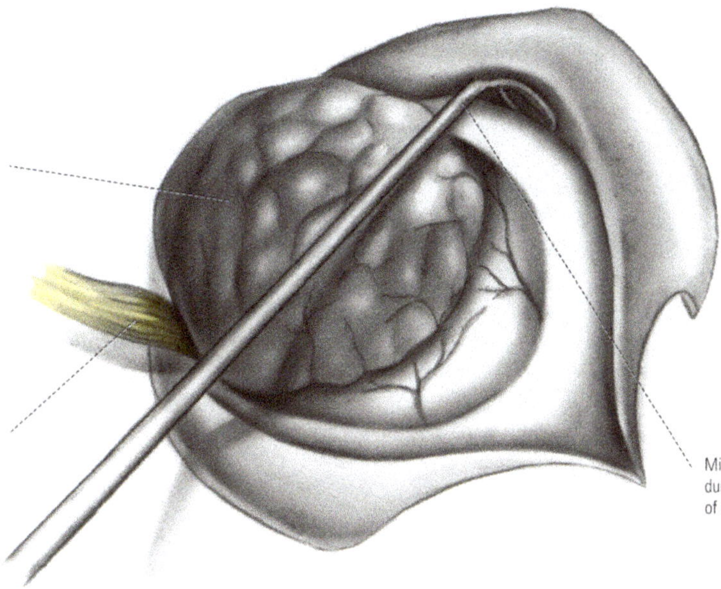

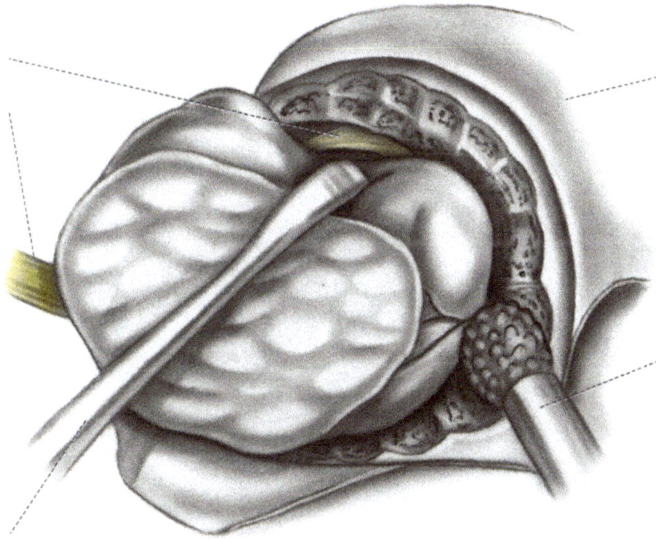

Figure 25-15. A, Elevation of meatal dura prior to drilling. B, Exposure of VIIth nerve in meatus. Note that the VIIth nerve is anterior and superior in the meatus even when it is anterior and ventral in the posterior fossa. Drilling is stopped before the lateral edge of the tumor is reached.

Figure 25-16. A, Drilling of posterior meatal wall. B, Intrameatal dissection after drilling posterior wall. C, Orientation of cranial nerves in right internal auditory meatus.

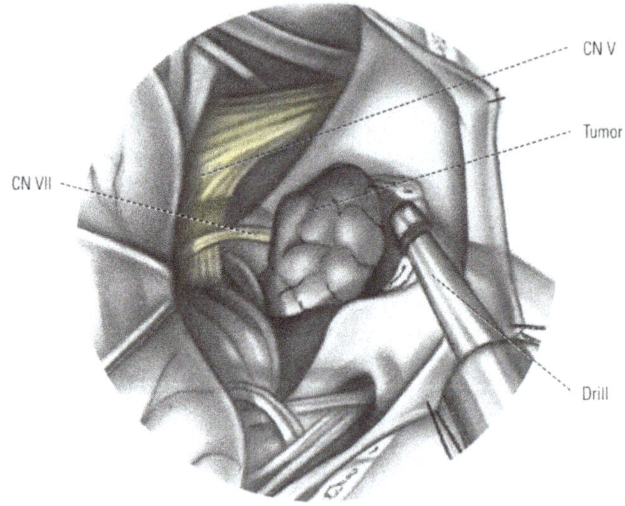

A

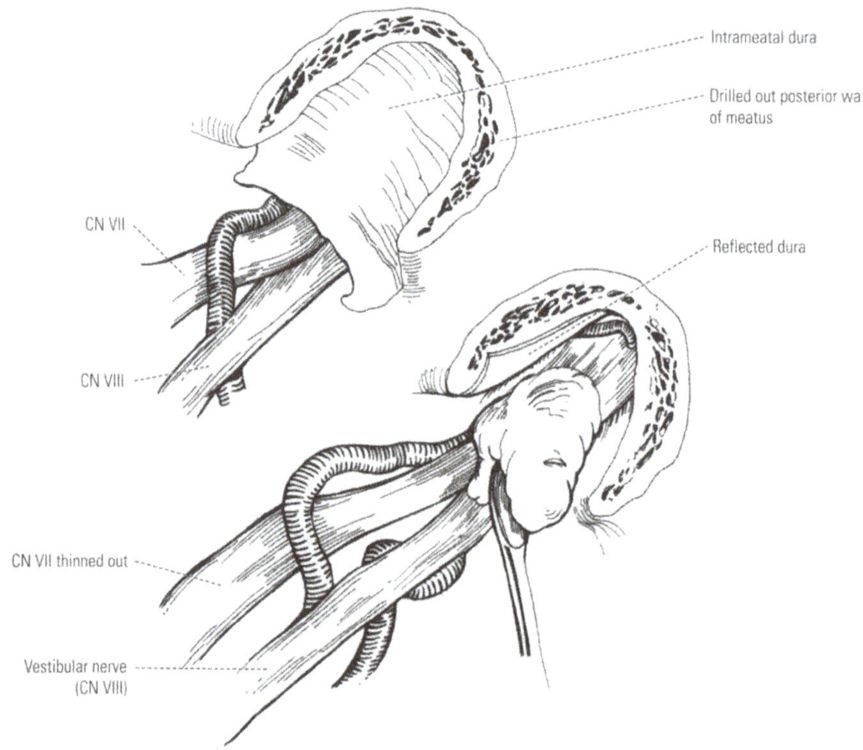

B

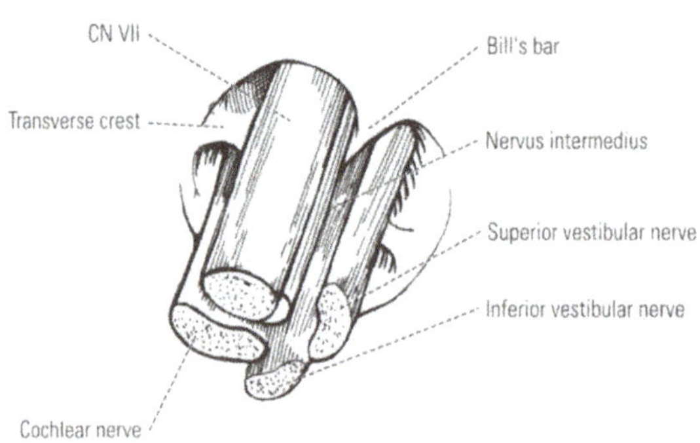

C

CHAPTER

26

Suboccipital Craniectomy: Retromastoid Approach for Trigeminal Neuralgia

Microvascular Decompression for Trigeminal Neuralgia

Microvascular decompression of the trigeminal nerve is the most frequently used open surgical procedure for the treatment of trigeminal neuralgia. It is most appropriate for patients with a 5-year expected survival who have had medically refractory trigeminal neuralgia for less than 8 to 10 years. The best results are obtained in patients who are neurologically intact without facial burning or numbness and in those who have not undergone a prior destructive procedure directed at the Vth nerve. The operation is carried out through a retromastoid suboccipital craniectomy, similar in many ways to the procedure described in chapter 25.

The patient is placed in the lateral decubitus position with an axillary roll under the dependent shoulder (see Fig. 25-1) and the head held in three-pin fixation. The neck is placed on stretch and the head slightly flexed forward and contralaterally. The same straight retromastoid incision is used as the one employed for small acoustic tumors, 10 cm in length from the top of the pinna to the mastoid groove, and one to two fingerbreadths medial to the groove (Fig. 26-1). The craniectomy is centered slightly higher because the trigeminal nerve relates to the junction of the tentorium and petrous ridge in the very apex of the cerebellopontine angle. Once again, exposure of the junction of the transverse and sigmoid sinuses is a useful landmark. After the dura is opened, it is sometimes necessary to slightly extend the head to open the space between the Vth nerve and the VIIth and VIIIth nerve complex. A rubber dam and large cottonoid are placed over the surface of the cerebellar hemisphere and the retractor blade is introduced into the superolateral corner of the exposure (Fig. 26-2). Cerebellar relaxation can be obtained by releasing cerebrospinal fluid inferiorly from the cistern around the IXth and Xth cranial nerves or by opening a previously placed lumbar catheter.

If the VIIIth nerve is exposed first, the Vth will be found deeply anterior and rostral to it; if the junction of the tentorium and the petrous ridge is exposed first, the superior petrosal vein and the Vth nerve will be deeply anterior and caudal to the tentorium. In the majority of cases, it is wise to electively cauterize and transect the superior petrosal vein before it causes troublesome bleeding in the cerebellopontine angle. The source of compression of the Vth nerve can be found by remembering that superior compression causes V3 trigeminal neuralgia, inferior vessel contact causes V1 neuralgia, and lateral or medial compression of the nerve is associated with pain in the V2 distribution. A loop of the superior cerebellar artery (SCA) is the most common culprit; small veins and arteries may also be responsible (Fig. 26-3). In 5% to 10% of cases, no obvious source of vascular compression is observed.

Large bridging veins and short arterial loops from the SCA and anterior inferior cerebellar artery are dissected free from the nerve with blunt probes and microscissors, then held away by small pieces of shredded polytef felt. Usually the arterial loops are ventral to the nerve (Fig. 26-4) and must first be carefully brought into a superficial position. If a long loop of the SCA is encountered, it must be extricated from beneath the nerve and mobilized into a horizontal position (Figs. 26-5) or "tacked" to the tentorium by a sling made from one or two long cigar-shaped pieces of rolled Teflon felt (Fig. 26-6). The closure is carried out as previously described for acoustic tumor surgery.

Nervus Intermedius Rhizotomy

Rhizotomy of the nervus intermedius may be done for geniculate neuralgia or intractable pain secondary to a malignancy. This operation has been recommended in the treatment of Horton's cephalgia (histamine headaches). In our experience the most common indication is intractable pain about the ear in patients with a malignancy who have been treated with irradiation.

The position of the patient, scalp incision, craniectomy and operative exposure are identical to that already described and illustrated for acoustic schwannoma. The retraction of the cerebellum, however, is different. In this operation the cerebellum is gently elevated rather than retracted medially (Fig. 26-7). Having exposed the VIIth and VIIIth cranial nerves in the cerebellopontine angle, magnification becomes essential to the successful completion of this rhizotomy. Magnification is not only helpful in preventing injury to the facial and auditory nerves and accompanying vessels, but is also of aid in identifying the nerve of Wrisberg (nervus intermedius). This nerve may consist of only two to four tiny fascicles. The nerve is usually, at least over part of its intracranial course, closely adherent to the vestibular nerve. A very fine blunt nerve hook is used to gently separate the VIIth and VIIIth nerve roots on their dorsal surface. When a plane has been developed so that the nerve hook "falls " between the nerves, the nerve hook is gently turned around and the nervus intermedius is "fished" out from this interval (Fig. 26-8). After ascertaining that no vessels are within this fine strand of nerve, it is coagulated and divided with a microscissors. Extreme care must be taken to avoid injuring the VIIth and VIIIth nerves.

Glossopharyngeal Rhizotomy

Glossopharyngeal neuralgia and intractable pain secondary to malignancy constitute the indications for glossopharyngeal rhizotomy.

The surgical exposure is identical to that used in acoustic schwannoma. The angle of retraction in this case is different. As in exposing the VIIth and VIIIth cranial nerves, the retractor blade should elevate the cerebellum. Correct initial position of this retractor is emphasized because the cerebellum can be very easily injured by repeated movement. The surgeon must have sufficient knowledge of the anatomical relationships within the posterior fossa so that the retractor can be placed definitively in one motion.

The glossopharyngeal nerve is easily identified as the most rostral nerve in the IXth, Xth and XIth group. Magnification aids in demonstrating that this nerve passes through a separate opening in the dura of the jugular foramen. The two rostralmost strands of the vagus nerve are included with the glossopharyngeal nerve in a blunt nerve hook. These fibers are elevated and separated from any vascular structure. Before the nerves are divided, the anesthetist is advised that the blood pressure may dramatically increase. This carotid sinus reflex is most striking in older individuals and in patients having bilateral rhizotomies. The nerves are divided using bipolar coagulation and a fine scissors (Fig. 26-8).

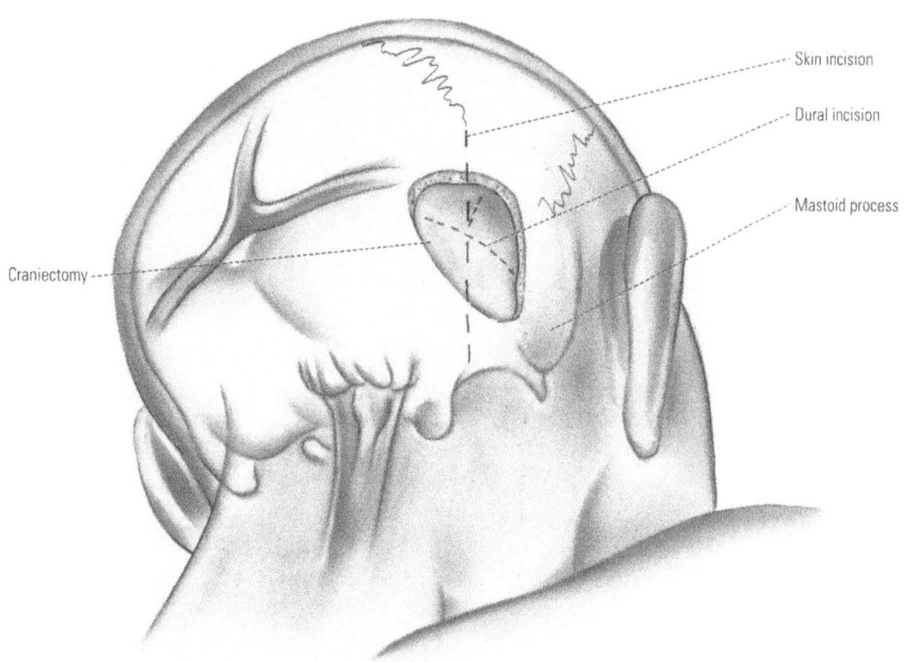

Figure 26-1. Retromastoid craniectomy for trigeminal neuralgia. Note extent of skin incision from above pinna to mastoid process.

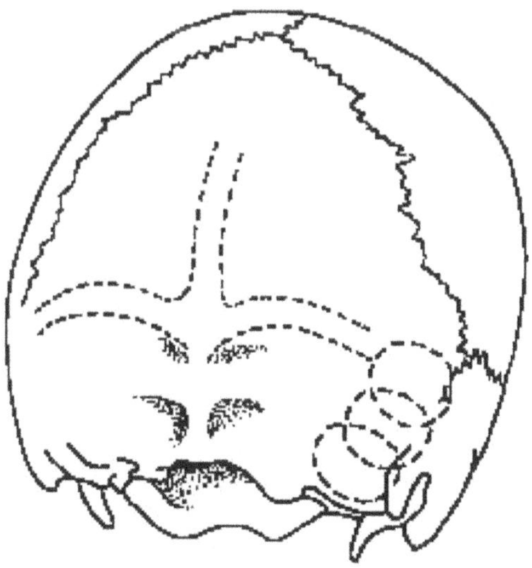

Figure 26-2. General orientation of retromastoid craniectomy for different cranial nerve procedures. Note upper circle for trigeminal neuralgia (CN V), middle circle for CNs VII and VIII, and lower circle for CNs IX, X, and XI.

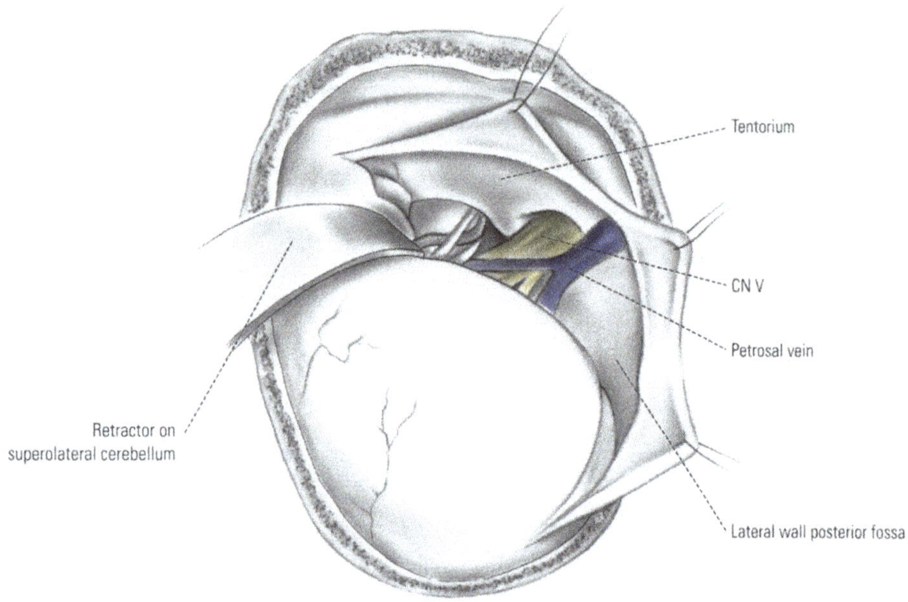

Figure 26-3. Initial approach for trigeminal neuralgia. Note superolateral retractor position.

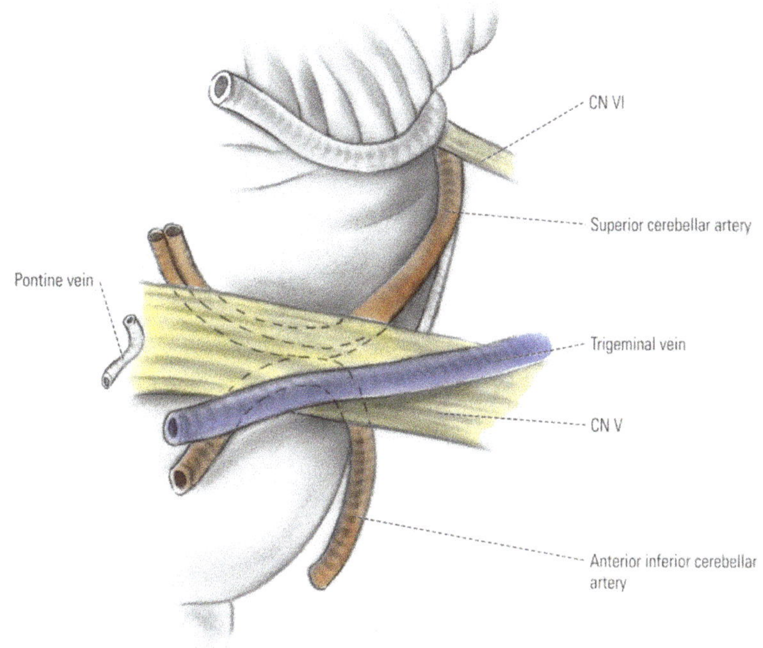

Figure 26-4. Common causes of vascular compression of trigeminal nerve. Arterial compression is more frequent than venous.

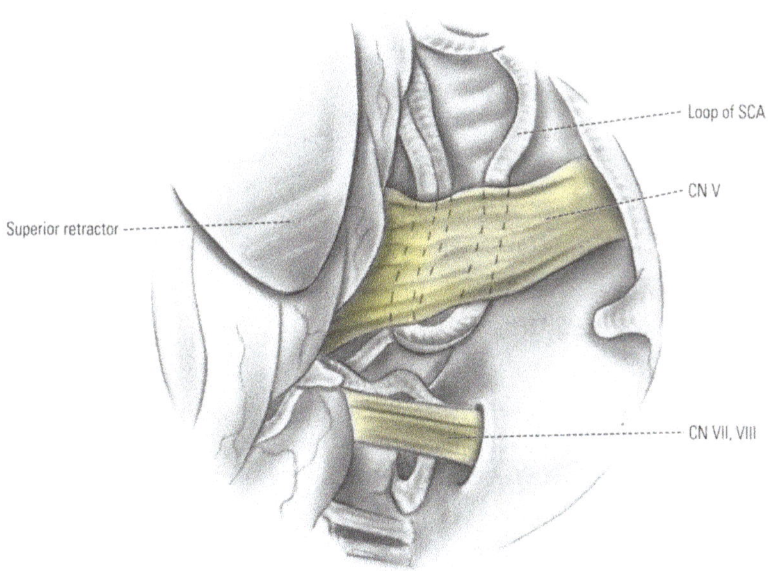

Figure 26-5. Trigeminal neuralgia caused by superior cerebellar artery (SCA) ventral to nerve.

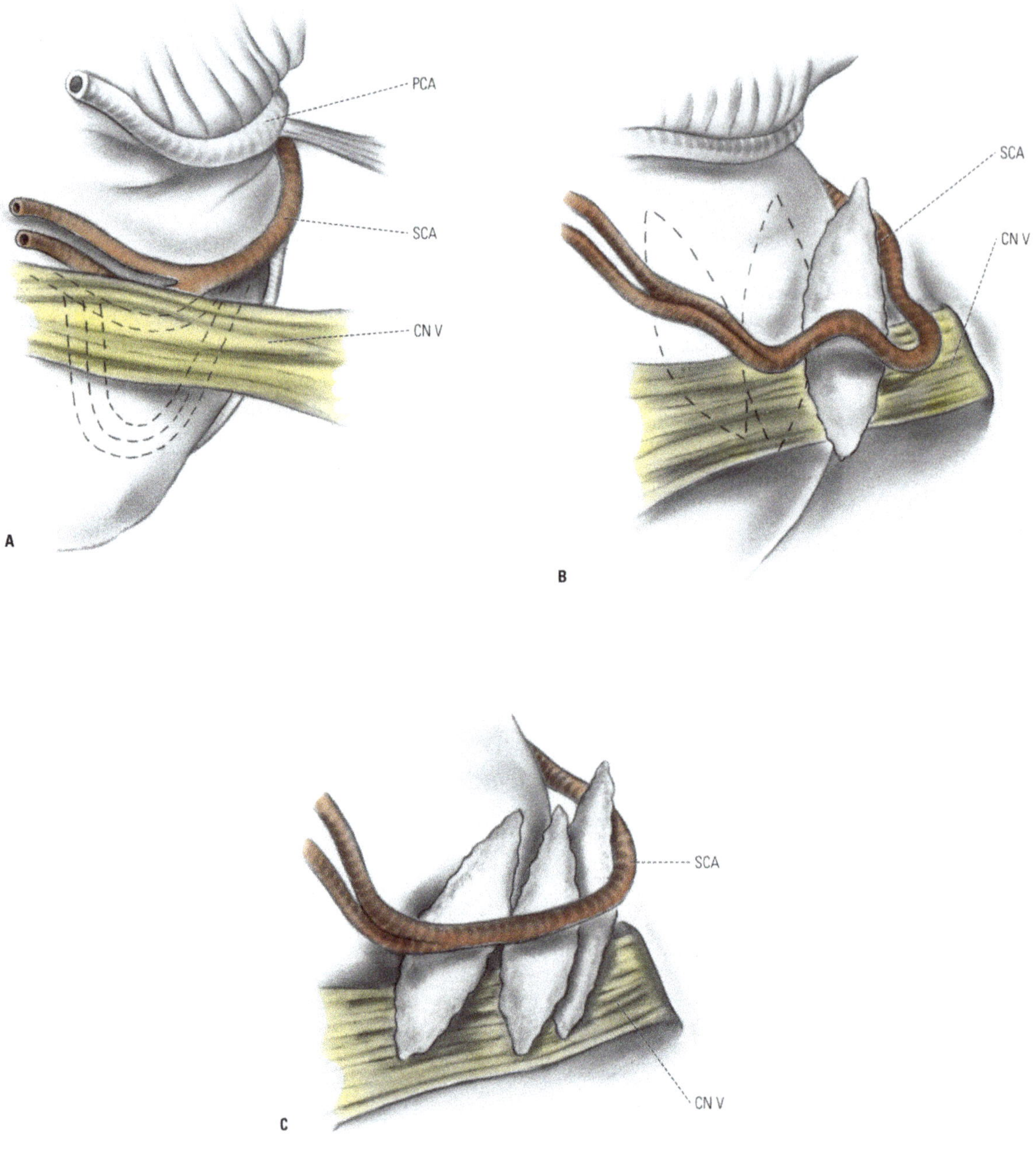

Figure 26-6. Treatment of superior cerebellar artery (SCA) compression. Vessel is fished out from behind nerve (*panel A*) and placed in horizontal position (*panel B*). Pieces of Teflon felt are slid from proximal to distal (*panel C*).

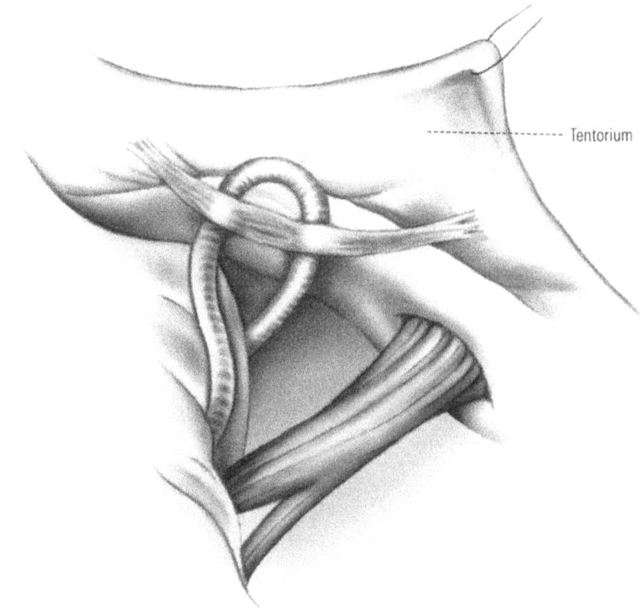

Figure 26-7. Securing vascular loop to tentorium by a "sling."

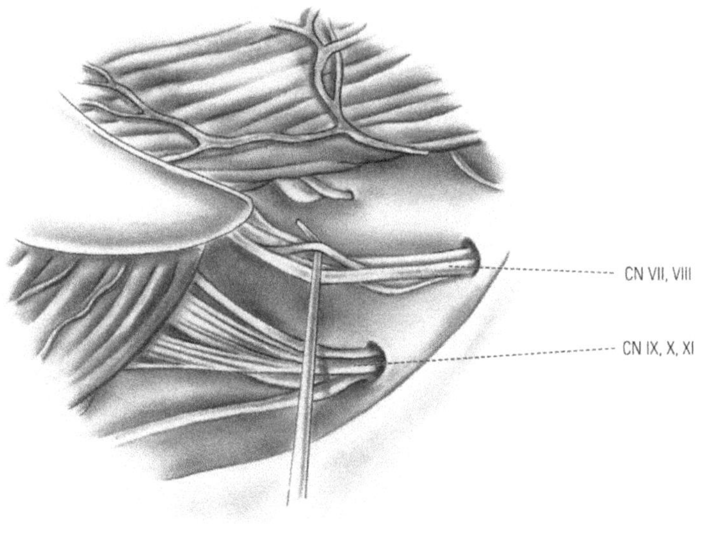

Figure 26-8. Nervus intermedius rhizotomy. Note nerve on small hook at interface between VIIth and VIIIth cranial nerves.

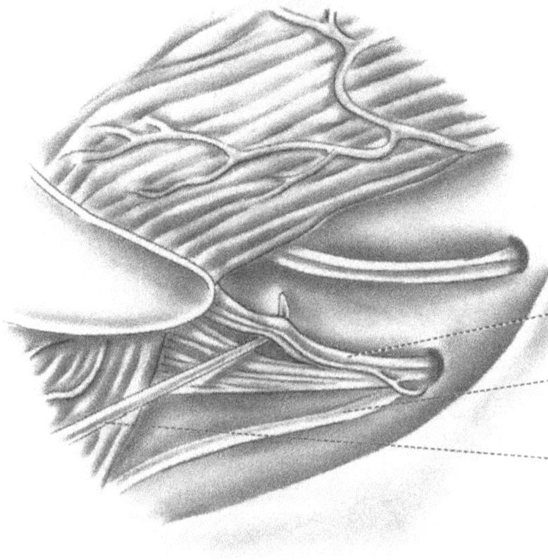

Figure 26-9. Glossopharyngeal rhizotomy. Note nerve hook picking up rostral-most fibers entering jugular foramen.

CHAPTER

27

Suboccipital Craniectomy: Midline and Paramedian Approach

Midline and paramedian suboccipital exposures are used for resection of midline tumors of the posterior fossa, removal of vascular malformations, and treatment of aneurysms and congenital anomalies. Whenever a lesion in the cerebellopontine angle appears to be too large for a routine retromastoid approach (see chapter 25), a paramedian exposure should be employed. In general, these procedures give wide exposure to one or both cerebellar hemispheres, the cerebellar vermis, one or both lateral sinuses and their confluence, the foramen magnum, and one or both mastoid processes. Formerly, midline and paramedian suboccipital craniectomies were carried out in the sitting position; at present they are most frequently performed in a lateral decubitus or prone position (see Chapter 25).

The Sitting Position

Certain precautions must be taken when using this position because of the danger of air embolism. The lower extremities must be wrapped with elastic bandages and elevated. An inflatable wrapping below the level of the diaphragm is an effective means of increasing the venous pressure thereby preventing air embolism. Bone wax must be used generously. Cut bone margins should be coated with wax even when not bleeding. Air emboli can be detected by an ultrasonic detector placed over the neck, blood-gas analysis and/or by a stethoscope placed over the precordium. Treatment must be rapidly carried out. The patient's head must be lowered, and the embolus aspirated via a catheter previously placed in the right atrium.

Proper position of the head is also crucial in the sitting position. As illustrated in Figure 27-1*A*, the head should not be flexed to the degree that venous drainage is obstructed. After positioning the head properly, the entire table is then tilted forward as shown in Figure 27-1*B*. The height of the table is very important. A common mistake is made in keeping the table too low with the result that the surgeon goes through back-breaking contortions especially in exposure of the cerebellopontine angle and tentorial incisura. The most comfortable height is achieved when the posterior rim of the foramen magnum is at the level of the surgeon's eyes. The arms will not tire at this level because the elbows can be rested on the back support of the operating table (Fig. 27-1*B*).

The patient's head must be draped in such a way that the occipital region as well as the suboccipital and cervical areas are exposed. It is wise to place a right occipital bur hole 4 cm lateral to the midline 6 to 8 cm above the external occipital protuberance so that the lateral ventricle can be tapped at any time during the procedure. When the suboccipital dura is tense, the lateral ventricle should be vented before proceeding any further.

Principles of Midline Exposure

A midline skin incision is made from two fingerbreadths above the inion to the midcervical region, but the musculature is cleared no lower than the spinous process and dorsal arch of C2 (Fig. 27-2). Self-retaining retractors are placed at either end of the wound and care is taken to stay strictly in the midline so that the incision is made along the avascular linea alba (Fig. 27-3). At the level of the superior nuchal line, the trapezius, splenius capitis, and semispinalis capitis muscles can be incised transversely a short distance below their insertion so that a good closure of this muscle layer can be obtained later. These muscles are stripped from the occipital squama with a periosteal elevator down to the posterior rim of the foramen magnum and laterally to the level of the mastoid processes. The mastoid emissary veins are encountered laterally and generous amounts of bone wax should be used to plug any bony venous channels. The arch of the atlas is palpated with an index finger to ascertain the level of the foramen magnum. In stripping the muscles from the suboccipital region, pressure in this area must be avoided. The rectus capitis posterior major and minor muscles are stripped from their insertion at the inferior nuchal line. The origin of the rectus capitis posterior and minor muscle from the arch of the atlas should be removed by sharp dissection. The periosteum of the arch of the atlas is incised in the midline and then stripped laterally (Fig. 27-4). Often the arch of C1 is removed with a Kerrison punch and small bone rongeurs (Fig. 27-5). The dense fibrous tissue in the deep suboccipital triangle can best be stripped laterally by grasping the muscle fibers and fibrous tissue with a pair of forceps and using a slightly opened straight scissors. The position of the vertebral artery laterally must be kept in mind during this maneuver, especially when using the cutting cautery to strip tissue down to the bone. Self-retaining cerebellar retractors are progressively inserted more deeply as each layer is exposed.

Multiple bur holes can be placed in the exposed suboccipital bone and the intervening bone removed by rongeurs. Alternatively, a single bur hole is placed and the bone uniformly thinned out with a large round cutting bur, after which the thin translucent shell is easily removed with a Kerrison punch. The bone must be removed superiorly until the transverse sinus comes into view for maximal exposure and so that the bridging cerebellar veins can be dealt with if necessary. In large midline procedures, the rim of the foramen magnum is removed and the lateral margins of the exposure go out to the mastoid air cells and both sigmoid sinuses (Fig. 27-6). In some cases, removal of the rim of the foramen magnum should be accompanied by resection of the arch of the atlas. The arch of C1 is removed using small sharp Kerrison punches after the bone has been thinned with a double-action rongeur (Fig. 27-5).

In most bilateral exposures, the dura is opened with a Y-shaped incision (Fig. 27-6), which crosses the marginal sinus but not the occipital sinus. Because the occipital sinus is located immediately over the falx cerebelli, it is not as easily clipped as the marginal sinus. The dura is reflected superiorly and laterally. The cerebellar hemispheres, vermis, and tonsils can be inspected through the intact arachnoid. Any deviation from the midline, discoloration, or asymmetry is noted. Almost invariably the tonsil will be lowest on the side of the cerebellar hemisphere containing a mass lesion. Symmetry, folial pattern, and vascularity of the hemispheres are observed. The arachnoid over the cisterna magna is opened and cerebrospinal fluid escapes (Fig. 27-7). This usually makes the pulsation of the intracranial structures much more obvious. The anesthetist is informed of the change in intracranial dynamics and reminded that from this point any change in the patient's vital signs must be reported immediately.

The cerebellar hemispheres are then gently palpated. An underlying cyst will give a boggy feeling, whereas a solid tumor will make the cerebellum feel firmer than the other hemisphere. If no abnormality is apparent at this point, the tonsils should be carefully separated to visualize the posterior end of the fourth ventricle (Fig. 27-8). A word is in order at this point regarding the use of retraction in the posterior fossa. This area, even more than other intracranial compartments, does not tolerate faulty insertion or application of instruments without disastrous sequelae. As in the previously mentioned exposure of the foramen of Magendie, the surgeon guides and holds the retractors on each side of the vallecula until the self-retaining retractor arms are locked by the assistant. When a retractor is held by an assistant he must be able to see what he is retracting. The position of a retractor is the responsibility of the surgeon even when he is not holding it; and, if it is incorrectly positioned, he must replace it. Tilting of a retractor is particularly hazardous. Even when retracting a cerebellar hemisphere, tilting can cause bleeding deep between the folia, which can be difficult to localize and disastrous for the patient. The surface of the cerebellum should always be covered with a rubber dam and a cottonoid subjacent to the retractor blade and irrigated frequently.

Having explored the distal fourth ventricle without discovering the pathology, the next step in a posterior fossa exploration is to split the vermis in the midline posteriorly (Fig. 27-9). Gentle retraction laterally then allows complete inspection of the remainder of the fourth ventricle up to the anterior medullary velum and distal aqueduct. Hemispheric tumors usually cause a deformity of the ventricular wall on the side of the lesion. If a cyst is known to be present from the preoperative magnetic resonance image or CT scans, it can be discovered with intraoperative ultrasound or by carefully tapping it with a ventricular needle inserted through the center of the inferior surface of a cerebellar hemisphere. The needle must be directed superior to the brain stem and lateral to the dentate nucleus. The use of such needles should be avoided in solid or well-vascularized lesions.

Attention is finally turned to the extra-axial subarachnoid space. The lateral recess of the medullary cistern and the posterior portion of the cerebellopontine angle are inspected. The ease of this exposure is directly related to the width of the craniectomy exposure at the posterior rim of the foramen magnum. Once again the position of the brain spatula and direction of retraction are important. Compare these two essential elements in Figure 27-10, where the posterior portion of the cerebellopontine angle is exposed, and in Figure 27-11, in which the anterior portion of the cerebellopontine angle is seen.

At the termination of any posterior fossa craniectomy in the sitting position, the anesthetist should be asked to compress the jugular veins so that hemostasis can be checked. If a tumor is totally removed and no swelling is present, the dura is closed. If only an incomplete excision is accomplished and decompression is required, a dural patch graft can be used to enlarge the space. Once the dura is closed, a thin absorbable gelatin sponge is placed over it to further prevent the seepage of blood from superficial layers of the wound into the subarachnoid space. When the lateral ventricle has been cannulated, the need for continued ventricular drainage must be considered. Usually the catheter is kept in place for at least 24 to 48 hours.

Suboccipital Craniectomy: Median Incision

Metastatic Tumor of the Cerebellar Vermis

To illustrate the midline incision in a suboccipital craniectomy, a metastatic tumor of the vermis and right cerebellar hemisphere has been chosen (Figs. 27-12 and 27-13). Solitary metastases within the central nervous system should be removed and radiated, especially in the posterior fossa where they may present an immediate risk to life. Adequately treated patients frequently die of their systemic disease and have no evidence of an intracranial lesion at autopsy. Many years of functional activity have been added to patients lives even when repeated operations are necessary to remove "solitary" lesions. The most common incision used in suboccipital craniectomies for intracerebellar pathology is in the midline (Fig. 27-14). The lateral decubitus or prone position as described in chapter 25 is used. The skin incision is made from 4 cm above the external occipital protuberance (inion) to the spinous process of C5. This length of incision is necessary for lateral exposure to the mastoid air cells on each side. The skin margins are freed from the deep fascia and retracted. A Y- or T-shaped incision is made into the deep fascia. The midline can easily be determined by intermittently palpating the inion and the spinous process of C2. The V portion of the fascial incision is elevated and suspended by a silk suture. The importance of this type of fascial opening will be apparent when it is time to close the wound. The incision is then continued in the midline down to the occipital bone and to the spinous process of C2. The median raphe is most easily split by using a straight scissors or the cutting cautery. By staying precisely in the midline, bleeding is kept at a minimum (Fig. 27-3). The insertion of the muscles to the occipital squama are stripped laterally by subperiosteal elevation. The spinous process of C2 is exposed using a sharp knife that can be kept against the bony contours of this bifid spinous process. The origins of the obliquous inferior and rectus capitus major muscles are transected, and the muscles are retracted laterally by a self-retaining retractor. The dorsal surface of the arch of the atlas is exposed by cutting the origin of the rectus capitus minor muscle and then stripping the fibrous tissue from the arch subperiosteally using scissors, the cutting cautery and straight curettes, or small periosteal elevators as previously described (Figs. 27-4). The bone in the suboccipital region and the arch of the atlas is removed (Figs. 27-5 and 27-6). A right occipital bur hole can be made at this point but cannulation of the ventricle should be avoided except in emergent circumstances.

After opening the dura, inspection of the cerebellum reveals an asymmetry of the cerebellar tonsils and hemispheres. The right cerebellar hemisphere is bulging across the midline and the right tonsil is larger and lower than the opposite one (Fig. 27-14). The arachnoid over the foramen magnum is opened and the cerebrospinal fluid is allowed to drain out. The vermis can be visualized only after the hemispheres are retracted laterally (Figs. 27-15 and 27-16). Flattening of the vermis indicates that the lesion extends across the midline. This means that the tumor should be approached by beginning in the midline and retracting laterally; that is, away from the brain stem. A midline pial incision into the vermis is made using bipolar forceps and a microscissor.

Because metastatic tumors are surrounded by edematous brain, a cleavage plane is easily developed around the tumor using suction, fine dissectors, and cottonoid pledgets. A small brain retractor blade is helpful to retract the tumor away from the fourth ventricle (Fig. 27-17). With any instrument in the posterior fossa, the direction of retraction or applied force must always be away from the brain stem and must never cause any pressure on this vital structure (Fig. 27-18). The tumor is removed with an ultrasonic aspirator, or a microbipolar and forceps.

Having totally removed the tumor and after obtaining meticulous hemostasis, the dura is reapproximated. The muscle and fascial layers are then carefully closed. The previously made Y- or T-shaped fascial incision allows a tight closure protecting the area from which the bone has been removed. Unless this type of incision is used, it is often difficult to close the superior aspect of the wound; incomplete closure may lead to cerebrospinal fluid fistula, pseudomeningocele formation, and serious infection.

Medulloblastoma

Most medullublastomas are midline lesions (Fig. 27-19). Characteristically this reddish-gray tumor protrudes between the cerebellar tonsils. Although the lesion may appear well demarcated, on closer inspection subpial extensions over the cerebellar folia or a tongue-like extension down along the medulla may be seen. Frequently, the most difficult aspect of the dissection is the tight adherence of the tumor to the floor of the fourth ventricle. Tumors that arise from the roof of the ventricle are frequently subjected to gross total removal.

The median incision is used with the patient in the lateral decubitus or prone position. Because medulloblastomas almost invariably block the cerebrospinal fluid pathways, a right occipital bur hole should be placed for possible cannulation of the lateral ventricle. As illustrated in Figure 27-20, a tumor protruding from the fourth ventricle is best approached by splitting the vermis. Even this initial step can be carried out under the microscope (Fig. 27-21). The blood supply of this tumor consistently comes from the choroidal arteries. As the margin of the tumor is exposed, large feeding branches can be identified and cauterized with the bipolar or clipped as necessary. Medulloblastomas are often so friable that they can be evacuated by suction (Fig. 27-22). As the tumor is removed, the choroid plexus of the fourth ventricle will be encountered along with arteries that feed the tumor and occasionally large draining veins. Because these vessels are so close to the floor of the fourth ventricle, they should be coagulated under irrigation (Fig. 27-23). The floor of the fourth ventricle should be protected by a wet cottonoid strip inserted beneath the caudal tip of the tumor; this helps the surgeon maintain the orientation of the dissection plane.

Sometimes portions of the tumor are too firm to remove by suction, and microdissectors and scissors must be used to remove it piecemeal. Traction on the tumor must be absolutely avoided. For this reason, the ultrasonic aspirator and the surgical laser are extremely useful adjuncts in shaving tumors down to the level of the floor of the ventricle and achieving a maximal resection. If the tumor invades the floor of the fourth ventricle, no attempt should be made to remove the tumor beyond this level. The objective of the surgery in these cases should be to remove the bulk of the lesion and, thereby, establish normal flow of cerebrospinal fluid. Although medulloblastomas are sensitive to both radiation and chemotherapy, length of survival and the chance for "cure" partially depend on the extent of surgical resection.

On occasion, following removal of a very large tumor, the cerebellar hemispheres appear in danger of collapsing into the tumor cavity. In this situation it is very important to deal with the bridging veins over the superior surface of the cerebellum (see Fig. 27-25). If these veins are coagulated but not divided, they will still serve to suspend the cerebellum but will not cause bleeding. While obtaining hemostasis in the posterior fossa, remember to have the anesthesiologist increase the venous pressure by a Valsalva manuever to check for further potential bleeding points.

If the dura can be closed, it should be closed completely. Small openings in the dural closure may provide sites for herniation of the cerebellum that can lead to strangulation and postoperative edema. As previously mentioned, the capacity of the posterior fossa can be increased by use of a dural graft and gelfoam.

Ependymoma

Figures 27-24 and 27-25 illustrate a typical ependymoma of the fourth ventricle. These tumors arise from the walls, roof, or floor of the ventricle. Even tumors that do not originate in the floor of the fourth ventricle may have a secondary attachment there. This tumor appears brownish-gray in color and firmly nodular in consistency. It may first be seen as a tongue-like protrusion between the cerebellar tonsils. This neoplasm is firmer to palpation than the medulloblastoma. It too receives its blood supply predominantly from the choroidal arteries.

Because of its intimate attachments to vital structures, this lesion must be removed piece by piece. Only when the tumor can be freely dissected from the floor of the fourth ventricle can a total removal be accomplished. Not infrequently the tumor appears to originate from the posterolateral surface of the restiform body on one side. Care must be taken to avoid digging into the medulla. Any tumor within or adherent to the medulla should not be removed (Fig. 27-25).

Juvenile Astrocytoma

The juvenile (piloid) astrocytoma is predominantly a tumor of childhood and adolescence. In the posterior fossa and elsewhere, its biology and clinical behavior are significantly different and more benign than the behavior of low-grade "ordinary" astrocytomas of the adult cerebral hemispheres. Many of the tumors are largely cystic and contain a reddish-brown mural nodule in an otherwise shiny, smooth white wall. Usually the cyst contains an amber-colored highly proteinaceous fluid that coagulates after removal. Most often these tumors are located near the midline within the posterior fossa or out laterally in a cerebellar hemisphere (Fig. 27-26).

Because this is a curable neoplasm, total excision is always the goal. Only rare adherence to, or invasion of, the floor of the fourth ventricle prevents complete removal; this usually occurs with predominantly solid variants of the lesion.

After exposing the inferior surface of the cerebellar hemispheres, asymmetry, flattening, and widening of the folia are noted on the side of the lesion. Gentle palpation with a wetted finger gives a boggy feeling in this area and may leave a dimple. A ventricular needle may be introduced into the lesion after coagulating the leptomeninges and making a 2-mm incision into the cortex. The cyst is aspirated. A cortical incision is made perpendicular to the long axis of the folia. The cyst wall is entered to reveal the solid mural nodule (Fig. 27-27). In hemispheric tumors near the midline, feeding vessels will arise from cortical arteries. These vessels can be coagulated and divided as they enter the solid portion of the tumor. Cure depends on removal of the mural nodule. The cyst wall can be removed in those areas where there is a good line of cleavage between it and the compressed cerebellum. Gentle retraction on the capsule along with blunt dissection outside the capsule usually allows total removal of the cyst wall as well as the more important solid portion of the tumor (Figs. 27-28 and 27-29). If there is any resistance, it is not necessary or advisable to remove small portions of the cyst wall from deep midline structures.

Some lesions, particularly when the base of the tumor reaches toward the center of the cerebellar hemisphere, may have indistinct planes of cleavage at the site of the solid tumor (Fig. 27-29). In these cases the neoplasm can be differentiated from the cerebellum by its response to suction. Unlike posterior fossa tumors that invade the floor of the fourth ventricle and thereby limit neurosurgical removal, deep penetration within the hemisphere should not be a deterrent to total removal when dealing with this relatively benign tumor. The ultrasonic aspirator and surgical laser are useful adjuncts in such cases.

Tumors located over the posterior vermis are fed by branches of the choroidal arteries, which should be coagulated before removing the tumor. In tumors extending to the superior surface of the vermis, large supplying vessels usually arise from the superior cerebellar arteries. Thin-walled veins may leave this type of tumor to empty into the superior petrosal sinus. Again, it should be emphasized that only bipolar coagulation should be used in the posterior fossa.

Hemangioblastoma

Cystic cerebellar hemangioblastomas may occupy a great variety of locations but commonly are located posteroinferiorly within the cerebellar hemisphere (Fig. 27-30). In lesions of the vermis, the tumor may reach into the fourth ventricle. Two of Kempe's 10 cases were located over the area postrema. When dealing with a hemangioblastoma, always remember that there may be more than one tumor.

After opening the dura, inspection through the arachnoid reveals asymmetry, increased vascularity, and discoloration over the hemisphere containing the tumor (Fig. 27-31). After opening the arachnoid, a ventricular needle can be inserted through an avascular area, and a large cyst aspirated under ultrasonic guidance. The fluid characteristically is yellow but may be any color from yellow to black, because spontaneous hemorrhage does occur within these lesions. The cyst is opened by coagulating the pia longitudinally in an area away from the dilated, tortuous surface vessels. The walls of the cyst may be white or yellow depending on whether or not hemorrhage has occurred (Fig. 27-32). The tumor is recognized by its bright color due to its rich vascularity. The neoplastic mural nodule must be totally removed. The base of the nodule contains all the feeding arteries and draining veins. Large vessels are clipped and smaller ones coagulated as the tumor is excised. Rarely, a tumor will be encountered in which the mural nodule is only a few millimeters in diameter.

The situation is quite different when this tumor is solid and in the midline. In this case the inferior vermis is divided in the midline. Such a tumor must be removed using magnification and bipolar coagulation.

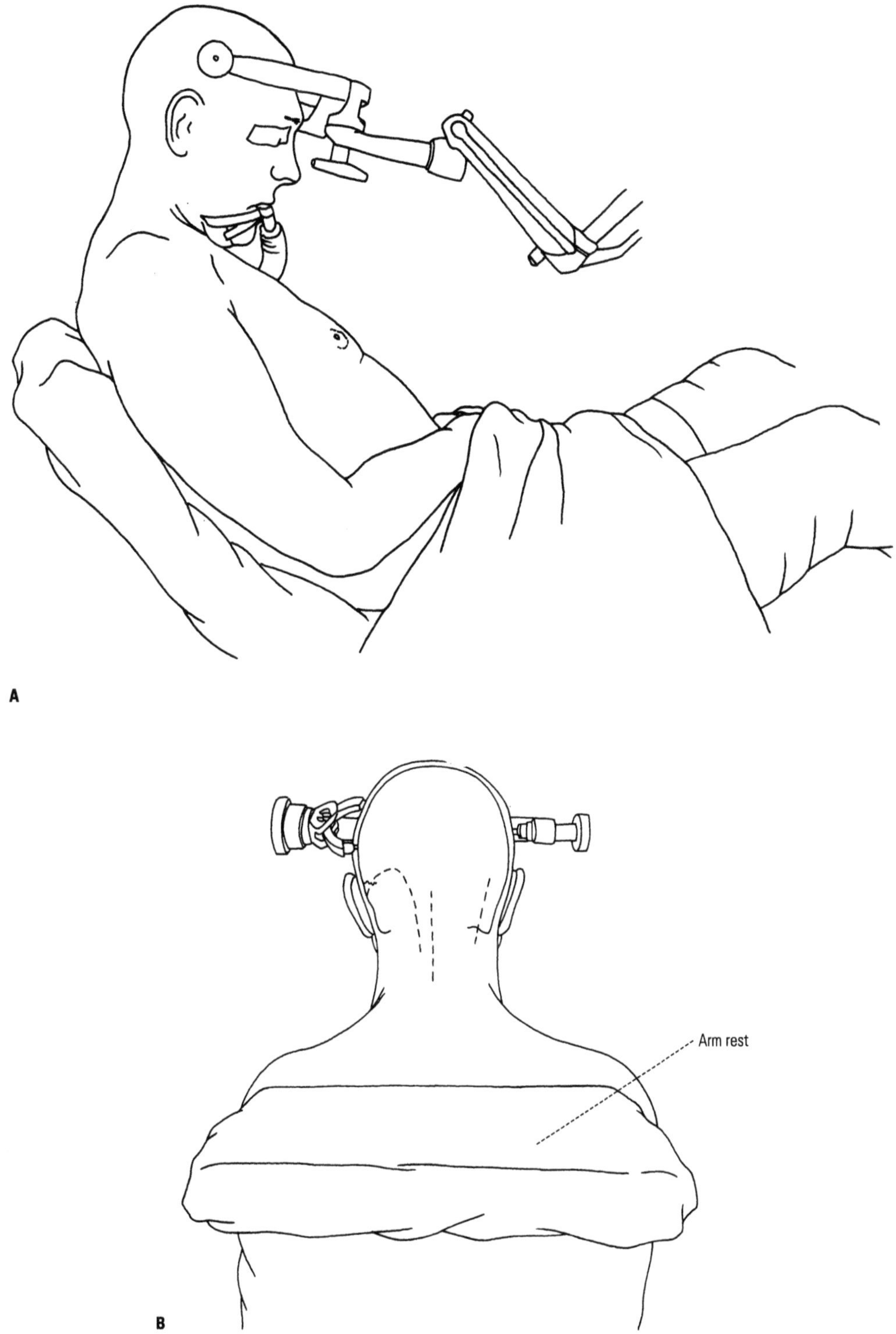

Figure 27-1. Sitting position. Note elevation of legs to height of chest (*panel A*) and use of head rest as arm brace for surgeon (*panel B*). Standard incisions are outlined.

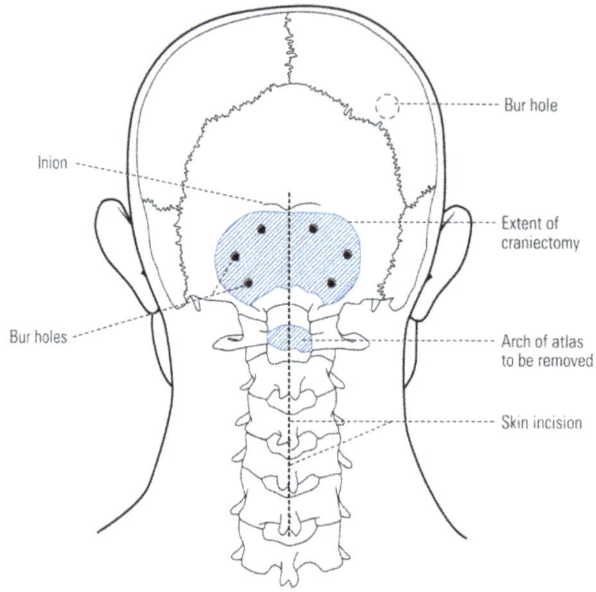

Figure 27-2. Midline incision for posterior fossa exposure. The *shaded area* indicates size of craniectomy and laminectomy. An occipital bur hole is made 6 to 8 cm above and lateral to inion.

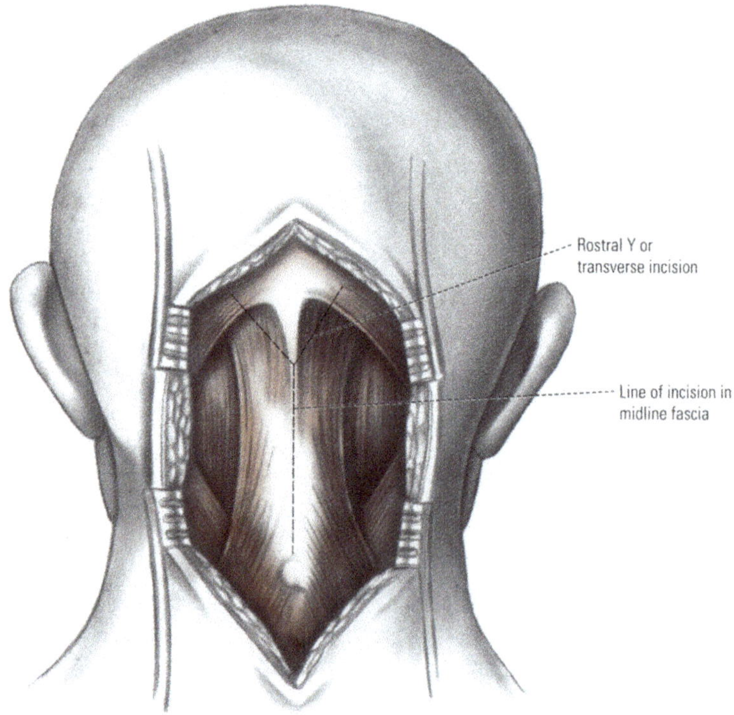

Figure 27-3. Midline fascial incision for posterior fossa surgery. Note line of incision of muscle and fascia below their insertion to facilitate closure.

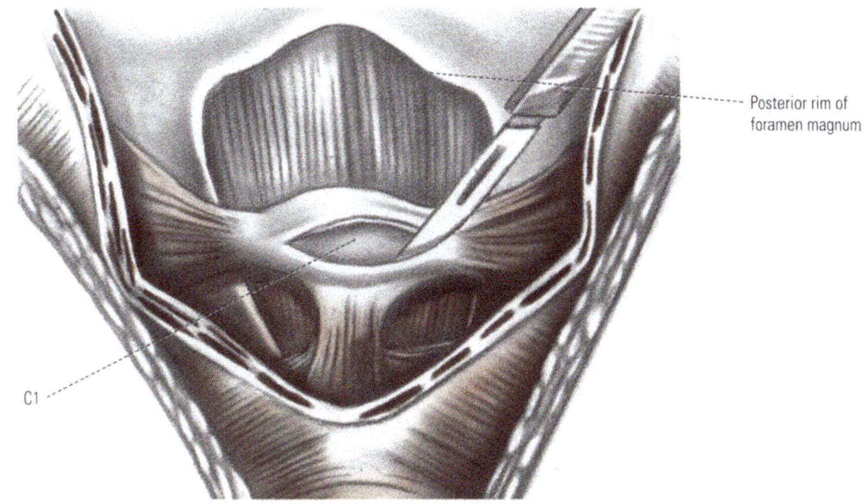

Figure 27-4. Subperiosteal exposure of arch of atlas.

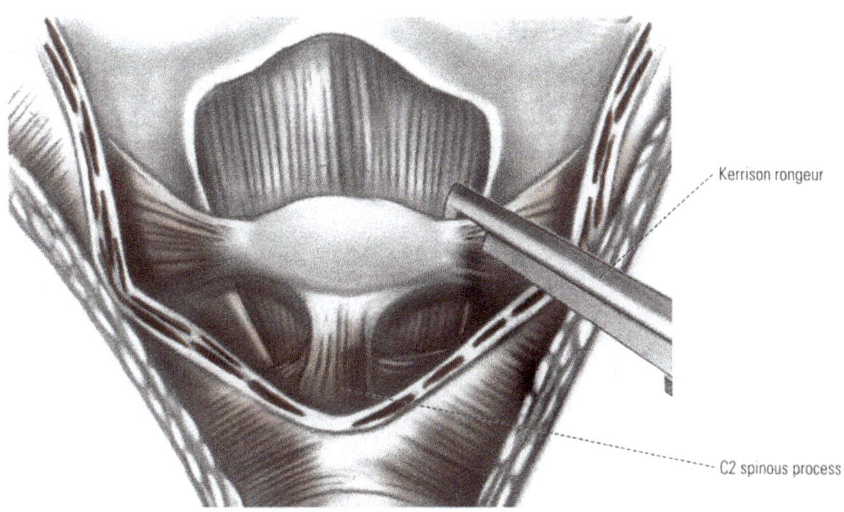

Figure 27-5. Removal of arch of the atlas.

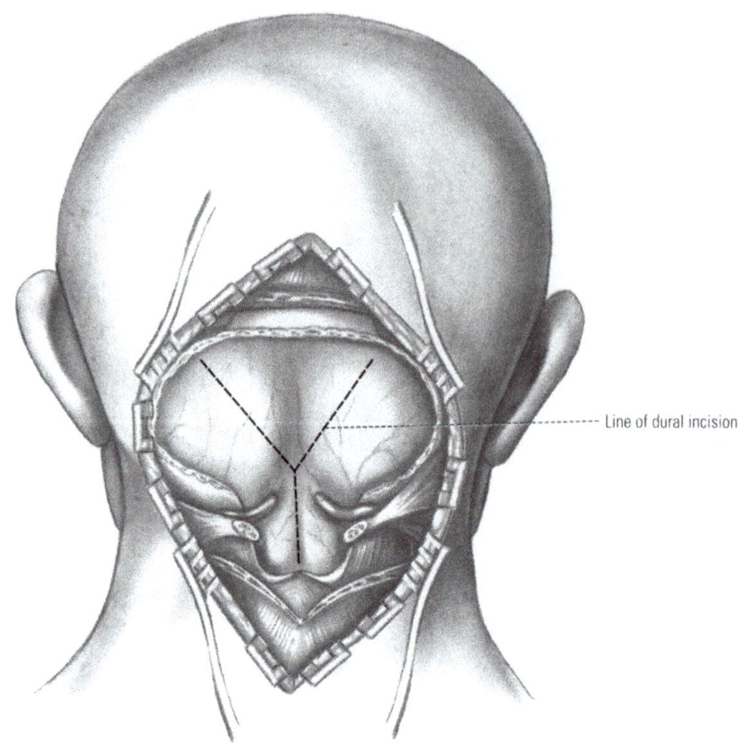

Figure 27-6. Midline craniectomy and dural incision. Note 1) extent of craniectomy to level of transverse sinus for control of bridging veins, and 2) *Y*-shaped dural incision avoids opening of occipital sinus: only the marginal sinus at the level of the foramen magnum will be traversed.

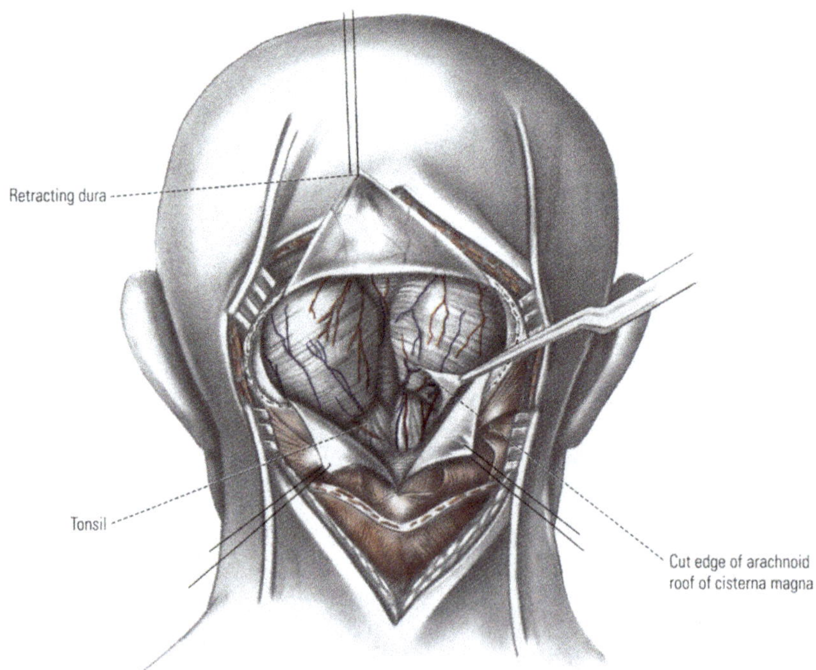

Figure 27-7. Operative exposure of cerebellum. Note 1) retraction of dura by sutures, and 2) opening of arachnoid over cisterna magna.

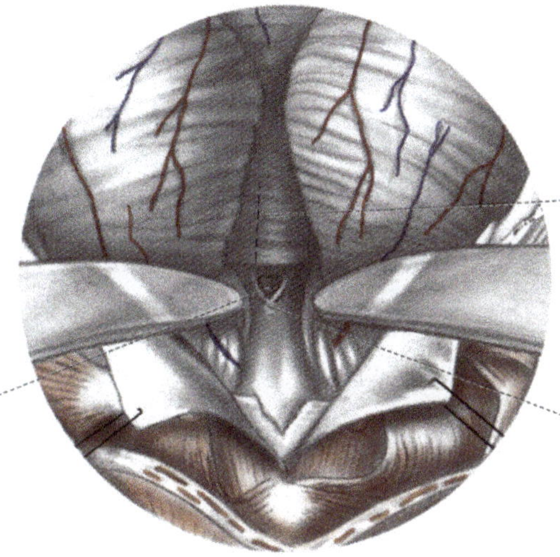

Figure 27-8. Posterior fossa exploration. Note 1) cerebellar tonsils retracted laterally to expose the obex and the foramen Magendie, and 2) extent of vermal incision necessary to inspect the fourth ventricle.

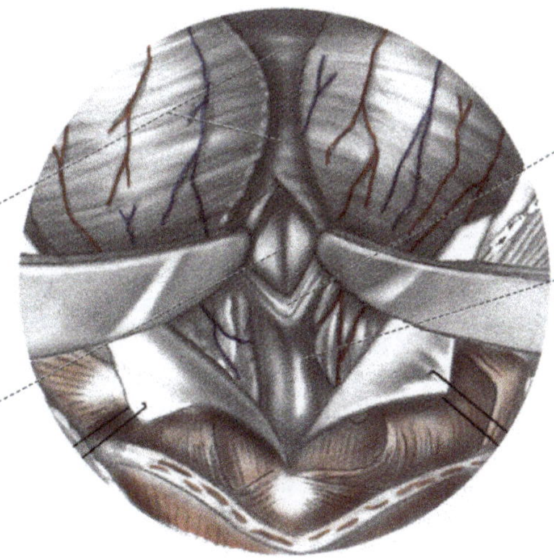

Figure 27-9. The floor of fourth ventricle as seen through a vermis-splitting incision. Normal anatomy of fourth ventricular floor is illustrated.

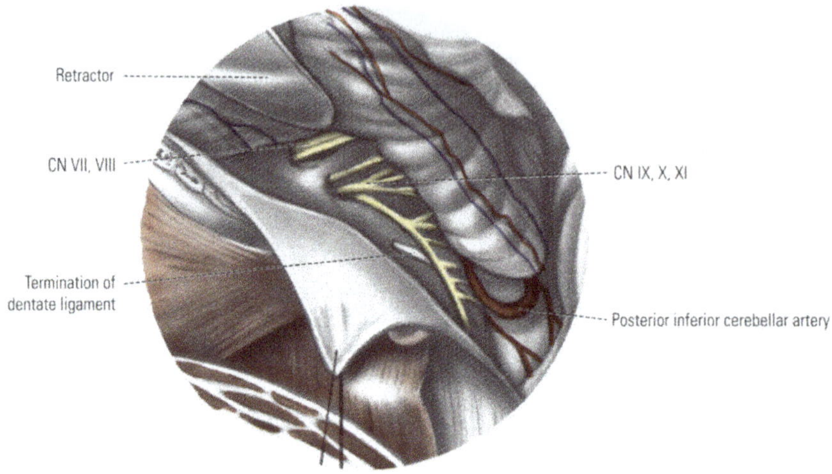

Figure 27-10. Inspection of lateral recess of medullary cistern and posterior portion of left cerebellopontine angle. Note 1) retraction is upward, away from the brain stem, and 2) exposure of nerves VII, VIII, IX, X, XI.

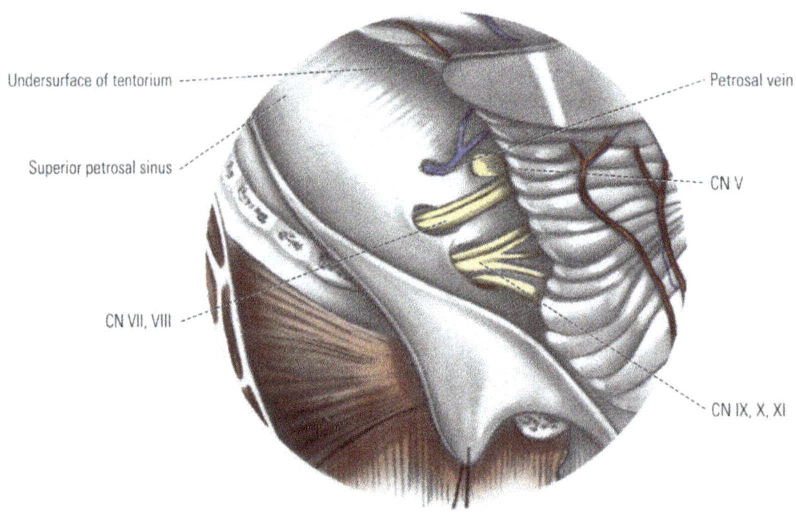

Figure 27-11. Inspection of entire cerebellopontine angle. Note that retraction is medial and superior. Compare position of brain spatula with that of Figure 27-10. Nerves V, VII, VIII, IX, X, and XI are exposed.

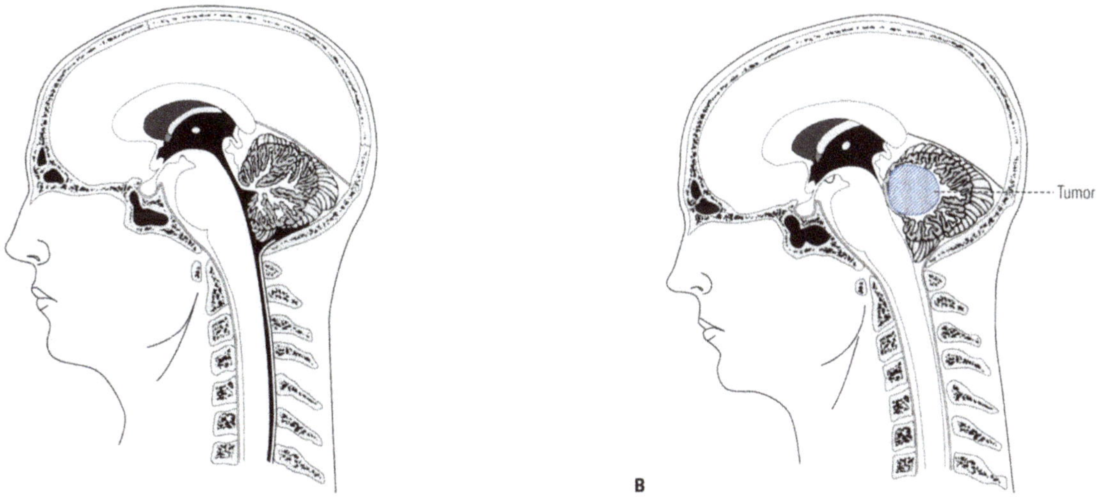

A B

Figure 27-12. Midline sagittal view of posterior fossa (*panel A*) and projected right hemisphere tumor (*panel B*).

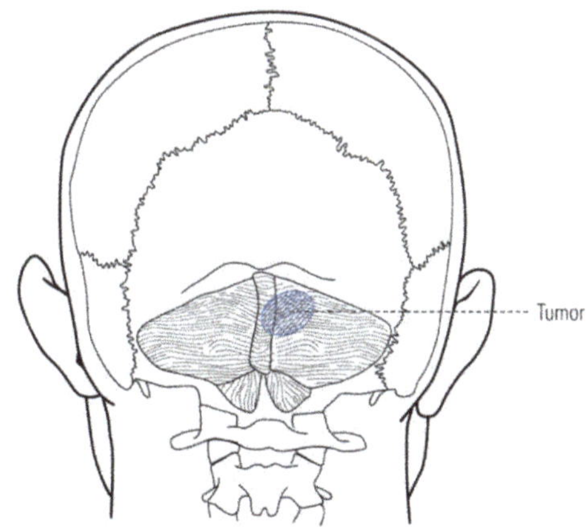

Figure 27-13. A metastatic lesion in vermis and right cerebellar hemisphere projected on an outline of head and spine in position for surgery.

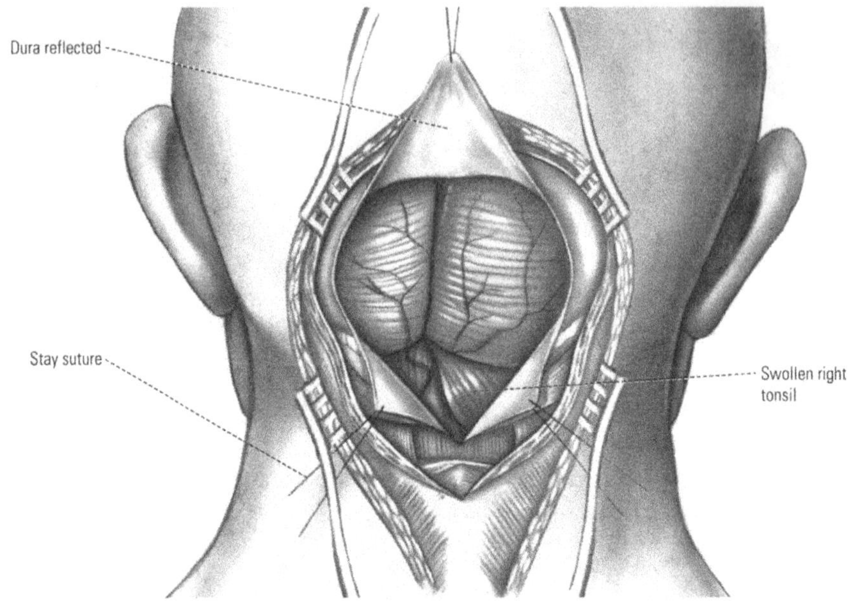

Figure 27-14. Suboccipital craniectomy for cerebellar tumor: inferior surface of cerebellum exposed. Note 1) the difference in size of cerebellar hemispheres and particularly of cerebellar tonsil on the side of the lesion, and 2) retraction of dura by stay sutures.

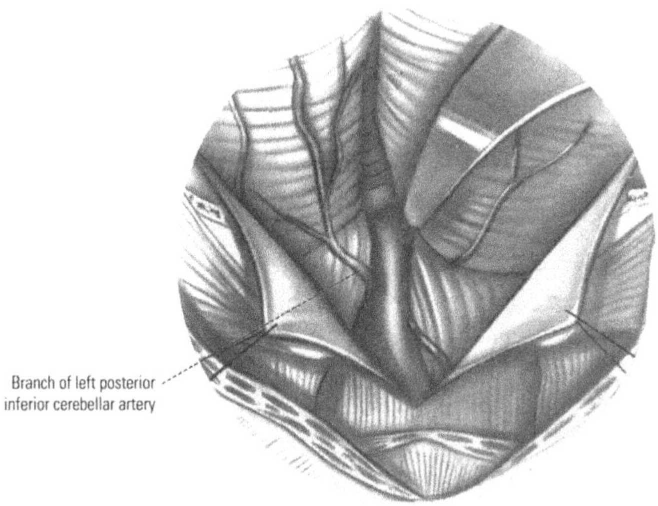

Figure 27-15. Exposure of the inferior part of the vermis.

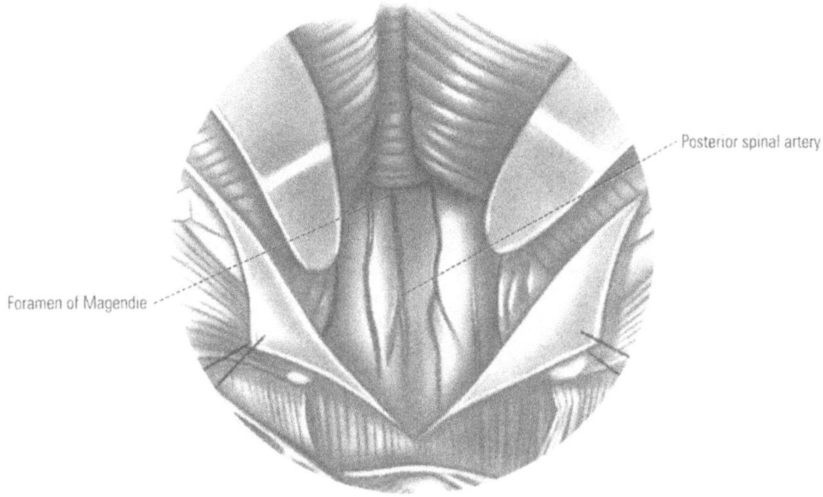

Figure 27-16. Exposure of the obex and the foramen of Magendie.

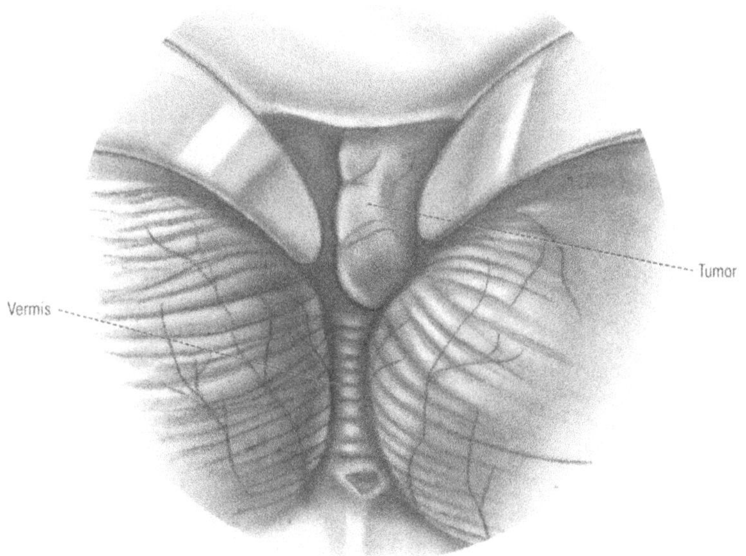

Figure 27-17. Retracting the cerebellar hemispheres to expose paravermal tumor.

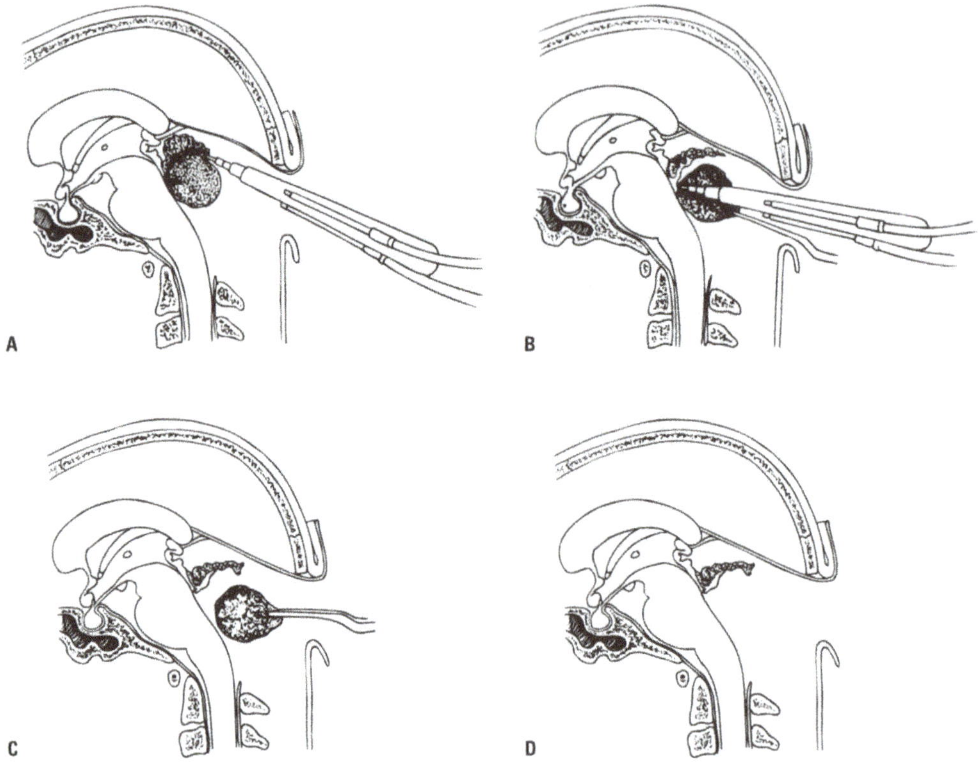

Figure 27-18. Use of ultrasonic aspirator and bipolar forceps in dissection and delivery of tumor (metastatic nodule). A, The instrument is moved up over the tumor without ever pressing the lesion anteriorly. B, The instrument has passed over superior extent of the tumor. C, Direction of movement is inferiorly and posteriorly. D, Tumor removed.

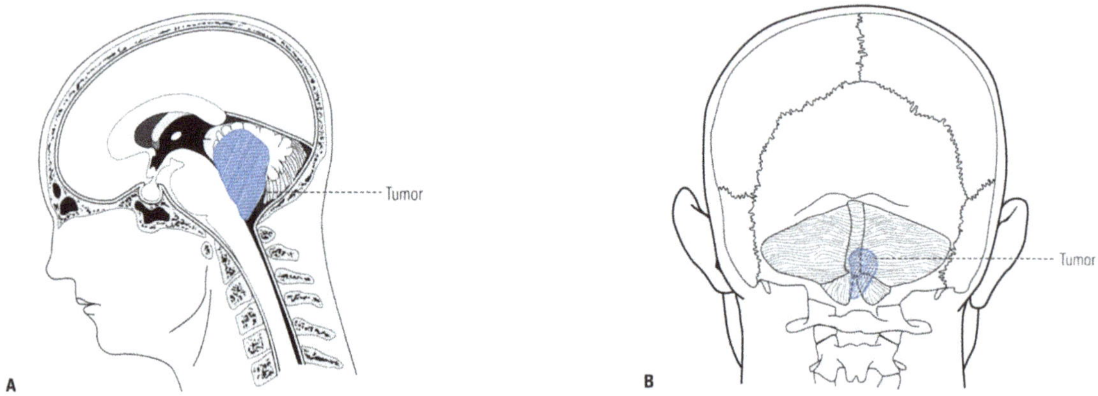

Figure 27-19. A, Median sagittal section of lower fourth ventricular tumor (cerebellar medulloblastoma). B, Lower fourth ventricular tumor projected on an outline of the head and spine in position for surgery.

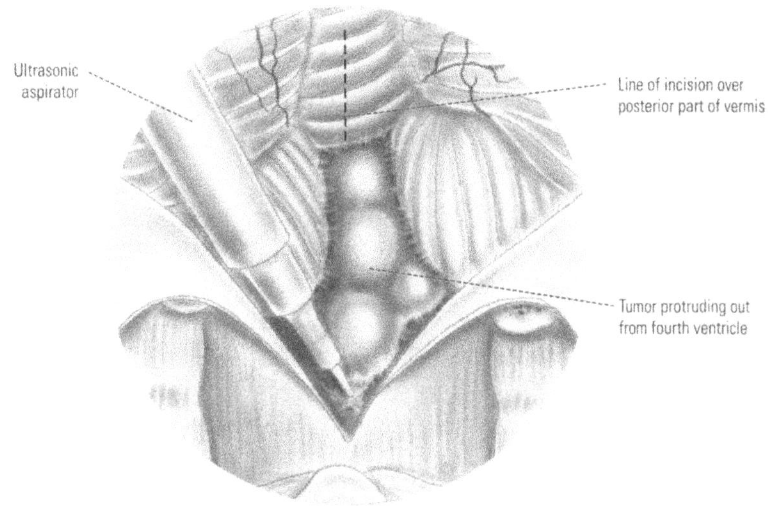

Figure 27-20. Medulloblastoma of the lower part of the fourth ventricle. Note 1) the arachnoid remains intact, and 2) tumor protrudes from beneath the vermis and between the tonsils.

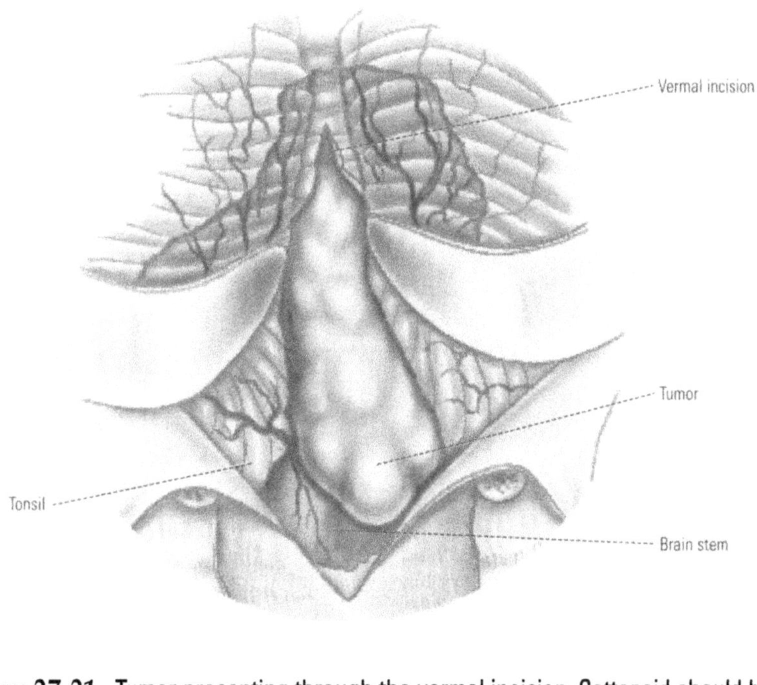

Figure 27-21. Tumor presenting through the vermal incision. Cottonoid should be placed ventral to caudal tumor and dorsal to brain stem.

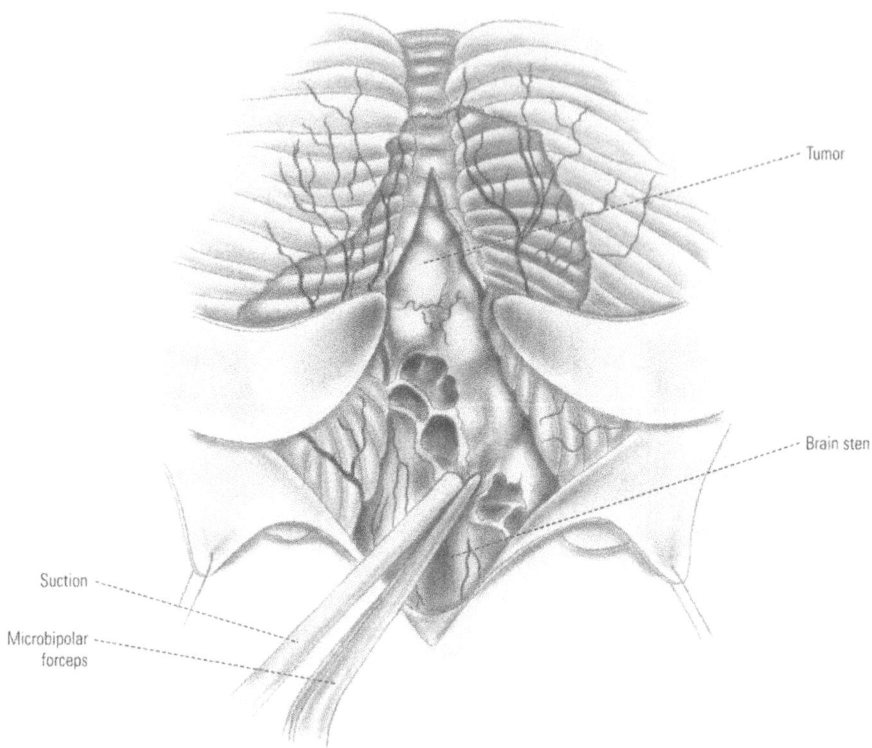

Figure 27-22. Medulloblastoma of the lower fourth ventricle being removed by suction and microbipolar cautery.

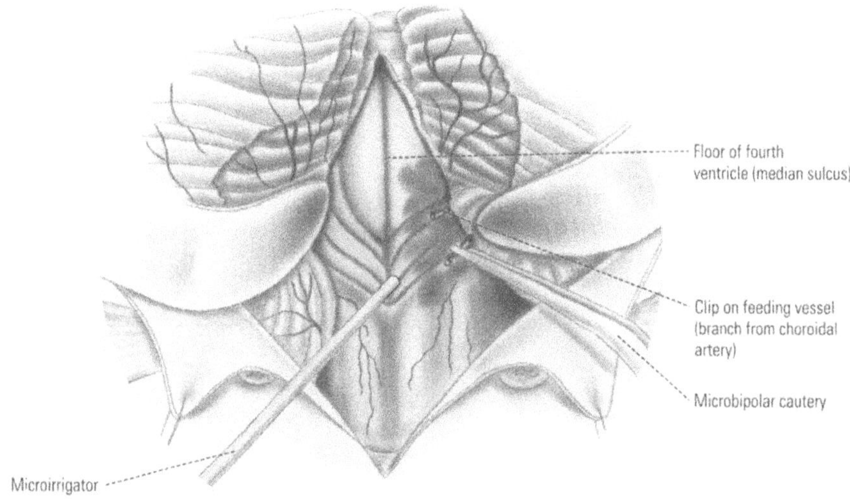

Figure 27-23. Control of feeding vessels, which are branches of the choroidal arteries, by clips and microbipolar cautery.

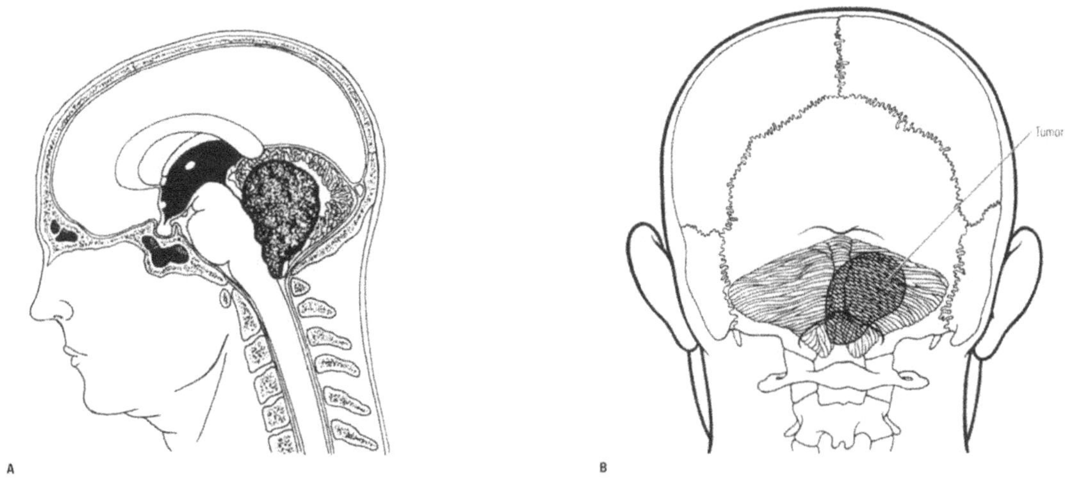

Figure 27-24. A, Fourth ventricle tumor (ependymoma): midline sagittal section. Note the attachment to the floor of the fourth ventricle.
B, Intraventricular tumor (ependymoma) projected on an outline of the head and spine in position for surgery.

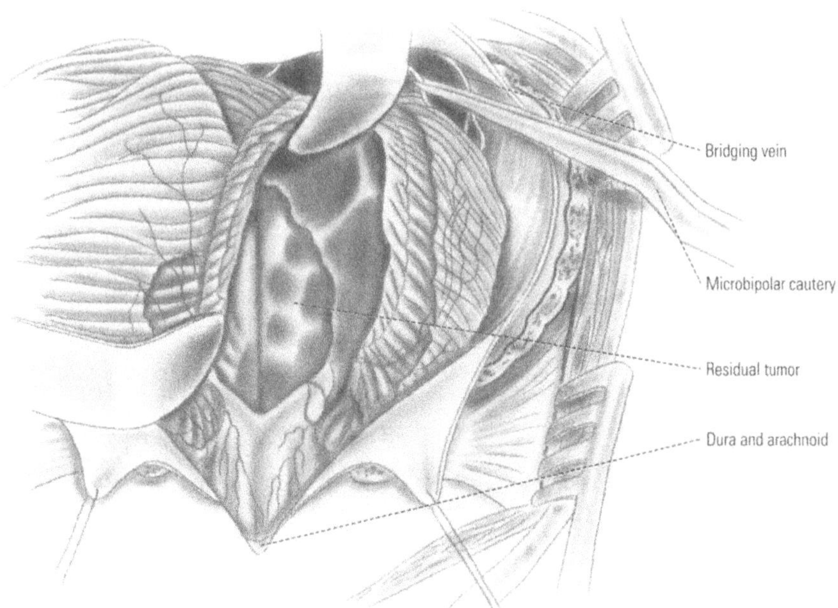

Figure 27-25. Subtotal removal of tumor leaving the part that is adherent to the floor of the IVth ventricle. Note that following removal of this large tumor, the right cerebellar hemisphere has collapsed. As a result the bridging veins must be coagulated and supported with gelfoam.

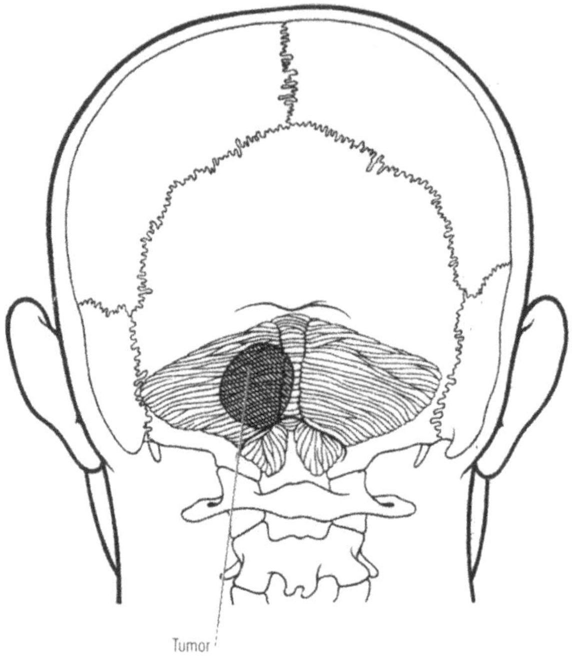

Figure 27-26. Left lateral cerebellar intrahemispheric glioma (juvenile astrocytoma) projected on an outline of the head and spine in position for surgery.

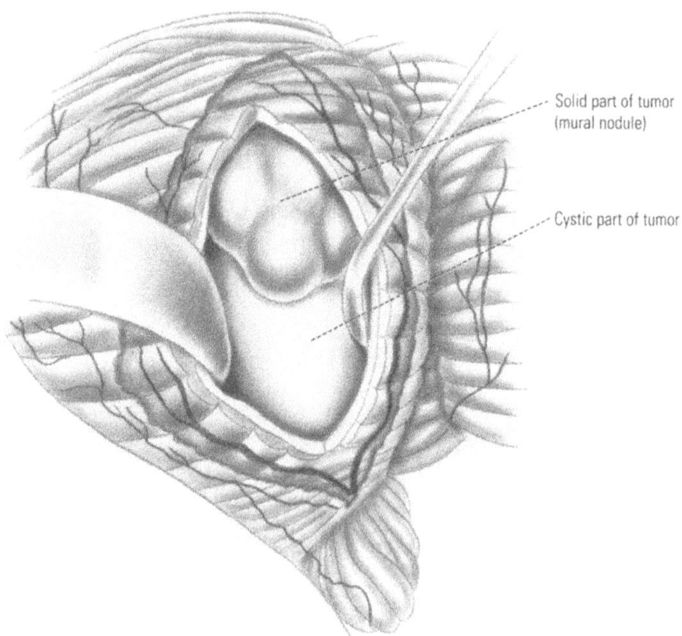

Figure 27-27. Cerebellar astrocytoma. Note that 1) the cyst has been entered to reveal mural nodule projecting into the cyst cavity, and 2) the cyst wall is white and smooth.

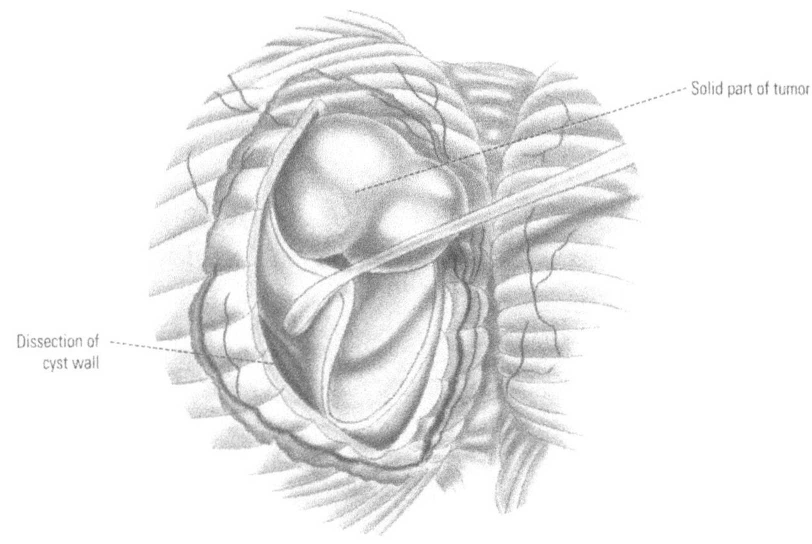

Figure 27-28. Removal of cystic cerebellar astrocytoma. The capsule of the cyst as well as the solid tumor is removed.

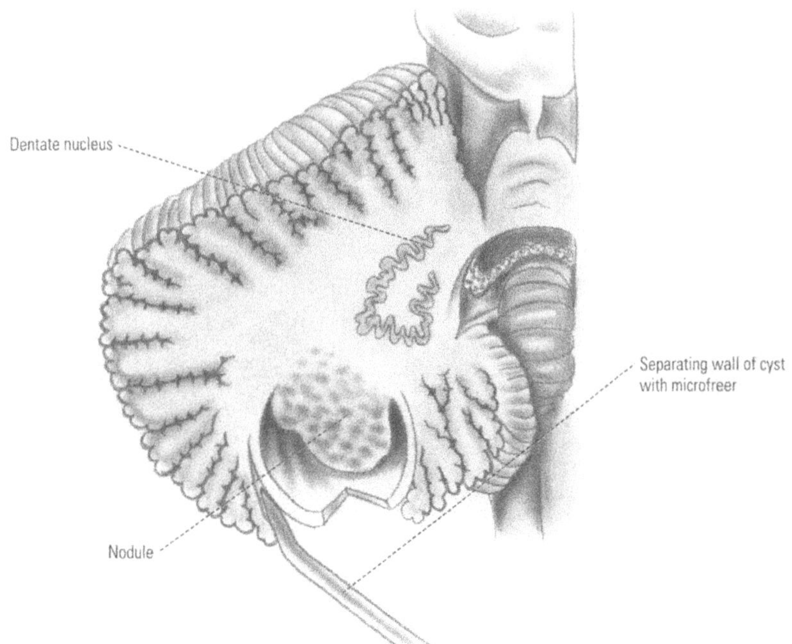

Figure 27-29. Oblique section through the cerebellar hemisphere and the tumor reveals indefinite border between solid tumor and normal brain tissue.

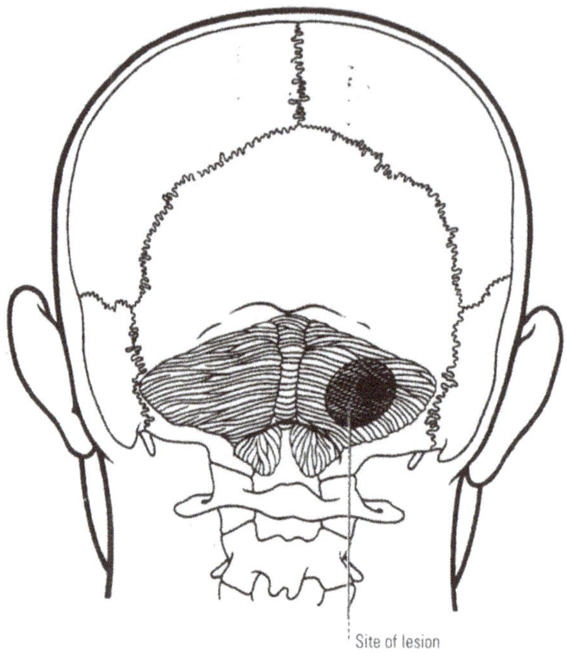

Figure 27-30. Hemangioblastoma of the right cerebellar hemisphere projected on an outline of the head and spine in position for surgery.

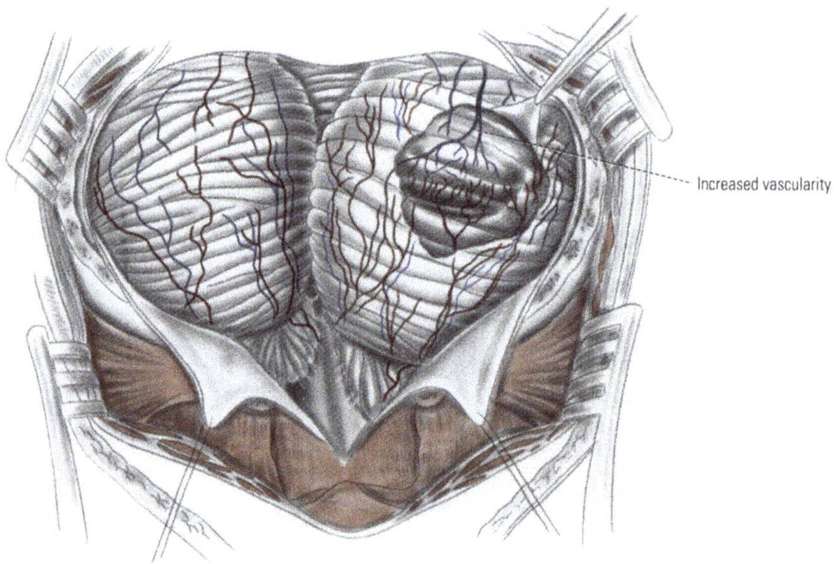

Figure 27-31. Hemangioblastoma of right cerebellar hemisphere: surface exposure. Note the increased vascularity and discoloration over the site of the lesion.

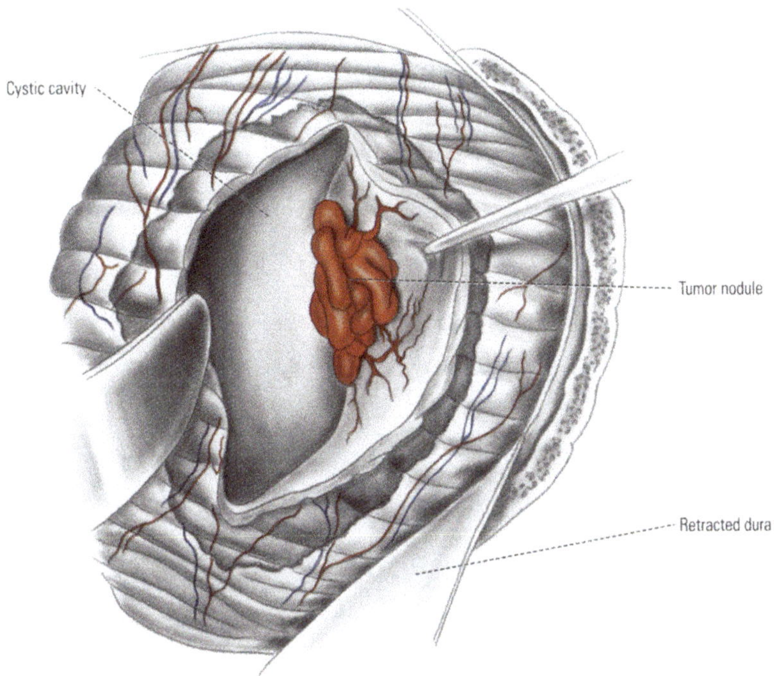

Figure 27-32. Cystic tumor with mural nodule. Note that the tumor is located close to the surface of the cerebellum.

CHAPTER

28

Combined Occipital-suboccipital Craniotomy

Meningioma of the Posterior Surface of the Petrous Bone

The most frequent location for meningiomas of the posterior fossa, in our experience, is on the posterior surface of the petrous bone (Fig. 28-1). The major blood supply to these very vascular tumors arises from short branches of the internal carotid artery as the blood passes through the carotid canal within the petrous bone. Additional vessels from the posterior branches of the middle meningeal artery and from meningeal branches of the vertebral artery feed the tumor. In medially placed tumors near the clivus, the blood supply may be identical to that for a clivus meningioma. These tumors are attached to the dura over the posterior surface of the petrous bone anterior and superior to the internal auditory meatus and to the undersurface of the tentorium. The tentorium may be perforated by the tumor just as the falx is often penetrated by meningiomas in that location.

Meningiomas in this location are most readily removed by a combined supra- and infratentorial approach. This operation can be done with the patient sitting or in the lateral decubitus position. All of the precautions against a sudden fall in blood pressure and air embolism must be taken.

A 20-cm curvilinear scalp incision is made beginning 5 cm above the lambdoidal suture, bisecting the superior nuchal line half way between the inion and the mastoid process, and then turning straight down the neck (Fig. 28-2). Extensive subgaleal and subperiosteal dissection then allows the bony exposure shown in Figure 28-3. Bur holes are then placed laterally just above the transverse/sigmoid junction in the occipital region, and superiorly and inferiorly in the suboccipital region. The craniotome is used to cut the bone flap after the sigmoid sinus is separated carefully both from the lateral bur hole in the occipital bone and through the medial bur hole just below the transverse sinus. The craniotome is used starting at the lateral bur hole in the occipital region, coming across the sinus to the inferior bur hole in the suboccipital region and then going into the foramen magnum. The craniotomy is restarted, after separating the dura from the foramen magnum, going upwards from the medial aspect of the foramen magnum to the superior suboccipital bur hole and then across the transverse sinus upwards and then laterally and then inferiorly to complete the craniotomy.

The occipital dura is opened so that the base of the dural flap is at the sinus (Fig. 28-3). A few occipital bridging veins are coagulated and the occipital lobe is elevated to expose the tentorium (Fig. 28-4). The superior surface of the tentorium is inspected for supratentorial extension of the tumor. If the tumor has perforated the tentorium, it should be incised so that the tentorial flap will be based at the superior petrosal sinus. At times it is better to expose the incisura from above and begin the tentorial incision at that point. In the case illustrated, the tumor did not perforate the tentorium; therefore, the small tentorial incision is based posteriorly (Figs. 28-5). Cerebellar veins may be draped over the tumor as they pass to the superior petrosal sinus. These veins must be coagulated and divided. The tumor capsule is coagulated and a window is made into the tumor. The tumor is then gutted using an ultrasonic aspirator or occasionally, in very vascular tumors, by laser or electrocautery loop (Fig. 28-6). Depending on the size of the tumor, the tentorium may be opened up to the transverse sinus, which gives a beautiful view of the cerebellopontine angle from above.

The dura over the posterior fossa is then opened as shown in Figure 28-3. Depending on the size of the tumor, it may be covered by only a shell of cerebellum or it may be so large that it is necessary to resect the lateral portion of the hemisphere. As the cerebellum is retracted, it must be covered by wet cotton pledgets; and when the cerebellum is dissected from the tumor capsule, cotton pledgets should be advanced into the line of cleavage. The cranial nerves, which are stretched by the tumor (Fig. 28-7), are also protected with a wet cottonoid as the tumor is morselized from below (Fig. 28-8). Feeding vessels from the superior and anterior inferior cerebellar arteries will become visible as the tumor is reduced in size and must be taken with the bipolar. It is often necessary to alternate back and forth between the supra- and infratentorial exposure as the tumor is gradually reduced in size. The facial nerve may be found displaced ventrally or it may be pushed superiorly toward the root of the trigeminal nerve. This means that the VIIth nerve must always be kept in mind since it can be found at any site around the tumor. The use of the nerve stimulator to locate the facial nerve has made preservation of the facial nerve much easier.

The outstanding hazard of this operation is the relationship of the tumor to surrounding vascular structures. The basilar artery may be adherent to or even enveloped by the tumor. This means that occasionally a small portion of tumor will have to be left behind. The superior petrosal sinus is usually obliterated by the tumor. After reducing the size of the tumor so that its dural attachments can be seen from above and below, it is excised. Perforating channels from the internal carotid artery in the carotid canal are plugged with bone wax. The tumor bed is thoroughly coagulated under continuous irrigation (Fig. 28-9).

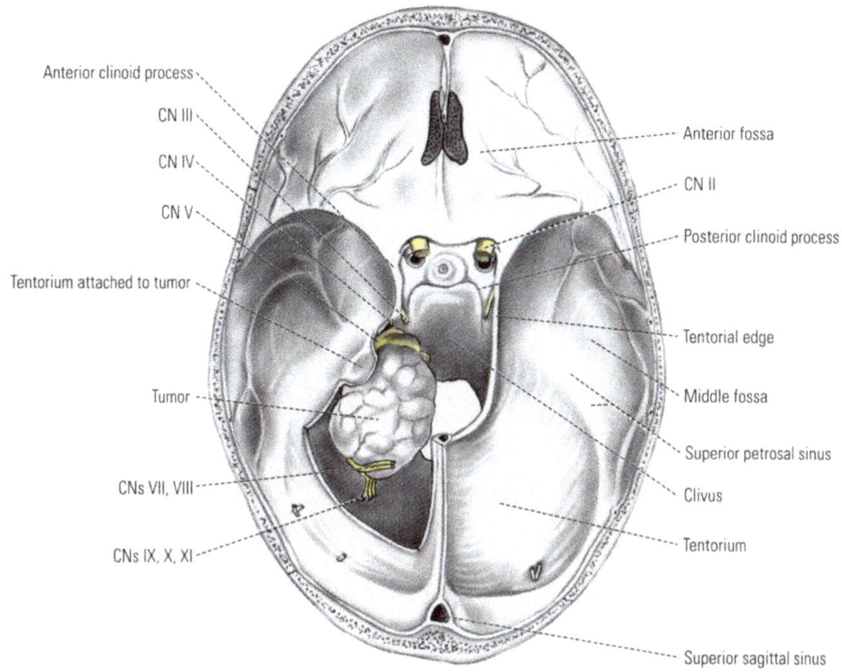

Figure 28-1. Anatomico-topographic demonstration of a meningioma over posterior surface of left petrous bone. Note 1) displacement and stretching of cranial nerves and 2) the tumor is also adherent to undersurface of the tentorium.

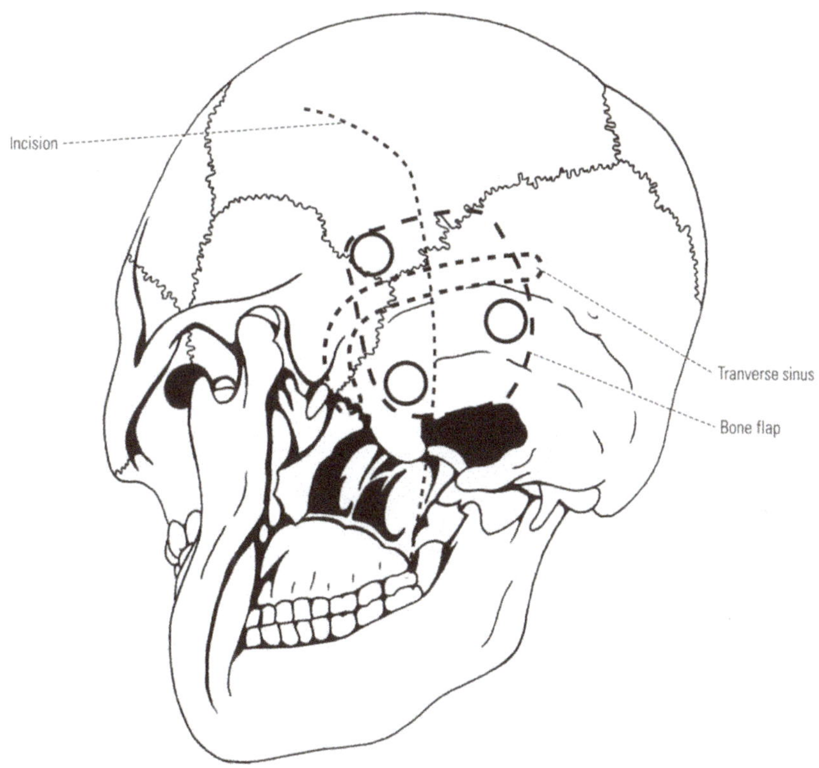

Figure 28-2. Unilateral occipital craniotomy and suboccipital craniotomy for meningioma of the posterior surface of the petrous bone. The bone flap extends above and below transverse sinus.

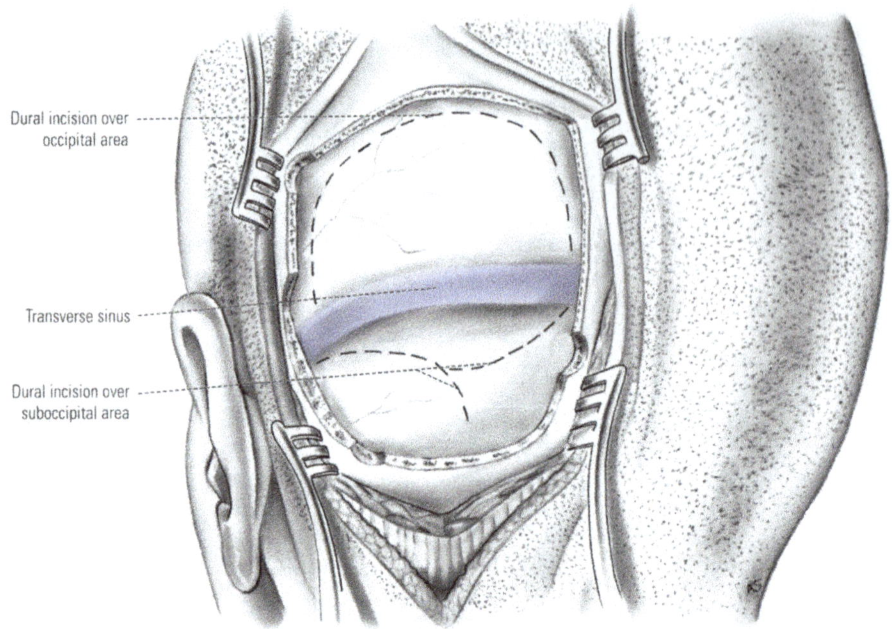

Figure 28-3. Unilateral occipital craniotomy and suboccipital craniectomy. Placement of dural incisions is indicated by the *dotted lines.*

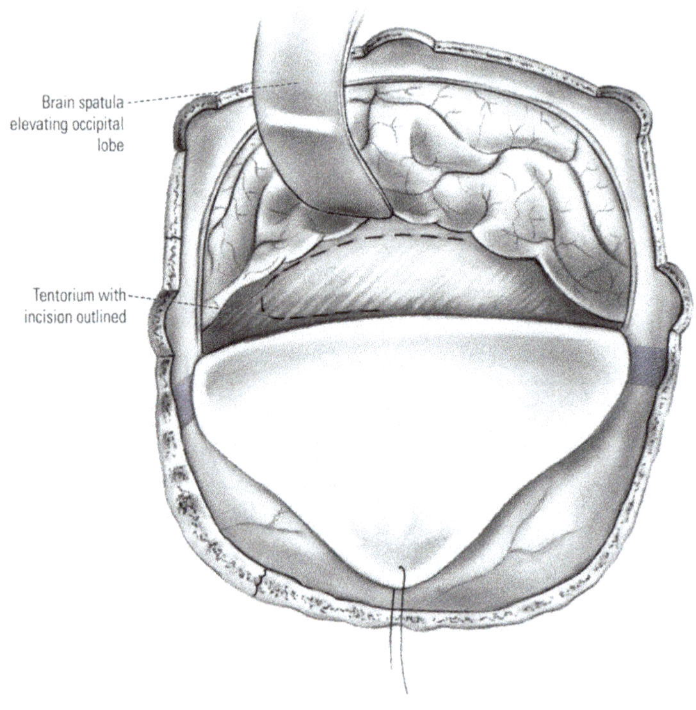

Figure 28-4. Transtentorial approach to a meningioma of the posterior surface of the petrous bone. Note that 1) the dura over the occipital lobe is reflected toward the transverse sinus, and 2) the occipital lobe is elevated exposing the tentorium. The *dotted line* indicates proposed tentorial incision.

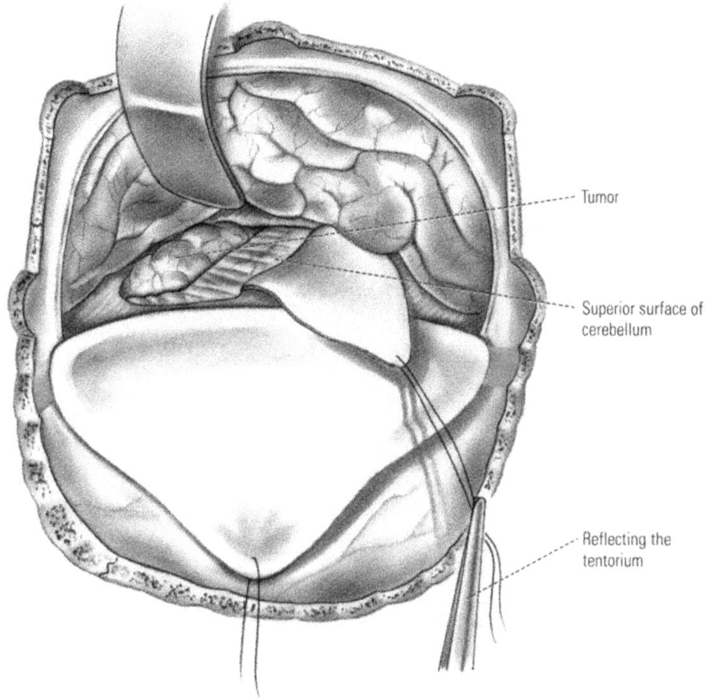

Figure 28-5. Note the tumor presenting through the tentorial incision.

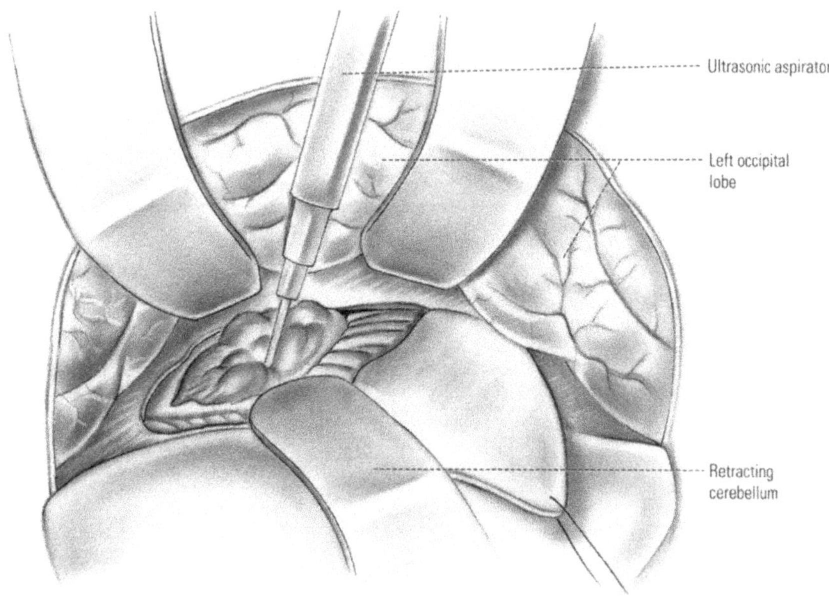

Figure 28-6. Reduction of tumor mass with ultrasonic aspirator. Review Figure 28-1 to visualize position of nerve V2. The petrosal vein, not shown here, may be seen stretched over the tumor at this site.

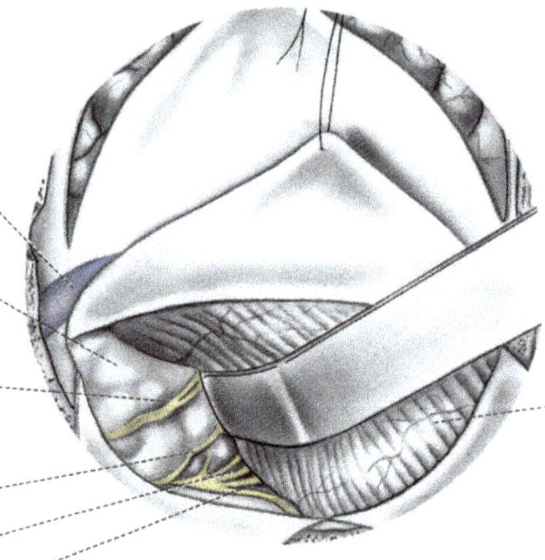

Figure 28-7. Exposure of inferior aspect of a meningioma of the posterior surface of the petrous bone. Nerves VII and VIII are coursing over the capsule of the the tumor.

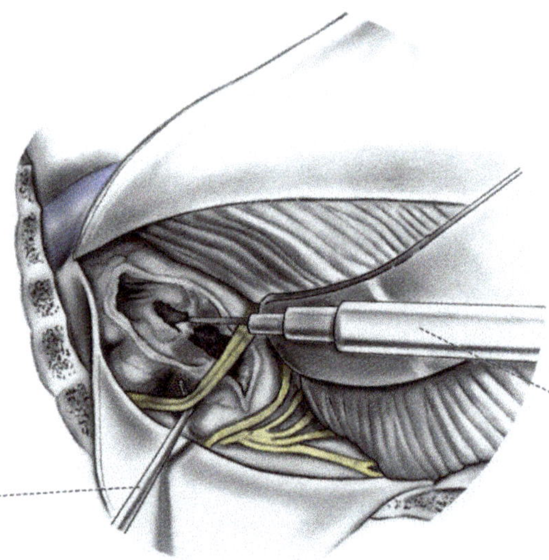

Figure 28-8. Reduction of tumor bulk using an ultrasonic aspirator.

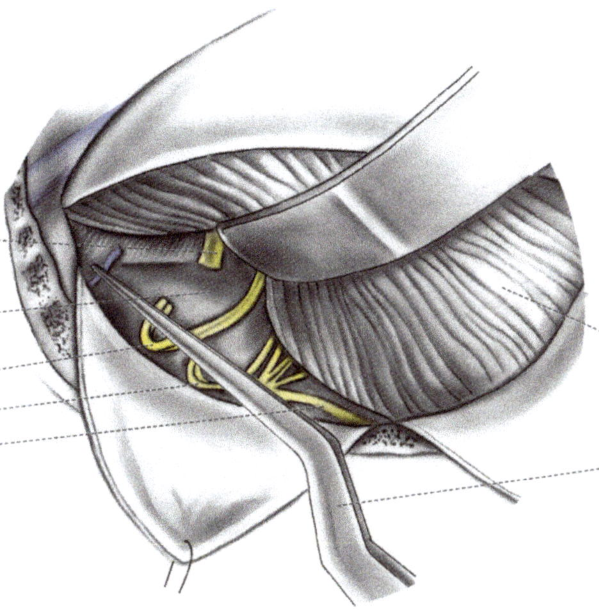

Figure 28-9. Operative field after total removal. Note the use of bipolar coagulation for hemostasis.

CHAPTER

29

Posterior Fossa Arteriovenous Malformation

The posterior fossa is not a common site for arteriovenous (AV) malformations. Only six of 92 AV malformations seen by Kempe were located below the tentorium. Of these, four were located laterally in the cerebellar hemisphere and cerebellopontine angle and two were situated in the vermis. Only one half of the patients presented with a history of hemorrhage (subarachnoid or parenchymal). Three of the patients with laterally located lesions presented with signs and symptoms suggestive of a mass lesion, *ie*, intermittent headaches, pain in the distribution of the trigeminal nerve, nystagmus, diminished hearing, and truncal ataxia. Two of these patients complained of tinnitus when lying on the side of the lesion. In only one of six cases was a bruit audible to the examiner.

The diagnosis is made by magnetic resonance scan and vertebral arteriography. Serial filming is essential and the subtraction technique is particularly helpful.

The principles of surgical technique in the treatment of supratentorial AV malformations as described in volume I, chapter 24 (pp 232–242) are equally applicable for infratentorial lesions. Pertinent points may be summarized as follows: 1) lesions that can be excised without causing significant neurological impairment should be removed; 2) total excision is the surgical goal (ligation of feeding vessels is like shoveling your sidewalk in the middle of a blizzard); 3) embolization does not seem to be applicable for posterior fossa AVMs; 4) except in small lesions, the sitting position is avoided in surgery of AV malformations of the posterior fossa; 5) the use of a very fine suction cannula is essential, which will prevent thin-walled vessels from being ruptured by the sucker; 6) bipolar coagulation also is essential in the posterior fossa; and 7) arterial feeders are always clipped, coagulated, and divided prior to occluding major venous outflow.

The lesion illustrated in Figures 29-1 through 29-5 is a laterally placed posterior fossa AV malformation. This type of lesion is supplied by branches of the posterior inferior, anterior inferior and superior cerebellar arteries (Figs. 29-1 and 29-2). In comparison, midline malformations are fed by medial branches of the posterior inferior cerebellar and superior cerebellar arteries.

Figure 29-3 demonstrates the relationship of the skin incision and craniectomy to the skull. The patient is placed in the lateral decubitus position on the side opposite the lesion. The head and trunk are elevated about 20° and the head is tilted so that the location of the lesion is uppermost.

A vertical 20-cm scalp incision is made midway between the inion and mastoid process beginning 4 cm above the superior nuchal line (Fig. 29-3). The suboccipital craniectomy should expose the lower margin of the transverse sinus superiorly and laterally the junction of the transverse with the sigmoid sinus. This exposure is necessary to give adequate exposure of veins draining the lesion into the transverse, sigmoid, and superior petrosal sinuses. After opening the dura as previously described, it often becomes apparent, particularly in patients who have had a previous subarachnoid hemorrhage, that the arachnoid is thickened and opacified. The arachnoid is opened beginning inferiorly at the junction of the hemisphere and tonsil. If large veins have been demonstrated draining the malformation into the sigmoid and superior petrosal sinus (Fig. 29-4), it will do no harm to coagulate a few small bridging veins posteriorly. This will give a clearer view of the extent of the lesion.

A cerebellar cortical incision is made a few millimeters medial to the margin of the malformation. After coagulating and cutting the pia, the fine sucker tip is used to remove brain tissue. In this manner each vessel leading to the malformation is exposed, clipped, coagulated and divided (Fig. 29-5). As the cortical incision reaches the superior surface of the cerebellum, branches of the superior cerebellar artery are expected and encountered. Having dealt with the arterial supply from the superior and posterior inferior cerebellar arteries, it is usually safe to transect the veins over the superior surface of the lesion draining into the transverse and straight sinuses. The cortical incision is deepened and feeding vessels from the anterior inferior cerebellar artery are clipped. This often results in a dramatic shriveling of the lesion to one half or even one quarter of its previous size. Lastly, the remaining veins draining into the superior petrosal and sigmoid sinuses are transected and the lesion is excised.

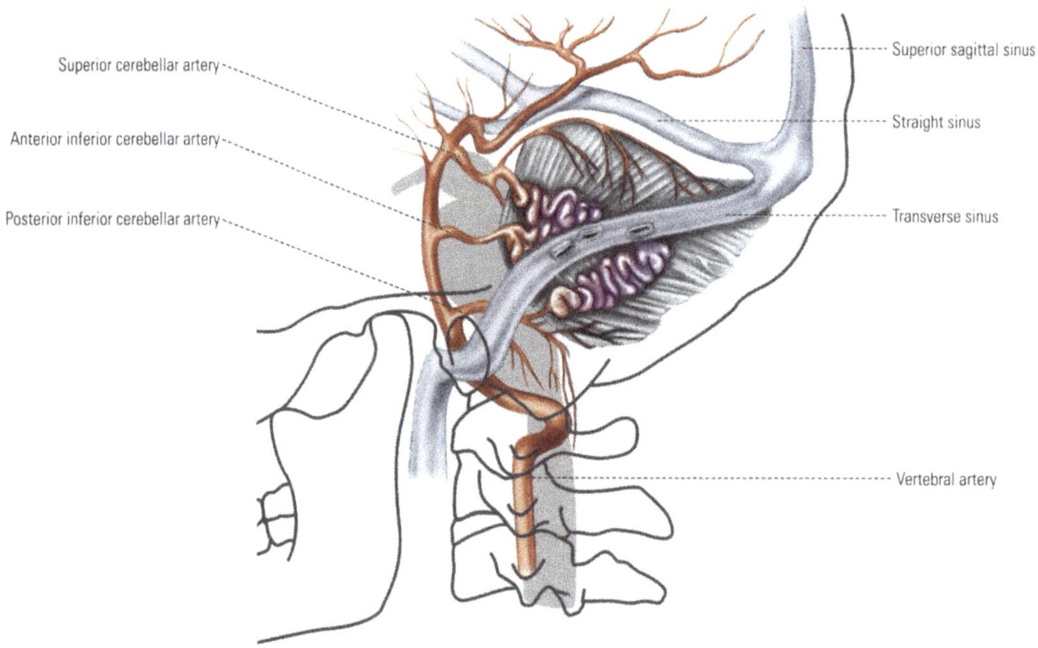

Figure 29-1. **An arteriovenous malformation over the left cerebellar hemisphere. Feeding arteries come from the major intracranial branches of the basilar and vertebral arteries.**

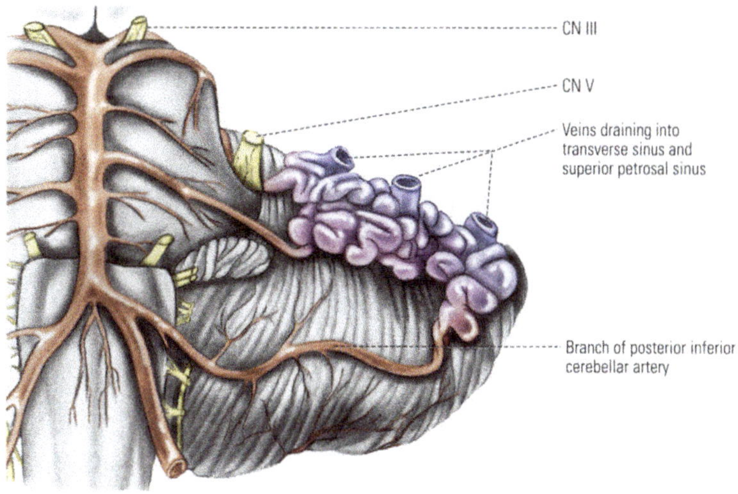

Figure 29-2. Ventral view of an arteriovenous malformation over the left cerebellar hemisphere.

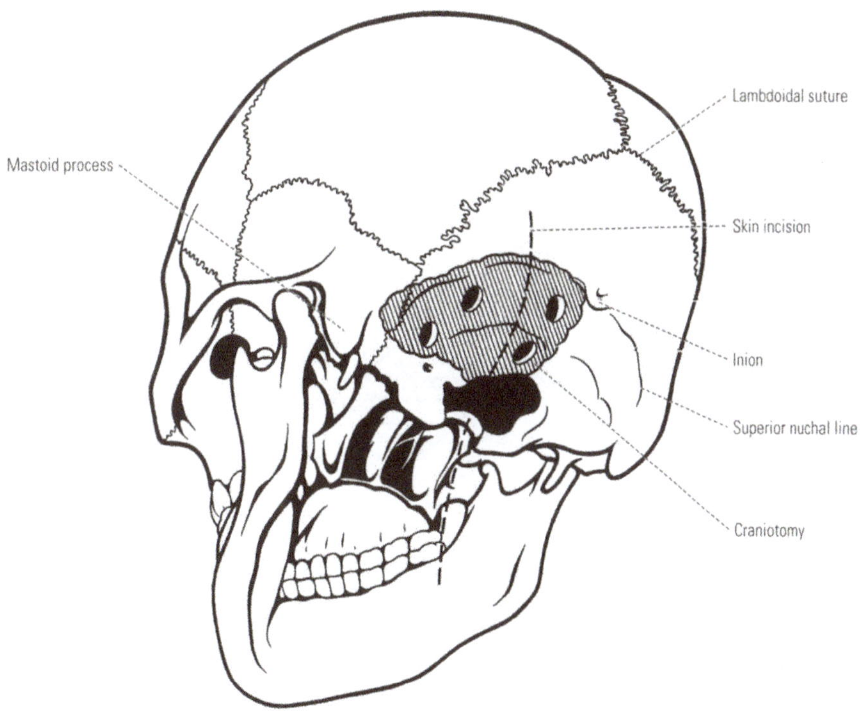

Figure 29-3. Skin incision and craniectomy for an arteriovenous malformation over the left cerebellar hemisphere.

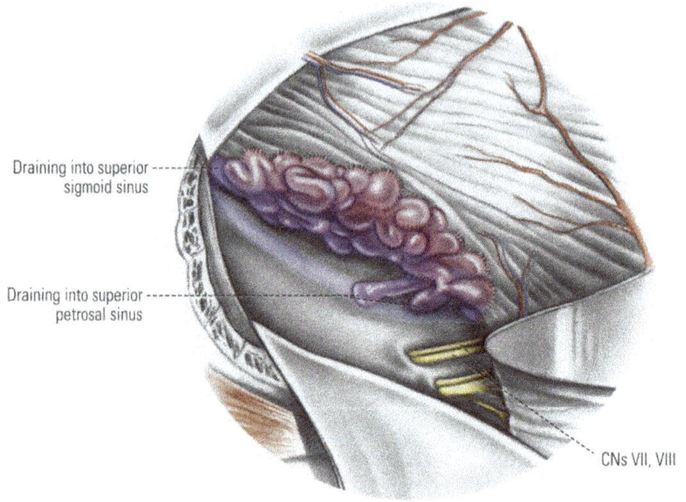

Figure 29-4. **Operative exposure of an arteriovenous malformation over the left lateral cerebellar hemisphere. Note venous drainage into superior petrosal and sigmoid sinuses.**

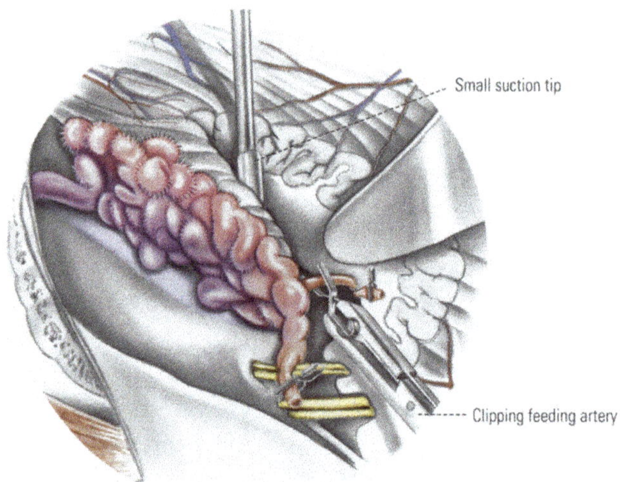

Figure 29-5. **Removal of an arteriovenous malformation of the left lateral cerebellar hemisphere. Note that 1) feeding arteries are clipped, and 2) draining veins are taken last.**

CHAPTER

30

Aneurysms of the Vertebral Artery

Aneurysms of the vertebral artery are commonly found at the origin of the posterior inferior cerebellar artery (PICA). Other locations include the distal PICA and the vertebral junction. Rarely, a more proximal vertebral artery aneurysm can present in the spinal canal and lie beneath the highest denticulate ligament, which has to be transected to expose the lesion. Vertebral-PICA aneurysms usually present with subarachnoid hemorrhage, but large lesions can compress the lower cranial nerves or brain stem (Fig. 30-1).

Aneurysms of the posterior fossa are diagnosed by computed tomography scan, magnetic resonance imaging, and by vertebral angiography. The subtraction technique is essential to demonstrate small lesions at the PICA origin. In addition to routine half axial and lateral series, a base view (submental-vertex) is often of value.

The posterior fossa is exposed with the patient in the lateral decubitus or park bench position by using a paramedian incision and a unilateral suboccipital craniectomy (Fig. 30-2). Further exposure from lateral and below can be obtained by resecting a portion of the occipital condyle (Fig. 30-3). It is important to remove the arch of the atlas so that the exposure will be low enough. The dura is opened in a gentle curve from the lateral suboccipital region to the spinal midline (Fig. 30-4). The arachnoid is opened over the foramen magnum. The cerebellar hemisphere is gently elevated at its junction with the tonsil. The arachnoid opening is enlarged toward the lateral gutter. The highest denticulate ligament is identified, transected, and reflected. This permits exposure of the vertebral artery as it enters the dura. The vertebral artery is followed rostrally, to the aneurysm (Fig. 30-5). A fenestrated clip is often required to encircle a loop of vessel or the lower cranial nerves.

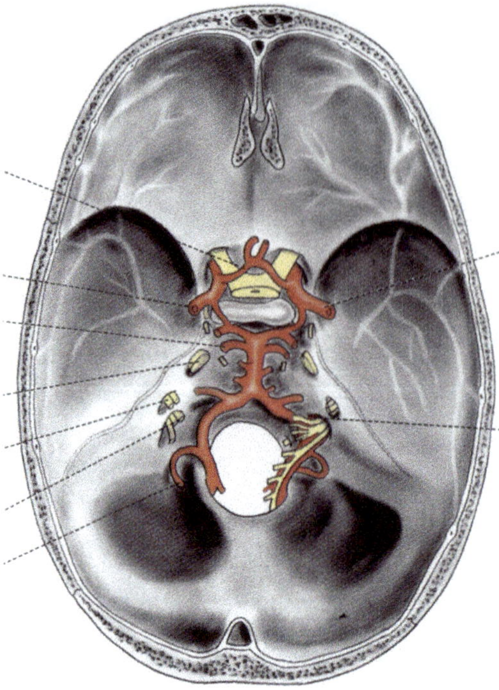

Figure 30-1. Anatomico-topographic demonstration of an aneurysm of the right vertebral artery at the origin of the posterior inferior cerebellar artery. Note the relationship of the aneurysm to nerves IX, X, XI.

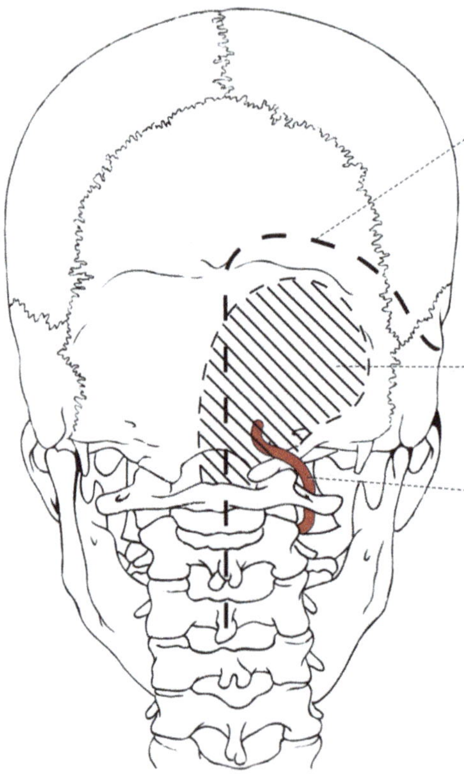

Figure 30-2. Exposure of the posterior fossa using a median incision and a unilateral suboccipital craniectomy.

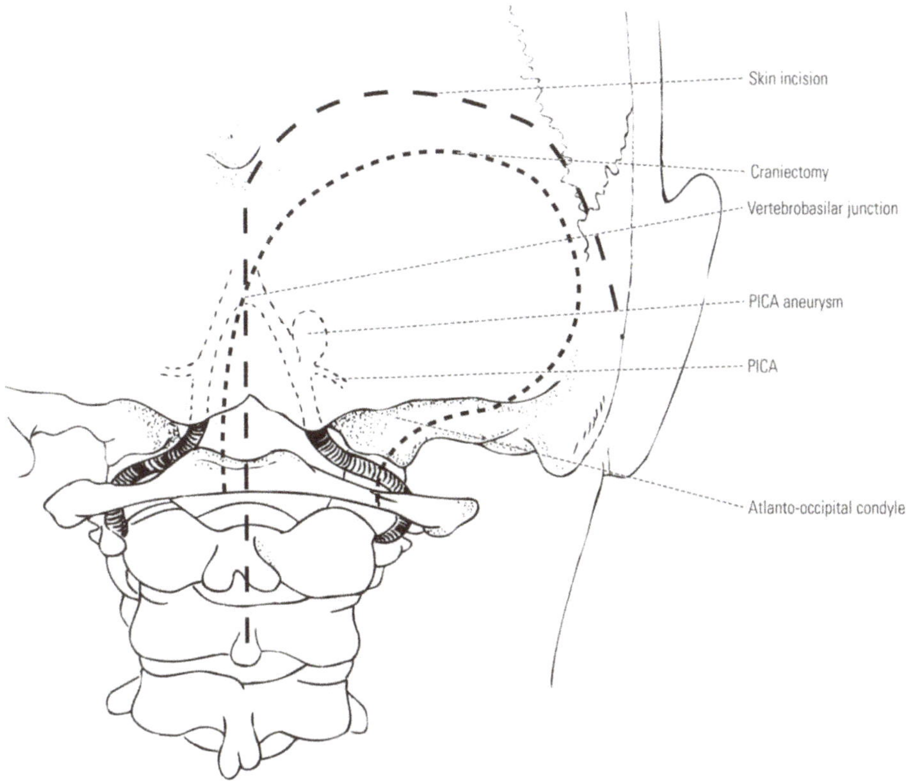

Figure 30-3. Position of the aneurysm in relation to the skin incision and craniectomy.

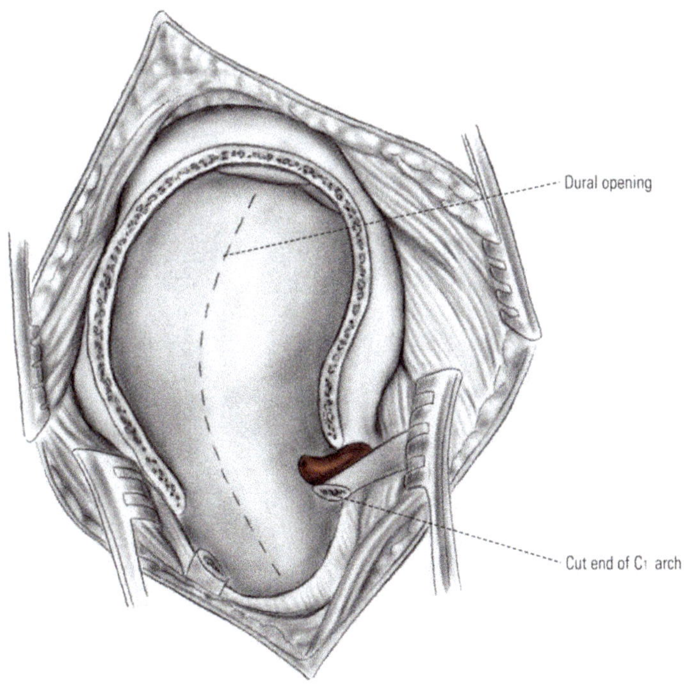

Figure 30-4. Dural opening after craniectomy.

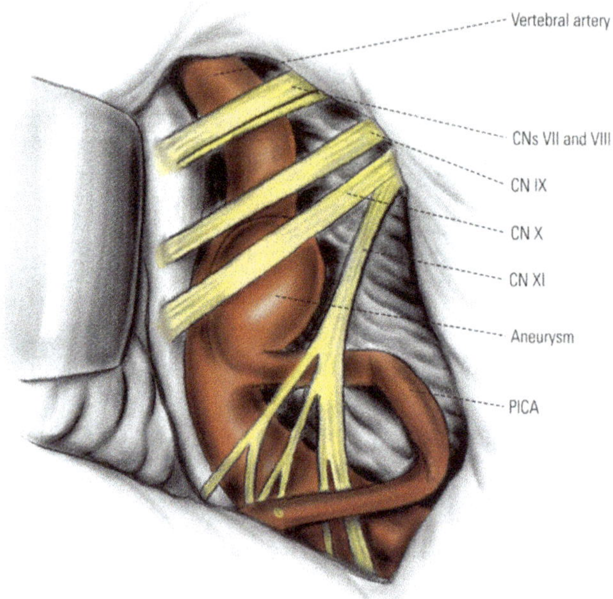

Figure 30-5. The IXth, Xth, and XIth cranial nerves are encountered as they lie stretched over the aneurysm.

References

1. Heros RC:Lateral suboccipital approach for vertebral and vertebrobasilar artery lesions. *J Neurosurg* 1986, 64:559–562.
2. Salcman M, *et al.*: Aneurysms of the posterior inferior cerebellar artery—vertebral artery complex: variations on a theme. *Neurosurgery* 1990, 27:12–21.

CHAPTER

31

Glomus Jugulare Tumor (Chemodectoma)

Glomus jugulare tumors have their origin from a small (0.25 to 0.5 mm) group of cells in the adventitia of the jugular bulb. These paraganglia have recently been identified in different places in the petrous bone such as in the tympanic branch of the glossopharyngeal nerve, in the canaliculus tympanicus, and in the submucosa of the promentory. Glomus jugulare tumors receive their blood supply from the ascending pharyngeal artery and other small branches of the external carotid artery; branches from the vertebral artery can also contribute to the vascularity of larger tumors. This is important because the majority of these tumors should be considered for preoperative embolization to reduce their vascularity and, frequently, their overall volume. This can make surgery of these tumors considerably safer.

These lesions tend to be locally invasive. They erode the petrous portion of the temporal bone. Glomus jugulare tumors often enter the internal jugular vein as well as the dural sinuses. The tumor may penetrate the dura to compress the posterior fossa structures. Characteristically, this lesion presents as a reddish-blue mass penetrating the tympanic membrane. When the otologist biopsies the tumor it usually bleeds profusely.

Preoperatively these patients are evaluated with computed tomography with bone windows and thin sections of the petrous bone and skull, with magnetic resonance imaging of the head and upper neck and, almost always, with selective angiography. Using arteriography or venography, the patency of the lateral and sigmoid sinuses and internal jugular vein should be ascertained. The development of the subtraction technique has greatly aided the quality of positive contrast studies in this area.

To illustrate the surgical technique for removing chemodectomas of this area, a relatively small tumor is presented. The lesion depicted in Figure 31-1 is filling the jugular bulb and could be expected to cause symptoms relative to the IXth, Xth, and XIth nerves.

The patient is placed in the prone or lateral decubitus position and the head turned so that the mastoid process and asterion on the side of the lesion are uppermost. The surgeon's view of the skull appropriately positioned for surgery is shown in Figure 31-2. The head and trunk are elevated slightly.

A skin incision is made beginning 3 cm above the lambdoid suture midway between the inion and the mastoid process and carried downward 12 cm (Fig. 31-3). In larger lesions, greater exposure is necessary. In this situation, a skin incision is made beginning in front of the ear and then passing posteriorly in the shape of a question mark and continuing inferiorly and then anteriorly across the sternocleidomastoid muscle.

The skin flap is taken down superiorly at a layer just superficial to the superficial fascia of the temporalis muscle. The suboccipital bone is exposed, after cutting through the muscle, by subperiosteal dissection. A cut is then made through the fascia and the periosteum starting anteriorly at the root of the zygoma and extending straight back. The temporalis fascia and muscle are then opened and taken forward, by subperiosteal dissection, as a free muscle flap. The suboccipital exposure is then carried forward, by subperiosteal dissection, to expose the mastoid all the way anteriorly to the posterior aspect of the external auditory canal. At this point, we prefer to proceed with a subtotal mastoidectomy using a high-speed air drill with a cutting bur and then, when only a thin layer of bone is left, with the diamond bur to expose the sigmoid sinus and the transverse/sigmoid junction, the superior petrosal sinus, and the presigmoid dura (Fig. 31-4). Drilling is then continued to remove the posterior aspect of the petrous bone until the anterior limit of the exposure, marked by the posterior semicircular canal, and the bone of the facial canal is reached. This portion of the drilling is carried out under the microscope under constant irrigation to prevent injury to the facial nerve and the bony labyrinth. Superiorly, the temporal bone plate is removed to expose the dura over the inferolateral aspect of the temporal lobe, to completely uncover the superior petrosal sinus and the junction of the superior petrosal sinus with the transverse/sigmoid junction posteriorly. Using the exposure already obtained by drilling, the dura is then separated in the temporal region and in the suboccipital region, and an L-shaped craniotomy, which includes a small portion of the temporal bone anterior and posterior to the transverse/sigmoid junction and about 2 or 3 cm of the suboccipital bone posterior to the sigmoid sinus, is cut with the high-speed air drill.

Depending on the size of the tumor and the extent of intracranial extension, the surgeon then has the option of working entirely infratentorially as described below or, in the case of a tumor with larger intracranial extension, using the full advantage of the subtemporal/presigmoid transpetrosal exposure to gain ample access to the anterolateral aspect of the posterior fossa. The latter exposure is obtained by making a vertical incision in the presigmoid region and connecting it to a small temporal incision that comes down to the superior petrosal sinus. The sinus is then divided and the tentorium transected, taking particular care to identify and spare the fourth nerve under the microscope. This allows the sigmoid sinus to be gently retracted posteriorly with the cerebellum to greatly enhance the exposure. The inferior aspect of the exposure can be optimized by extending the suboccipital craniotomy into a "far lateral" exposure by drilling the lateral rim of the foramen magnum and drilling into the condyle, removing the medial half of the condyle while protecting the vertebral artery, as has been described in detail (see Chapter 30).

Figures 31-3 through 31-8 illustrate the technique for removing a smaller tumor, which can be done strictly through an infratentorial exposure without exposing the temporal region or dividing the petrosal sinus and the tentorium. For these types of tumors, the skin incision and craniotomy are shown in Figures 31-3 and 31-4. After the craniotomy is completed and the sigmoid sinus and presigmoid region are exposed by drilling as described above, small dural flaps are elevated anteriorly and posteriorly to the sinus just above the tumor (Fig. 31-5). Since these dural incisions flank the sigmoid sinus, rather than the transverse sinus, they will both be below the tentorium. The sinus is ligated with 00 silk and opened longitudinally below the ligature. A tongue of tumor will be seen in the lumen of the sinus. The soft tumor is removed by suction and curettage (Fig. 31-7). Additional bone is removed as necessary (Fig. 31-5 and 31-6). No tumor should be left within the mastoid air cells. The internal jugular vein is followed inferiorly through the skull after drilling the bone of the jugular tubercle. The vein then passes just in front of the transverse process of the atlas. This transverse process is exposed subperiosteally and removed taking particular precautions to expose and protect the vertebral artery as it runs posteriorly and then medially from the transverse foramen of C2 to the sulcus arteriosum of C1 Fig. 31-8). The jugular vein and its tributaries are ligated at this level. In doing this, care must be taken to avoid injuring the VIIth, VIIIth, IXth, Xth, and XIth nerves. The vein is opened longitudinally above the level of the ligature and the tumor removal is completed.

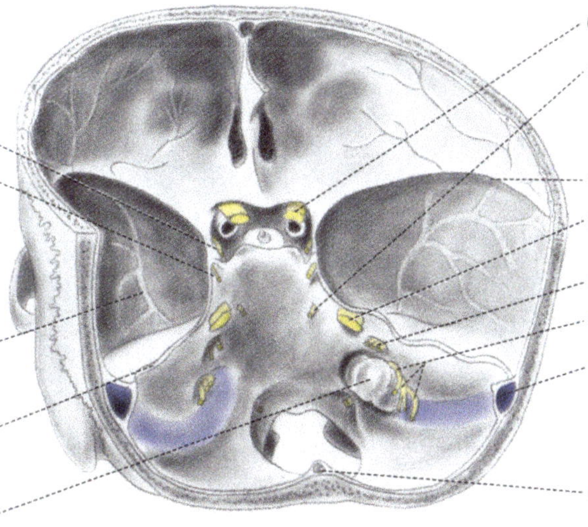

Figure 31-1. **Anatomico-topographic demonstration of a right glomus jugulare tumor. Note that dura remains intact over the tumor.**

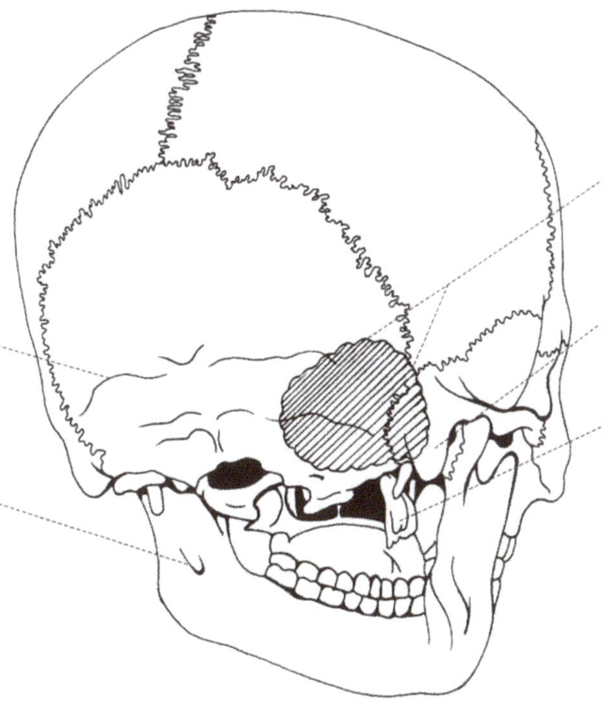

Figure 31-2. **Craniectomy for a moderate-sized right glomus jugulare tumor.**

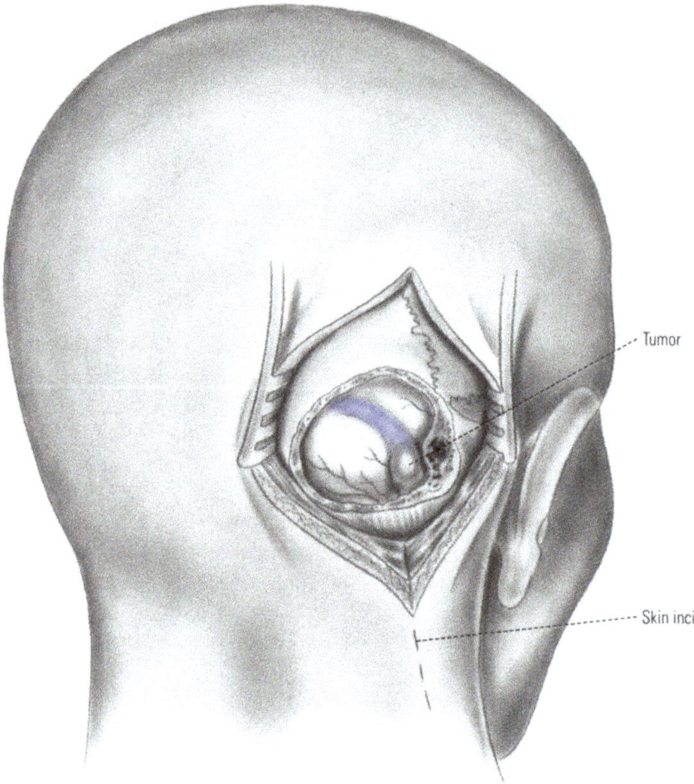

Figure 31-3. Operative exposure of glomus jugulare tumor. Note that sigmoid sinus is occluded by the tumor, and the extent of bone removal.

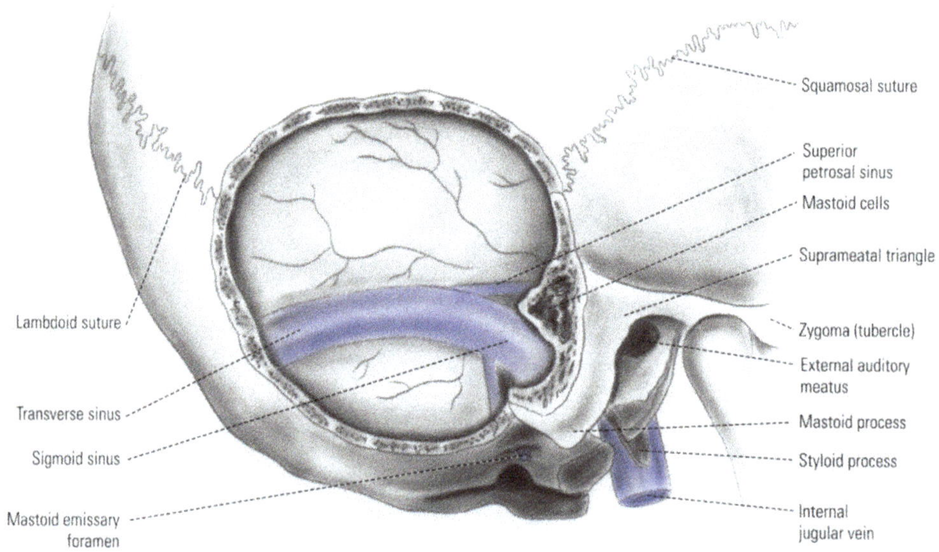

Figure 31-4. Anatomic relationships of the right sigmoid sinus and internal jugular vein to the superior petrosal sinus, mastoid emissary vein, and petrosal bone.

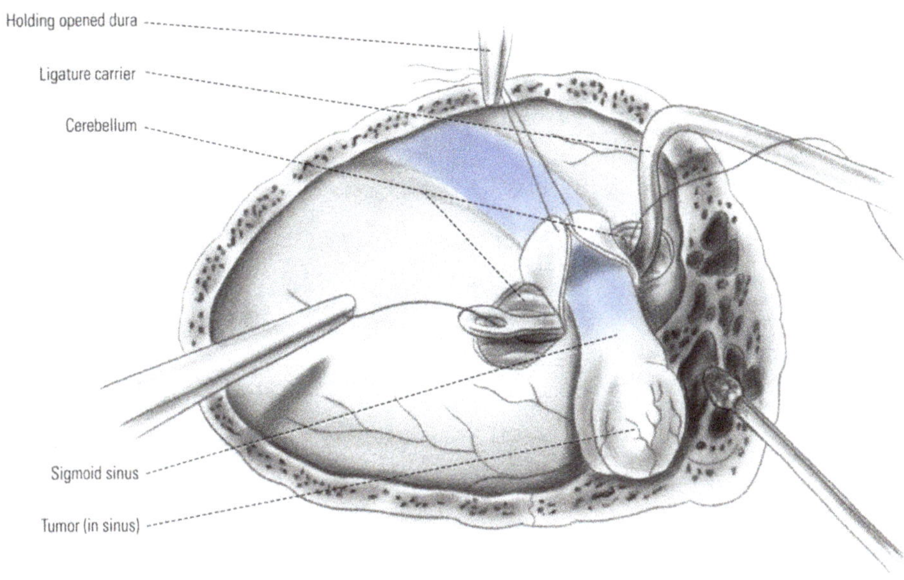

Figure 31-5. Ligation of the sigmoid sinus and further removal of petrous bone.

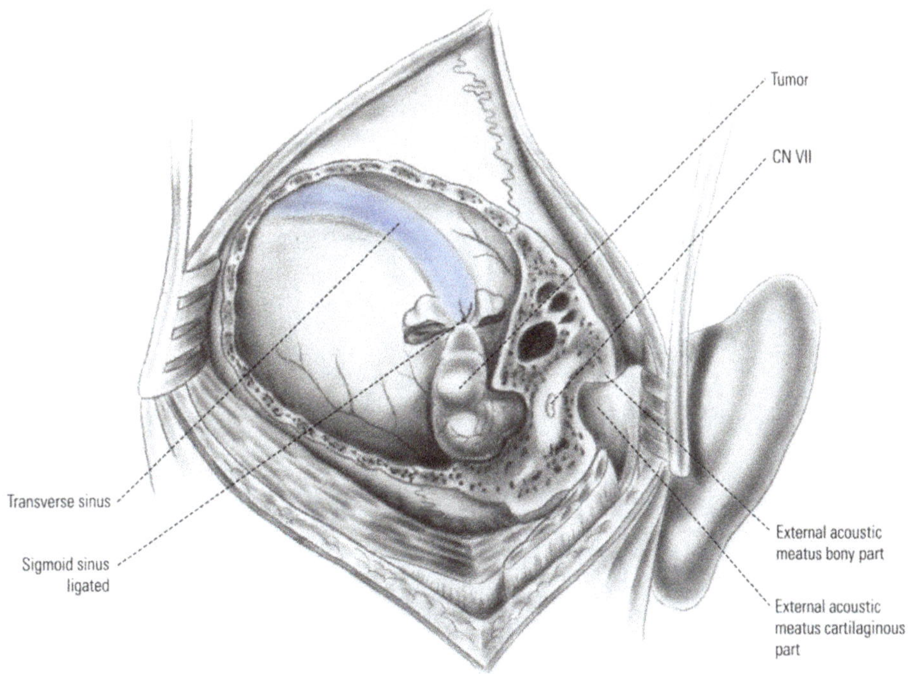

Figure 31-6. Extent of petrous bone removed.

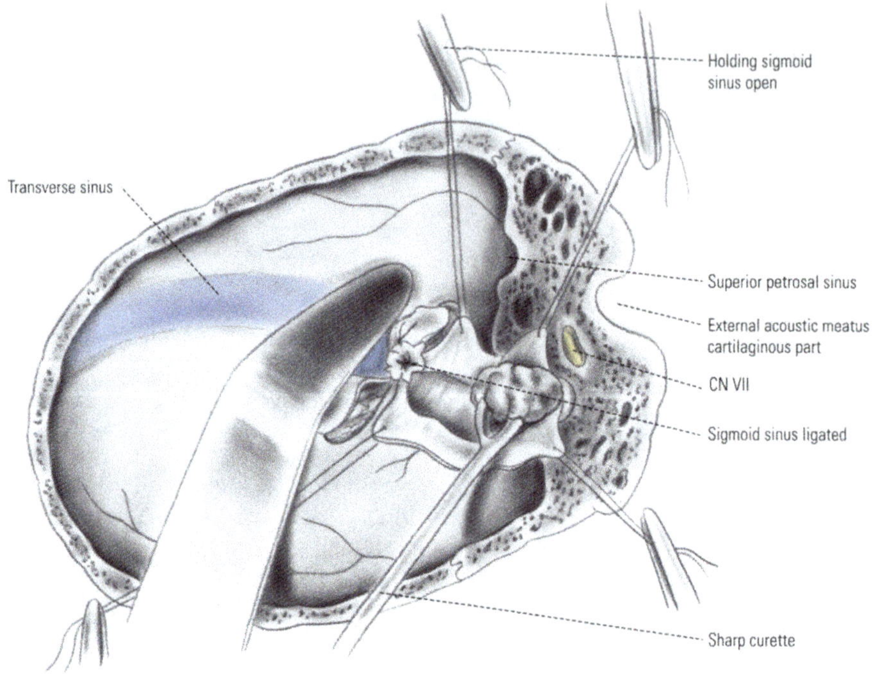

Figure 31-7. **Ligated sigmoid sinus is opened to remove tumor which has grown within the lumen of the sinus.**

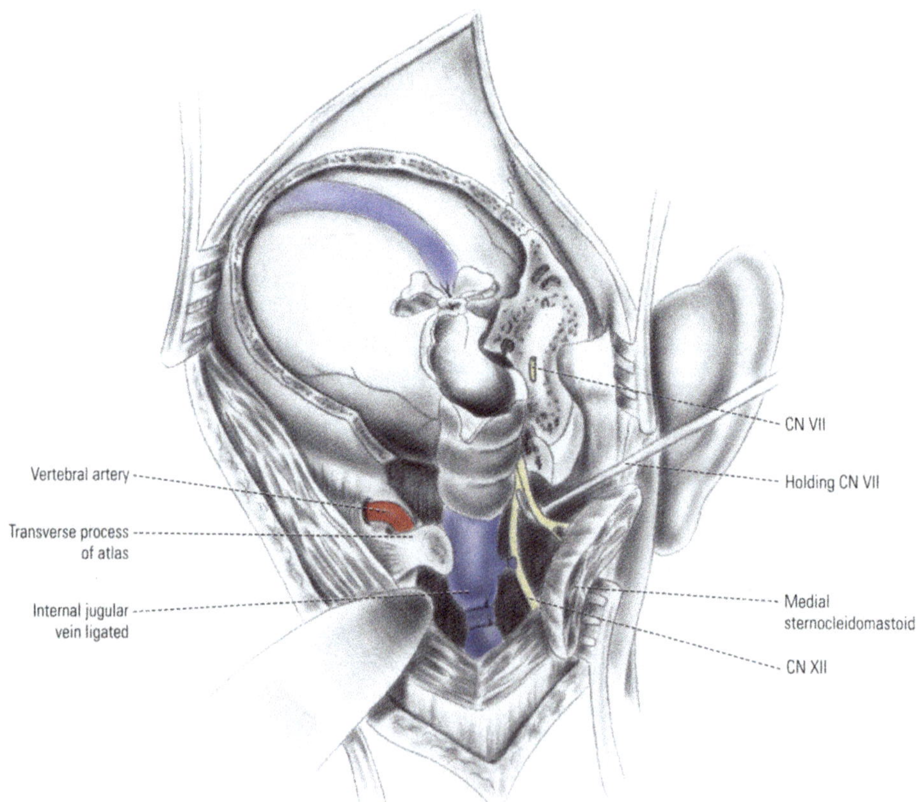

Figure 31-8. **Further removal of petrous bone and the transverse process of the atlas exposes the internal jugular bulb and vein. Ligation of the internal jugular vein is also shown.**

CHAPTER

32

Meningioma of the Foramen Magnum

The second most frequent location for meningiomas of the posterior fossa is on the anterior rim of the foramen magnum. These tumors may extend for a considerable distance up the clivus or down into the spinal canal. These slow-growing tumors may cause remarkable distortion and compression of the cervicomedullary region. The vertebral artery and its branches, as well as the lower cranial nerves, may be completely enveloped by the tumor (Fig. 32-1).

These patients should be studied with both magnetic resonance scanning and vertebral arteriography. The intimate relationship of these firm tumors to the vertebral arteries mandates preoperative information in regard to vascularity and arterial position as well as a three-dimensional concept of the extent of the lesion.

The patient is placed in the prone or lateral decubitus position and all precautionary measures, as outlined previously, are observed. If the tumor is somewhat lateral in its location, an incision is made from above the inion to C5. The lamina of both C1 and C2 are removed and an ipsilateral or bilateral suboccipital craniectomy completes the exposure (Figs. 32-2 and 32-3). The dura is incised in the shape of a *Y* and reflected. Figure 32-4 illustrates the operative exposure after opening the arachnoid. The tumor depicted descends into the spinal canal on the right side. The highest denticulate ligament is stretched over the tumor. This ligament helps locate the level at which the vertebral artery enters the intrathecal space. In this patient it means that the tumor is covering the right vertebral artery. The dorsal root of C2 and the highest denticulate ligament are transected, separated from the tumor, and reflected medially. The spinal accessory nerve is gently elevated off the tumor capsule (Fig. 32-5). The tumor capsule is opened inferiorly and gutted. We prefer to use an ultrasonic aspirator with irrigation or a combined suction–bipolar cautery to morcellate the tumor. The tumor is thus gradually reduced in size. The inferior cerebellum is elevated and the tumor capsule gently dissected free of adhesions and feeding vessels. The tumor is removed piecemeal until only the anterior dural attachment remains. This area is then curetted and cauterized using bipolar coagulation with constant irrigation.

In large tumors with midline clival extensions, as seen in Figure 32-1, this exposure is inadequate. These types of lesions should be approached with a combined foramen magnum–cerebellopontine angle exposure or even occasionally with a supratentorial exposure added to it. Examples of this exposure are given in the chapters on combined supratentorial and infratentorial craniotomies for tentorial meningiomas and chemodectomas. In dealing with meningiomas in front of the brain stem, remember that an already-distorted brain stem does not tolerate additional retraction without disastrous results. Extensive bone resection not only gives more room but also helps in identifying and protecting important vascular structures and cranial nerves.

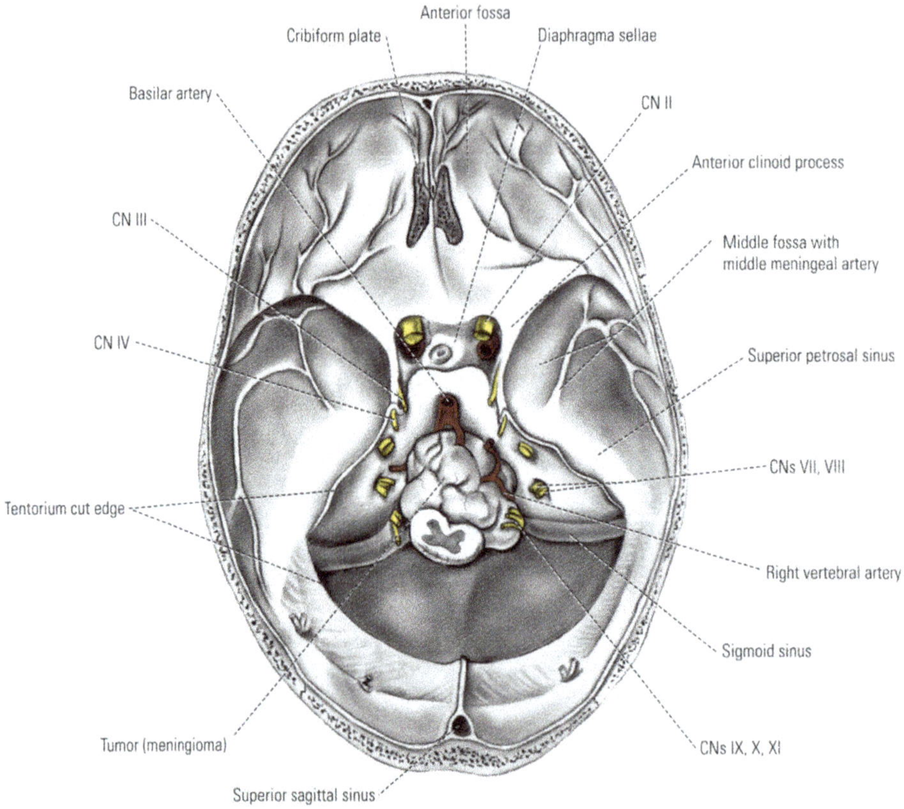

Figure 32-1. Anatomico-topographic demonstration of a meningioma of the foramen magnum. The attachment of the tumor is at the anterior rim of the foramen magnum. The tumor extends halfway up the clivus. Its inferior extension reaches to the level of the arch of the atlas (see Figs. 32-3 and 32-4).

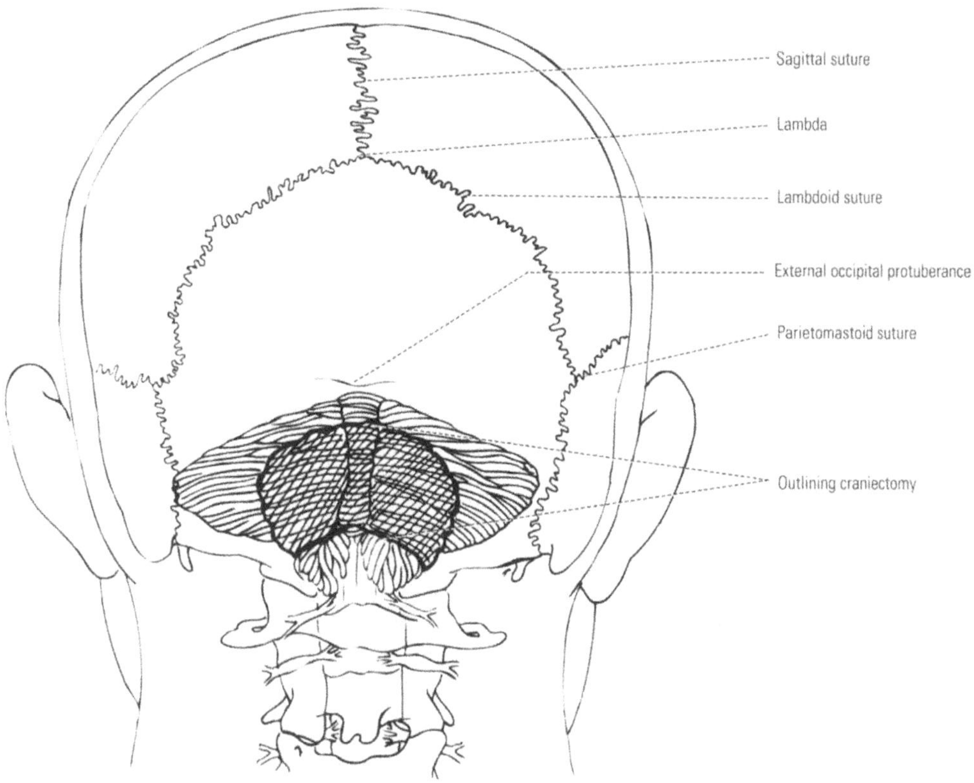

Figure 32-2. Craniectomy for a meningioma of the foramen magnum. Laminectomy of C1 and C2 is also performed.

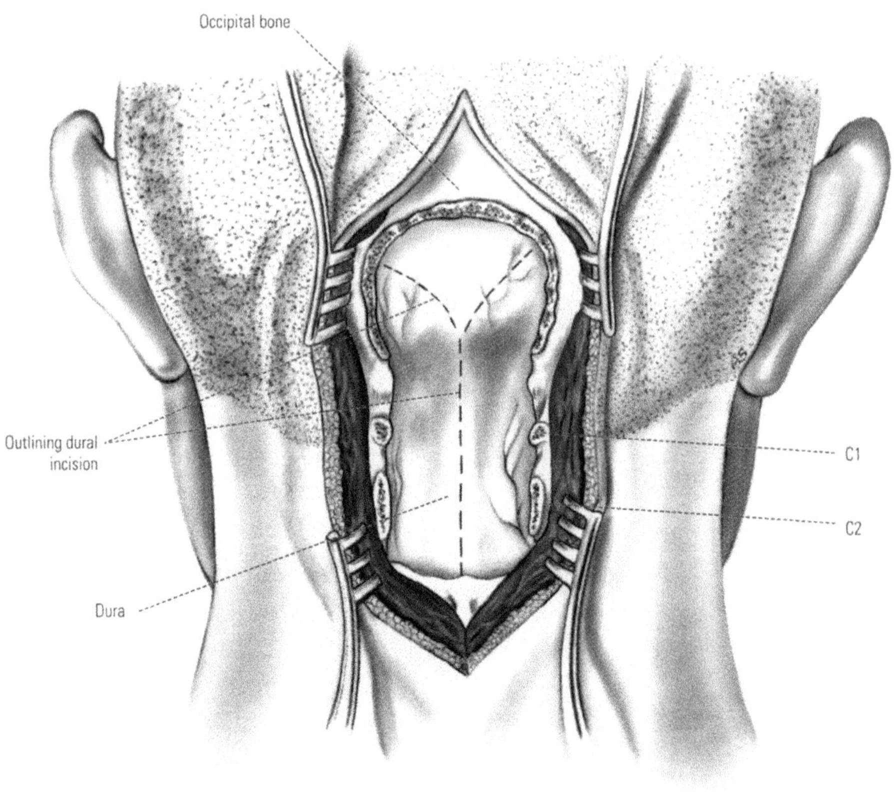

Figure 32-3. Dural incision.

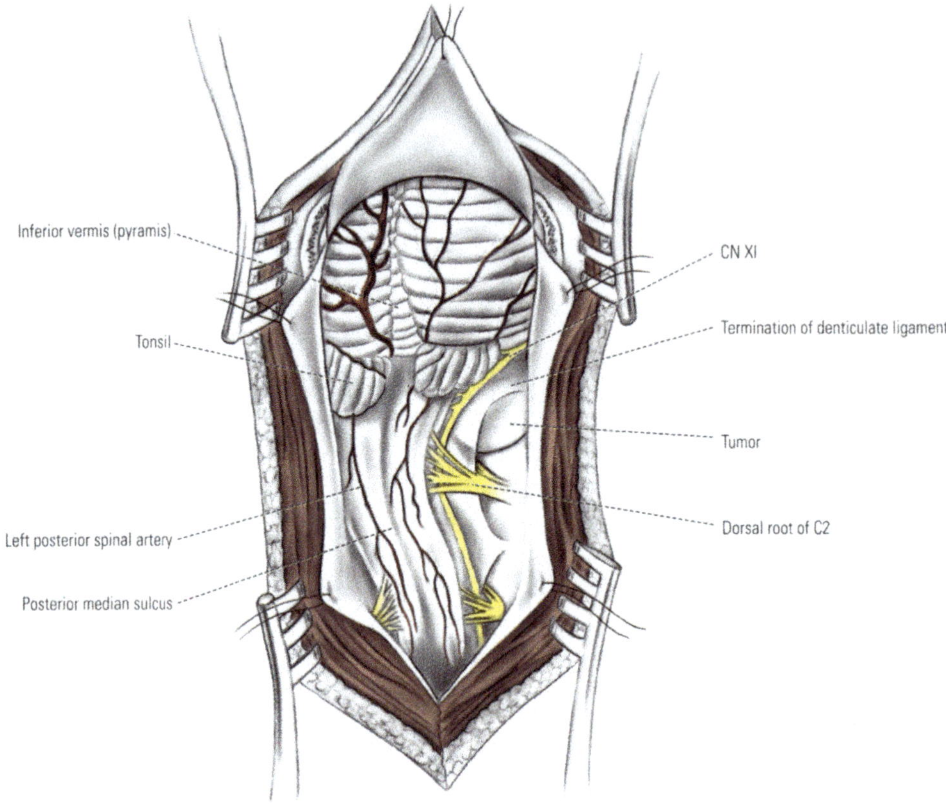

Figure 32-4. Operative exposure.

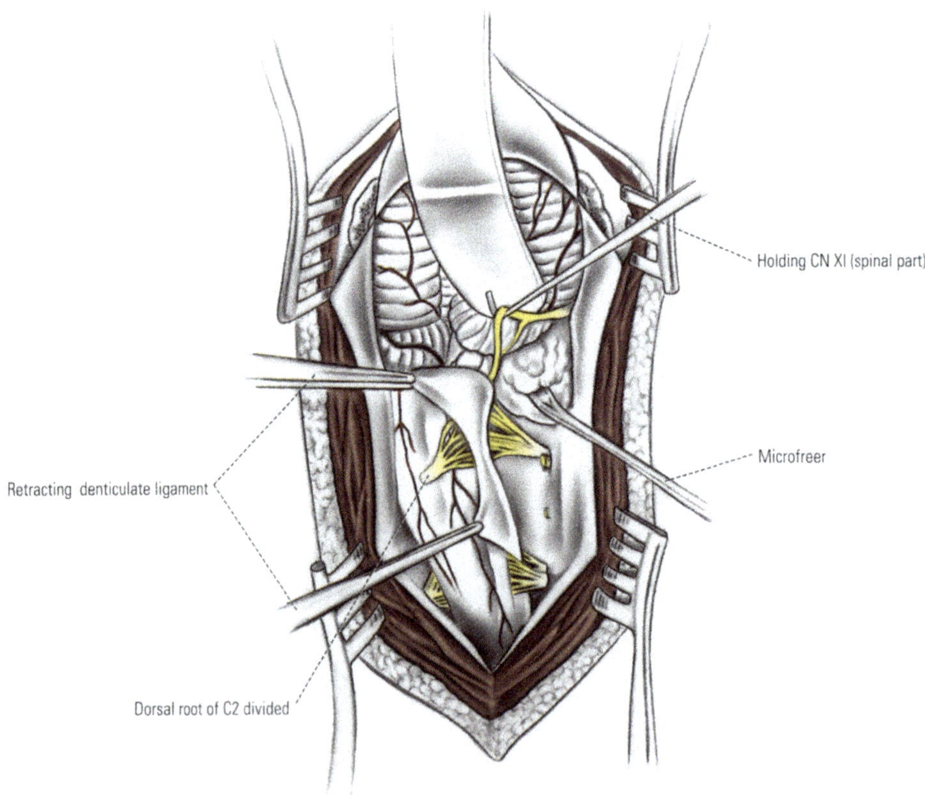

Figure 32-5. Inferior extent of the tumor is being removed.

CHAPTER

33

Cervical Cordotomy

Interruption of the spinothalamic tracts is a neurosurgical procedure for the treatment of intractable pain (Fig. 33-1). Because the level of analgesia may fall gradually, this procedure is most effective for treating intractable pain associated with malignant diseases. Although methods have been developed to interrupt these pain pathways percutaneously, the open operation still has a place in the neurosurgical armamentarium. Open cordotomy may be preferred for patients with deformities or congenital malformations of the cervical spine for craniovertebral junction patients who are unable or unwilling to cooperate with the intraoperative physiological testing needed for the percutaneous procedure, and for patients in whom a previously attempted percutaneous procedure could not be completed.

A high cervical cordotomy results in more complete and longer lasting levels of analgesia. Consequently, it is preferable to proceed with a unilateral cordotomy at the level of C1-C2. When a bilateral cordotomy is indicated, it is performed either at a lower level (high thoracic) or in stages. A simultaneous bilateral high cervical cordotomy may cause respiratory difficulties, postural hypotension, or both. When a bilateral cordotomy is performed, the second lesion is placed 8 mm above or below the first incision.

Although local anesthesia is preferable, neuroleptanalgesia should be considered because it can be useful for establishing whether the desired level of analgesia has been obtained. After the patient is placed in a prone position, a 15-cm vertical midline incision is made beginning at the level of the inion (Fig. 33-2). The spinous process of C2, the arch of the atlas, and the posterior rim of the foramen magnum are exposed unilaterally. The interlaminar space between C1 and C2 is identified and enlarged by doing a hemilaminotomy (Fig. 33-3). The ligamentum flavum, which is very thin at this level, is incised. Under the microscope, a longitudinal dural incision is made from the lamina of C1 to the lamina of C2 in the lateral one third of the dural exposure. Care must be taken to avoid opening the epidural veins in the lateral gutter. The dural margins are retracted with stay sutures (Fig. 33-4). The arachnoid is opened and cerebrospinal fluid is aspirated.

The dentate ligaments are identified, sectioned at their lateral dural attachment site, and then grasped with a fine-tipped needle holder. The spinal cord is rotated gently, and an avascular area between C1 and C2 is selected as the site for the cordotomy (Fig. 33-5). The attachment of the dentate ligament to the pia of the cord must be precisely defined because this is the exact level at which the knife blade is inserted. Because sacral fibers are most posterior in the spinothalamic tract, this area will be missed if a cordotomy is not extended to the exact point at which the dentate ligament inserts. If the cut extends too far posteriorly, however, the corticospinal tract will be injured. A cordotomy knife or knife blade that has been marked previously at a depth of 5 mm is inserted with the cutting edge down. The incision usually extends anteriorly only as far as the exiting nerve roots (Fig. 33-6). In patients with upper extremity pain, the incision is extended anteriorly another millimeter to within 2 mm of the anterior spinal artery.

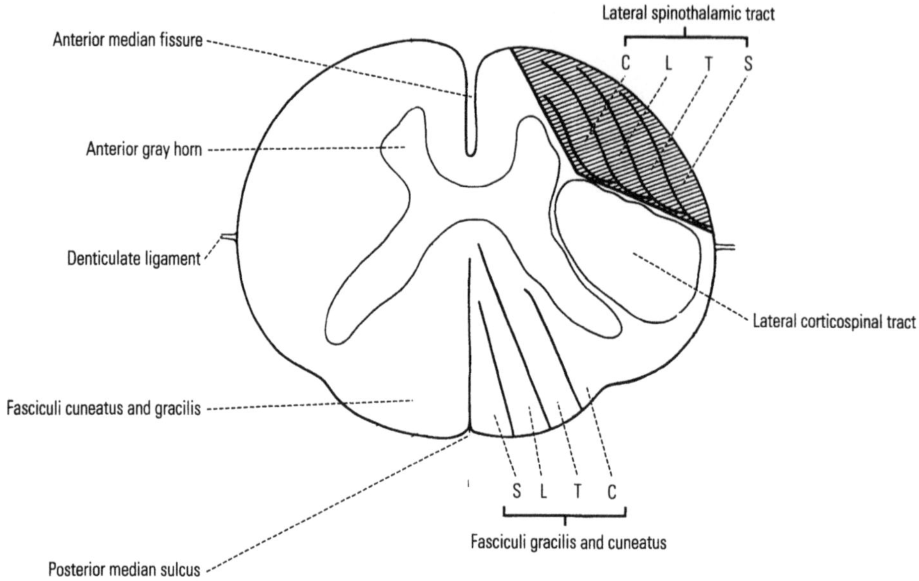

Figure 33-1. Cross-section of the upper cervical spinal cord. C—cervical; L—lumbar; S—sacral; T— thoracic.

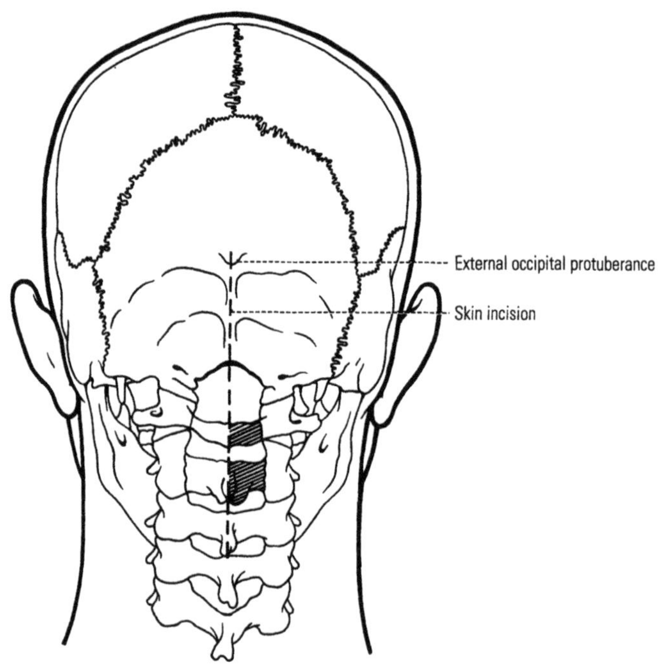

Figure 33-2. The skin incision and hemilaminectomy. A hemilaminectomy of C1 and C2 is performed.

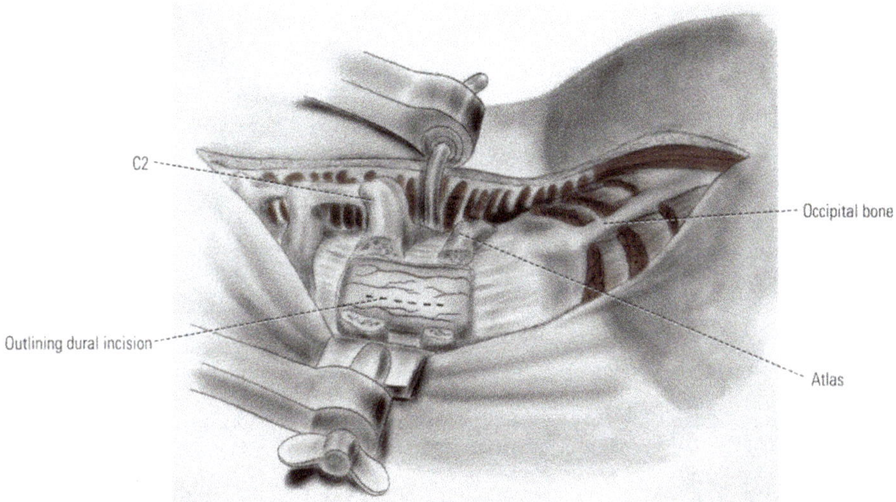

Figure 33-3. Operative view after the muscle has been stripped from the sub-occipital squama and a hemilaminectomy of C1 and C2 performed.

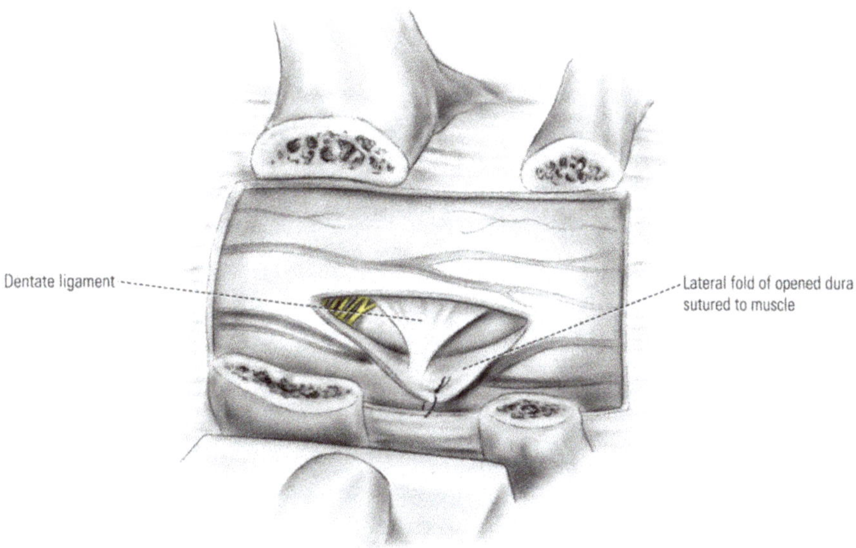

Figure 33-4. Operative exposure after the dura between C1 and C2 has been opened. The lateral fold is over an epidural vein. The dentate ligament is attached to the pia and dura.

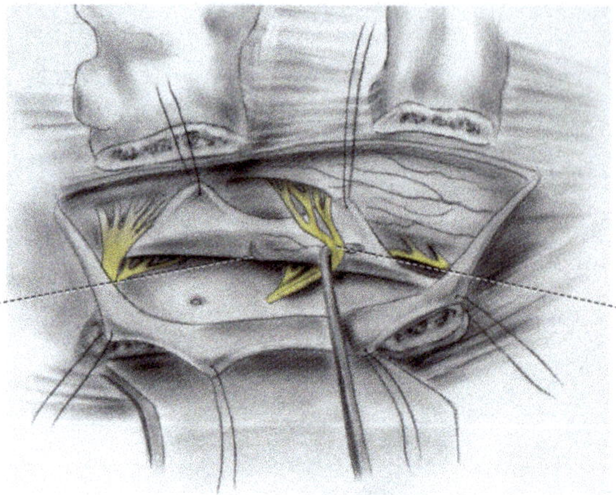

Figure 33-5. Operative view showing that spinal cord is incised at the insertion of the dentate ligament.

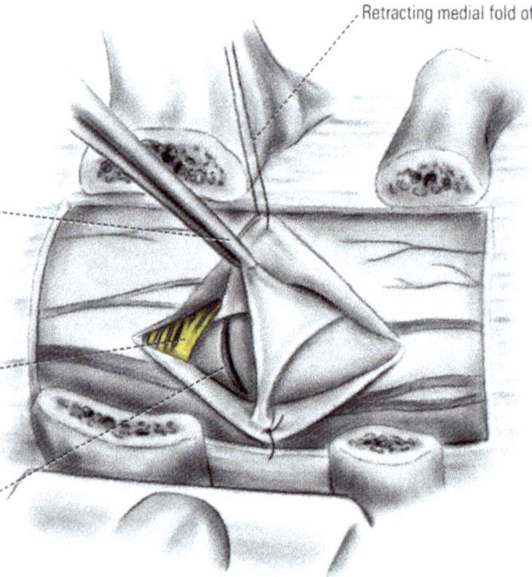

Figure 33-6. Close-up view of the operative field after the incision has been made.

CHAPTER

34

Cervical Laminectomy

This chapter describes the technique of cervical laminectomy, which is indicated for a variety of disorders. Syringomyelia is used as an example of an indication for cervical laminectomy. Duraplasty as a treatment for cervical syringomyelia is also described. The procedure illustrated in this chapter is a total laminectomy of C2 through C5 and a partial laminectomy of C6.

Syringomyelia

Spinal cord pathology, including syringomyelia, is most often diagnosed by magnetic resonance (MR) imaging. If a tumor is suspected in the cervical spine, MR imaging with contrast enhancement is indicated. Cervical laminectomies are most often performed with the patient in a prone position with the head fastened to a Mayfield headholder. As in all surgical procedures, the patient is padded appropriately. In patients with myelopathy, somatosensory evoked potentials are routinely monitored.

A vertical midline incision is made from 2 cm below the inion to below the vertebral prominence of C7. Figure 34-1 illustrates the extent of the skin incision relative to the topography of the area and the underlying bony landmarks. Because of the downward inclination of the cervical spinous processes, the vertebral bodies are considerably rostral to them. The incision is continued from the midline down to the spinous processes. Repeated palpation of the bifid spinous processes of C2 through C6 serves as a guide to the midline. It is easier to stay in the midline if self-retaining retractors are not placed beneath the cervical fascia until the spinous processes have been reached (Fig. 34-2). Retractors tend to pull fibers from one side to the other and thereby obliterate the median plane.

After the spinous processes have been reached, self-retaining retractors are inserted to maintain the exposure. Beginning inferiorly at C6, a knife or Bovie is used to transect the muscle attachments of the spinous processes (Fig. 34-3). Instruments are always kept against the bone. Once the spinous process is exposed, the remaining muscle insertions are elevated by stripping the spinous process and lamina subperiosteally with continued sharp dissection (Fig. 34-4). Periosteal elevation proceeds laterally to the facet, and an open gauze sponge is inserted to aid in the blunt elevation of the paravertebral muscles. This maneuver also helps tamponade small bleeders (Fig. 34-5).

The spinous processes are removed with a Leksell or cutting forceps (Fig. 34-6). Beginning in the midline, the lamina is gradually removed piecemeal with a rongeur. Extreme care must be taken to avoid pressing the inferior lip of the rongeur against the dura and spinal cord. The rongeur is held with two hands. It is preferable for the lamina to be removed without placing the lip of the rongeur underneath it (Fig. 34-7). One hand maintains pressure on the instrument away from the spinal cord so that if the rongeur slips off the bone, it will always slip away from the spinal cord. The rongeur is a cutting tool and should not be twisted in an attempt to cut through the lamina, or the articular facet could be broken or some of the twisted bone pushed onto the spinal cord. The lamina is removed laterally just short of the facet joints bilaterally. The ligamentum flavum, which becomes very thin in the upper cervical levels, is excised along with the lamina.

An alternate technique for doing a cervical laminectomy, especially when a laminoplasty is considered, is to remove the lamina and the spinous processes en bloc. This procedure is performed by sharply dissecting the interspinous ligament between C1 and C2 and C6 and C7 and slightly enlarging the interlaminar space between C6 and C7 on both sides with a high-speed drill. The high-speed drill with a footplate is then used to cut the lamina along a line between the lamina and the lateral mass of the cervical spine (Fig. 34-8). Both sides are incised. The option of replacing the lamina after the spinal operation is maintained.

Bone wax is applied to the cut lamina with a number 1 Penfield dissector to reduce bleeding. Bothersome epidural veins are always encountered laterally and can be controlled by bipolar coagulation or placement of gelatin sponges or other hemostatic material. The area should be covered with moist cottonoid strips and dura reflected over it to preserve hemostasis throughout the operation.

The dura is opened in the midline over the entire length of the laminectomy without opening the arachnoid. Violating the arachnoid can easily be avoided by placing a 5-0 suture in the superficial layers of the dura, which is then tented, and a small incision is made next to the suture with a number 15 scalpel blade. Next, a grooved Woodson tool is placed under the dura and over the arachnoid, and a number 15 blade is used to follow the underlying (Fig. 34-9). Multiple stay sutures are placed in the dural margin bilaterally after the arachnoid has been dissected free of the dura. Although it is not mandatory, opening the dura separate from the arachnoid provides a beautiful picture of the underlying pathology.

At this point, the enlarged spinal cord is exposed and multiple options are available for treating the syringomyelia. One option is to shunt the syrinx cavity to the subarachnoid space. Alternatively, a small cordotomy can be performed under the microscope over an avascular area of one of the dorsal columns just lateral to midline or where the dorsal column is obviously thinned. The cordotomy is performed by coagulating a 2- to 3-mm area and cutting it sharply with a number 11 blade. The cyst is found by using a number 6 Rhoton microdissector. Once the cavity has been entered, clear fluid gushes from it (Fig. 34-10).

The cordotomy is optional. A duraplasty, however, is mandatory to establish normal pathways for the cerebrospinal fluid. The duraplasty is performed by suturing substitute dura into the two dural edges after the stay sutures have been released (Fig. 34-11). Watertight closure is preferred.

The wound is closed in layers. A few sutures in the muscle decrease the amount of dead space, but the fascia must be closed meticulously. The subcutaneous tissue is closed with an inverted suture, and the skin is approximated appropriately. To relieve the patient's discomfort, an orthosis is often applied but is not necessary.

Trauma

Immobilization is the *sine qua non* of managing cervical spinal cord injuries. Initially, the patient is examined in the emergency department. Patients with multiple traumatic injuries should wear a hard collar until a cervical injury is ruled out. Once a cervical spinal cord injury is diagnosed, a detailed neurologic examination and standard cervical radiographs are obtained. If an injury might benefit from cervical skeletal traction, it is applied.

The application of skeletal traction should reflect the type of fracture found on the patient's radiographs. When a cervical fracture is not associated with slippage, the tongs are placed directly above the ear (Fig. 34-12). For a hyperextension injury with posterior subluxation, the tongs are inserted 2 cm behind the ear (Fig. 34-13*A*). For a flexion injury with anterior subluxation, the skeletal tongs are inserted 2 cm in front of the ear (Fig. 34-13*B*). Pins must be inserted an equal distance above the ear on each side to provide traction on the long axis of the spine. Gardner-Wells tongs, which are easily and quickly applied, are preferred. As an alternative, especially if a patient's injury might be appropriately treated with a halo vest, a halo ring can be applied.

Once the traction is in place and the patient has an injury that might be reduced, weights are applied progressively starting with approximately 5 pounds per level. If reduction does not occur, the traction is increased by approximately 5 pounds every 15 to 30 minutes. The process is monitored closely by lateral radiography. Occasionally, 60 pounds or more of traction may be required.

When proper alignment is achieved, the weight of traction is reduced to 10 to 15 pounds. At this time, diagnostic tests such as CT and MR imaging can be performed. Whether reduction should be performed before the diagnostic imaging studies is controversial. If an imaging study can be obtained within 30 to 60 minutes, obtaining it before traction should be considered.

The indications for cervical laminectomy in patients with cervical spine and spinal cord trauma remain controversial. It is not within the scope of this book to consider this debate except to state that if posterior compression exists, which is relatively uncommon, cervical laminectomy and fusion should be considered. This section illustrates and discusses cervical laminectomy performed for closed fractures of the posterior column of the cervical spine.

Patients with cervical spinal cord injuries are administered systemic high-dose methylprednisolone for 24 to 48 hours. Low blood pressure in patients with cervical injuries may reflect either neurogenic shock or associated hemorrhagic shock. Appropriate treatments are instituted.

When operative treatment is indicated, the patient is anesthetized while lying supine with skeletal traction in place. The patient should be intubated without movement of the neck, and endoscopic intubation is often required. The patient is then turned prone while light traction is maintained on the skeleton traction and the spine is kept in a completely neutral position.

The procedure for laminectomy of the cervical spine down to the bony elements is similar to that described for syringomyelia. Once the bony elements are encountered, care must be exerted to avoid pushing fragmented pieces of bone into the spinal canal (Fig. 34-14). Consequently, at all times pressure is directed laterally (Fig. 34-15). After the soft tissue has been cleared from the bony elements (Fig. 34-16), a laminectomy is performed and bony fragments pressing the spinal cord are removed (Fig. 34-17). One or two levels above the injury are usually exposed, and they should be inspected for ligamentous and bony injury.

Preoperative diagnostic tests will guide the surgeon on how aggressively he must evaluate the instability and to decompress the injury. Because the injury involves the posterior column, posterior cervical fusion is often also indicated. This procedure is described below. Once the decompression and fusion, if needed, have been performed, the dura is closed in a watertight fashion (Fig. 34-18). If an injury of the anterior and middle columns is also suspected, the patient wears an external orthosis until the injury can be diagnosed and treated appropriately.

Posterior Cervical Fusion Technique Using Lateral Mass Plates

Multiple procedures are used to stabilize the posterior lower cervical spine (C3–C7), including sublaminar wiring, facet-to-process spinous wiring, facet-facet wiring, interspinous wiring, and clamps. All of these procedures are excellent techniques. Most of them, however, require some portion of the posterior bony elements (*ie*, the lamina or spinous process and facets) to be intact. Sublaminar wiring carries the risk of injuring the spinal cord because the wires are passed under the lamina. Facet-to-spinous process wiring helps control rotational instability, but the spinous process must be intact and the facets often are quite small. Likewise, clamps require the lamina to be intact. Facet-to-facet wiring does not require intact midline structures, but it does not provide immediate stability nor does it guarentee bone fusion.

In contrast, lateral mass plating offers immediate stability and eventual lasting bone fusion. Except for facet wiring and lateral mass plates, most other procedures require harvesting autograft (usually from the hip) with its associated morbidity. In the two exceptions, however, either no bone is required after the facet has been roughened or bone taken from the base of the spinous process and placed in the facet joint is adequate to obtain permanent fusion. Lateral mass plating should be performed in unstable spines if the spinous process, lamina, or facets are fractured or if instability is present after a laminectomy has been performed for decompression or tumor resection.

During intubation, care is taken not to extend the neck. Fiberoptic intubation is often required. Somatosensory evoked potentials are recorded before the patient is turned and after he or she is placed in the prone position in the Mayfield head tongs with the neck in a neutral position. A cross-table lateral radiograph is obtained, and the patient's position is adjusted if needed. Pharmacologic paralysis with neuromuscular blocking agents should be undertaken with great caution or avoided entirely in patients with cervical instability. Even under profound anesthesia, the cervical musculature maintains some resting tone, functioning as a physiologic splint that contributes to the overall maintenance of alignment. If axial cervical traction was used preoperatively, it is typically continued during the operative procedure.

The dorsal aspects of the subaxial cervical spine are exposed via a posterior midline approach as previously described (Fig. 34-1). The midline incision is carried sharply to the ligament nuchae, and self-retaining retractors are gently placed. The ligament is divided with monopolar electrocauterization. The underlying paraspinous musculature is dissected from the spinous process and lamina in a subperiosteal manner and retracted laterally. Sharp dissection techniques are preferred to avoid inadvertent manipulation of the cervical region (see Figs. 34-15 and 34-16).

Caution must be used when the dorsal cervical spine is exposed, particularly in the presence of laminar fractures. The dimension of the cervical exposure is dictated by the extent of the pathology and the type of fixation. When fixation with lateral mass plates is used, lateral exposure must be extensive to uncover the lateral masses fully at the levels to be fused. Once adequate exposure has been achieved, the offending pathology can be addressed and corrected.

Plates of identical lengths are selected to span congruous segments on either side of the spine. When possible, plates should be implanted bilaterally and symmetrically. The shortest plate that will allow screw purchase in each lateral mass to be instrumented should be selected. If the posterior elements are intact, approximating these structures with a clamp or interspinous wiring often enables the application of a plate that initially appears to be too short. This maneuver also may confer biomechanical advantages because preload constructs compress the facet joint and may enhance the possibility of successful fusion. The maneuver, however, should only be performed after the facet has been roughened and pieces of cancellous bone obtained from the inferior spinous processes have been placed in the facet (Fig. 34-19).

Ideally, alignment of the instrumented cervical spine should approximate the normal lordotic posture. If lordosis cannot be achieved by preoperative traction or gentle intraoperative manipulation, the cervical spine can be instrumented in neutral alignment. It is more appropriate to modify the plate to fit the patient than to attempt to alter the patient's anatomy to conform to the plate. The lateral mass plate should never be bent into kyphosis. If an irreducible kyphotic deformity is encountered, anterior reconstruction should be considered instead of or before posterior stabilization.

Once the plate is selected and custom contoured, holes can be drilled into the lateral masses in preparation for screw placement. The center of the lateral mass is identified as the midpoint between the superior and inferior facet rostrocaudally and the lateral edge of the lamina (*ie,* where the lamina meets the inner edge of the lateral mass [Fig. 34-20]) and lateral edge of the lateral mass. An awl is used to mark the point for drilling 1 mm medial to the center of the lateral mass.

A variable-speed drill with a 3-mm diameter bit premeasured to penetrate 13 to 19 mm (depending on the size of the lateral mass) is employed. The hole is drilled 20° to 30°

superiorly (Fig. 34-21) and 20° to 30° laterally (Fig. 34-22). Angling the drill superiorly, almost in the plane of the facets, avoids penetrating the facet joints and aligns the screws anatomically with the lateral mass. It also directs the screw away from the nerve root located just beneath the pedicle. Angling the drill laterally avoids penetrating the foramen transversarium and puncturing the vertebral artery, which lies directly ventral to the lateral edge of the lamina (*ie,* where the lamina interfaces with the lateral mass).

In this manner, several screws can be placed from C3 to C6. At C7, the screw trajectory is often somewhat altered because of the relatively small size of its lateral mass. If a lateral mass fixation at C7 must be performed, a slightly more lateral and cephalad trajectory accommodates this anatomic constraint. Because the lateral mass is small, it is often preferable to perform pedicle fixation at C7 and T1. The pedicle of C7 can be entered 1 mm caudal to the facet joint and directed 25° to 30° medially (Fig. 34-23).

Each screw hole must be positioned optimally in its lateral mass. Thus, the holes are oriented with reference to the patient's anatomy; they are not placed according to the lie of the plate. To minimize this latter tendency, the holes can be drilled before the plate is placed. While the holes are drilled, toggling, which can cause irregular, oversized holes, must be minimized. Bicortical screw purchase in the lateral mass is desirable but not mandatory. If the anterior cortex is penetrated before the predetermined depth set by the drill stop has been reached, drilling should cease immediately.

Screw holes should be placed ipsilaterally in all lateral masses to be instrumented before the contralateral side is addressed. When a three- or four-hole plate is placed, the rostral and caudal holes are usually drilled first. If a three-hole plate is used to bridge a fractured facet or pedicle, no screws should be placed at the site of the injury. If the corresponding contralateral elements are intact, the center hole should be drilled and the screw placed on that side. The primary screw, 3.5 to 4.5 mm in diameter and 13 to 19 mm long, is usually sufficient to fixate the lateral masses. Typically, safe bicortical fixation is obtained with 3.5 × 15 mm screws.

Cancellous screws provide better purchase than those with cortical threads. The screws may or may not be self-tapping. If a screw is not self-tapping, the posterior cortex of the lateral mass should be tapped before the screw is placed.

After all lateral masses to be instrumented on the ipsilateral side have been drilled, the plate is secured with appropriate screws and tightened to about 80% of final torque in a sequential fashion. The contralateral lateral mass is then drilled, and the corresponding plate is applied and secured with partially tightened screws. Final tightening of the screws on both sides may then be performed. The screws will set into the plate and become snug with two-finger torque (Fig. 34-24). Overtightening should be avoided because it can strip the screw bed.

If the purchase is inadequate, a salvage technique must be used. The primary screw is removed and can be replaced by a rescue screw of a slightly larger diameter to improve bony purchase. Alternatively, the stripped screw hole can be filled with methylmethacrylate and the primary screw reinserted. After the fixation is completed, the wound is reapproximated in anatomic layers with absorbable sutures. If irradiation is anticipated, nonabsorbable sutures should be considered.

After the patient is placed in the supine position, the Mayfield clamps are removed and anesthesia is reversed. A detailed neurologic examination is mandatory. New neurologic deficits must be investigated promptly with imaging studies, surgical exploration, or both. After surgery, the patient typically is placed in an external orthosis (*eg,* a hard collar) for 4 to 6 weeks.

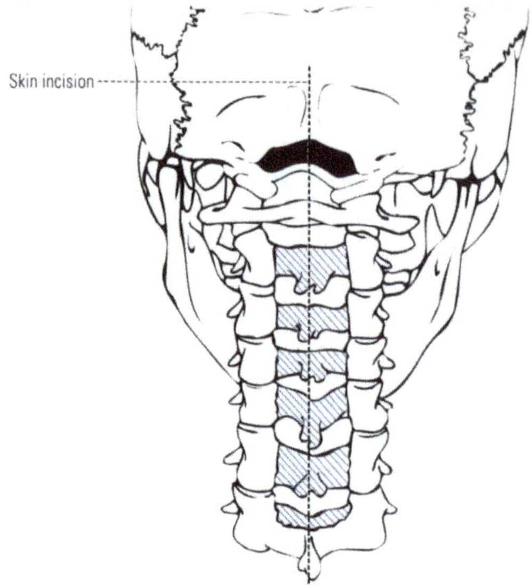

Figure 34-1. The incision for a cervical laminectomy is indicated, and the planned laminectomy of C2–C6 and the partial laminectomy of C7 are shown.

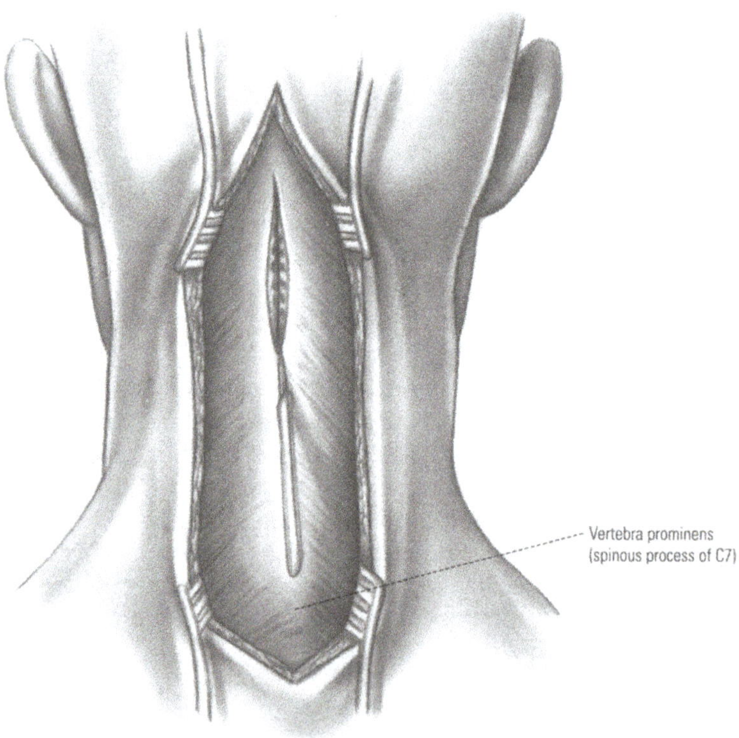

Figure 34-2. The skin has been opened and the superficial fascia has been incised sharply, staying within the relatively avascular nuchal ligament over the suboccipital and upper cervical area.

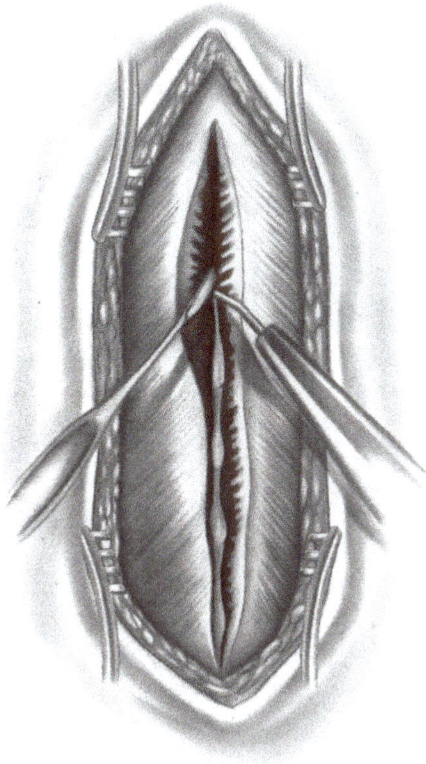

Figure 34-3. A Bovie and a periosteal dissector are used to dissect muscle from the spinous processes.

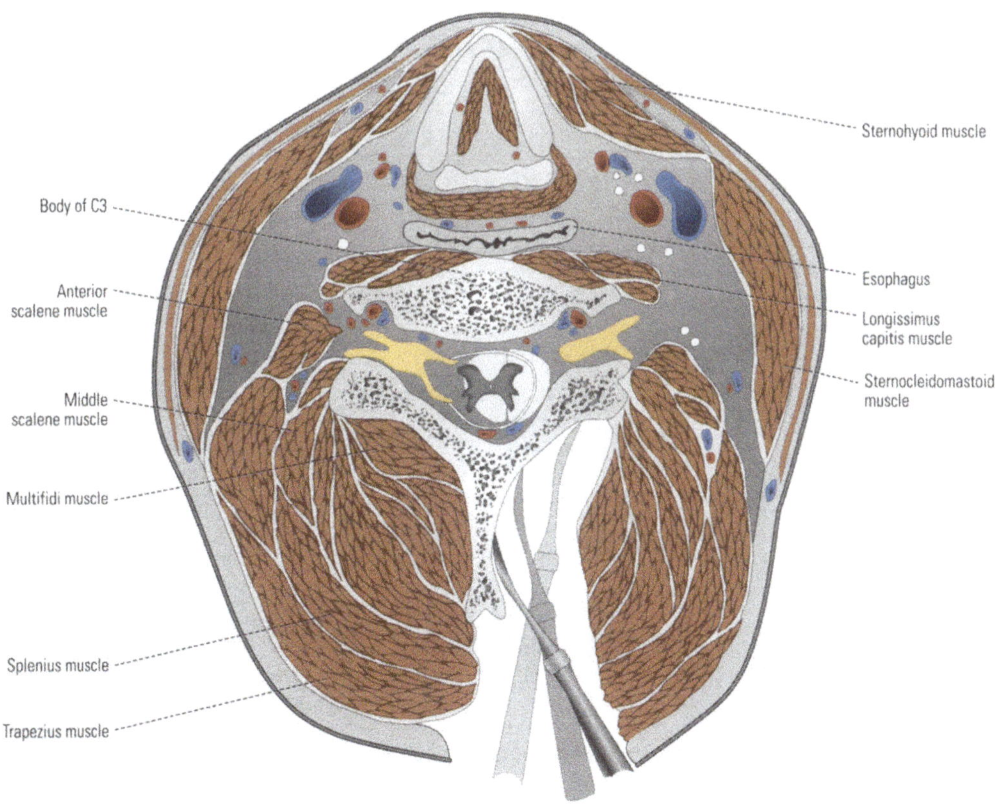

Figure 34-4. Cross-section of the neck demonstrates subperiosteal stripping of the spinous processes and lamina.

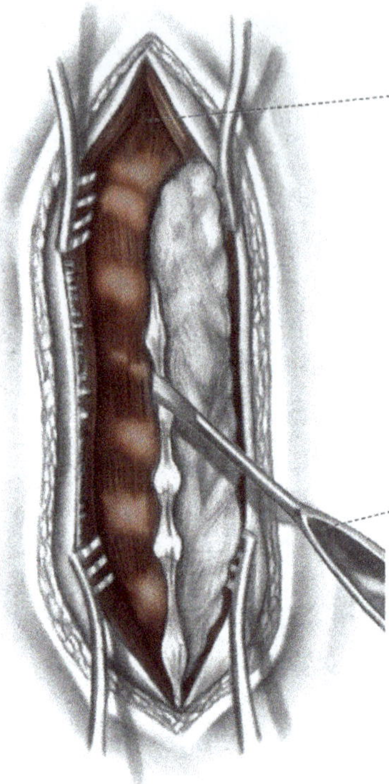

Figure 34-5. Operative view of muscle stripping. Bleeders are tamponaded with a sponge.

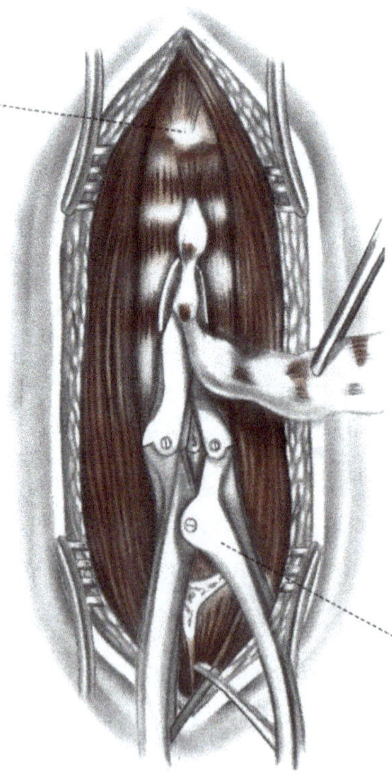

Figure 34-6. The cervical spinous process is removed with a Leksell rongeur.

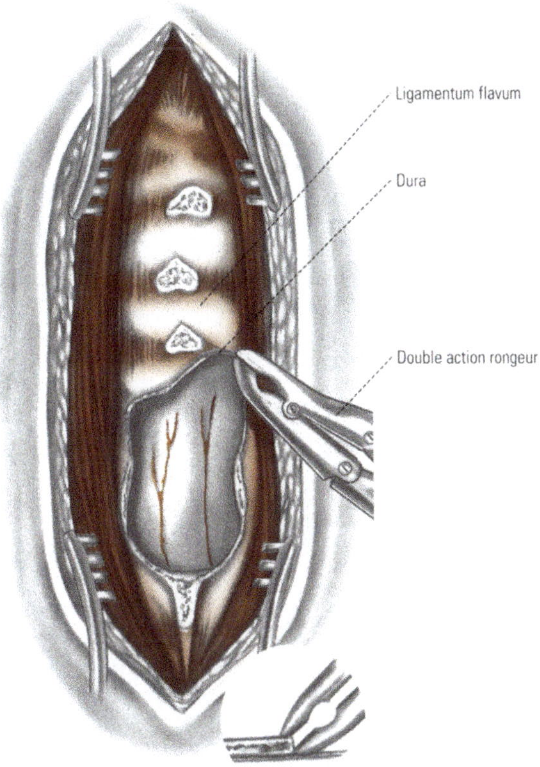

Figure 34-7. The lamina is removed without placing the lip of the rongeur beneath the lamina.

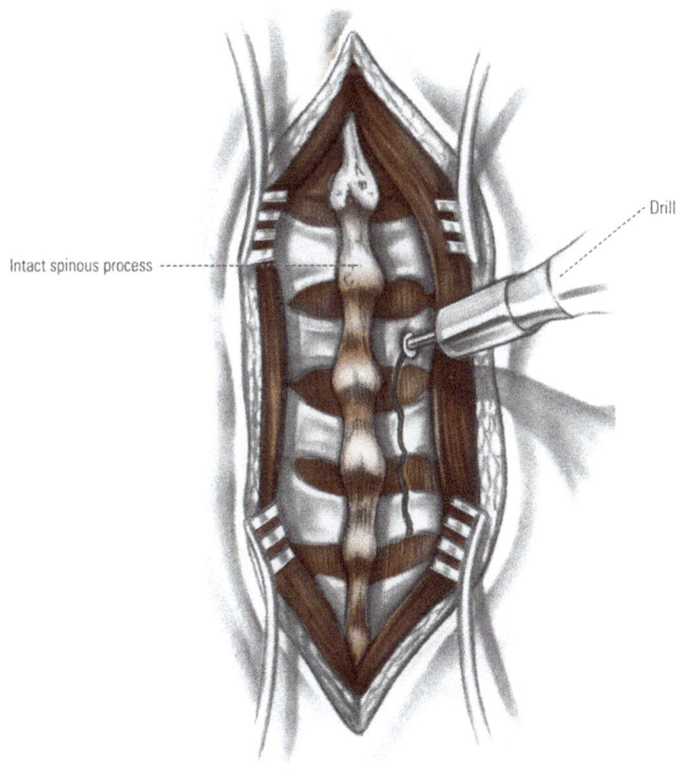

Figure 34-8. A high-speed drill is used to cut the lamina along a line between the lamina and the lateral mass.

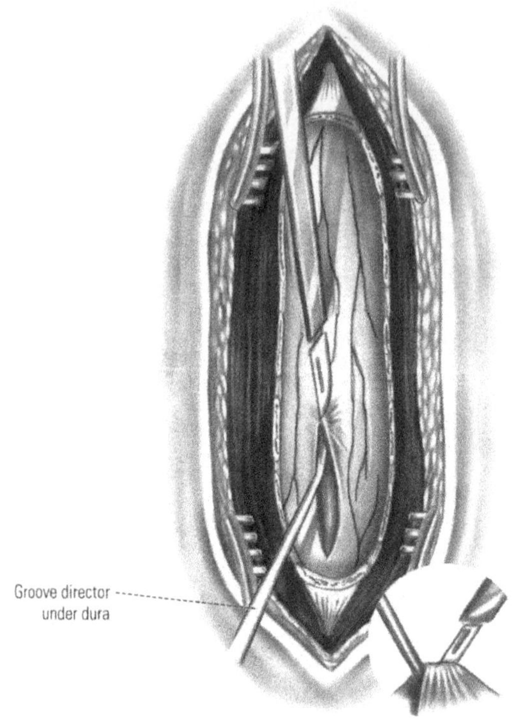

Figure 34-9. The dura is cut with a Woodson tool placed under the dura and a number 15 blade placed over the dura (see inset).

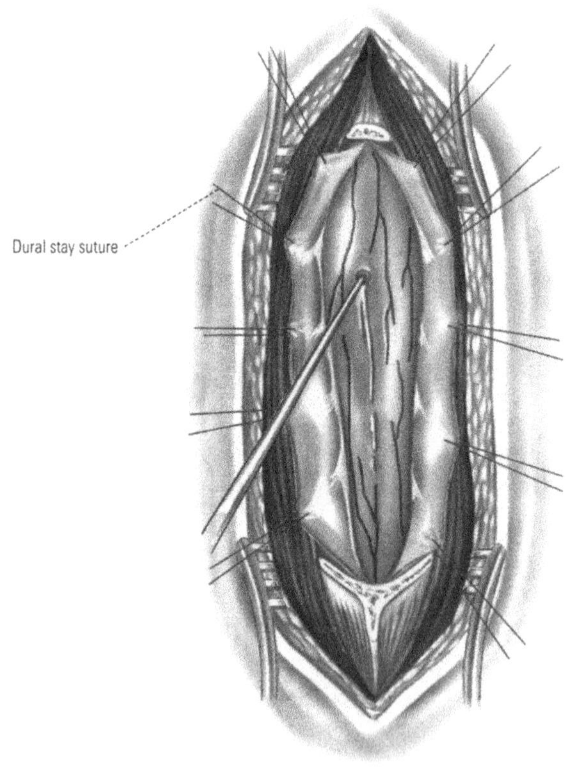

Figure 34-10. After a cordotomy is made with a number 11 blade, a number 6 Rhoton dissector is used to drain and enlarge the syrinx.

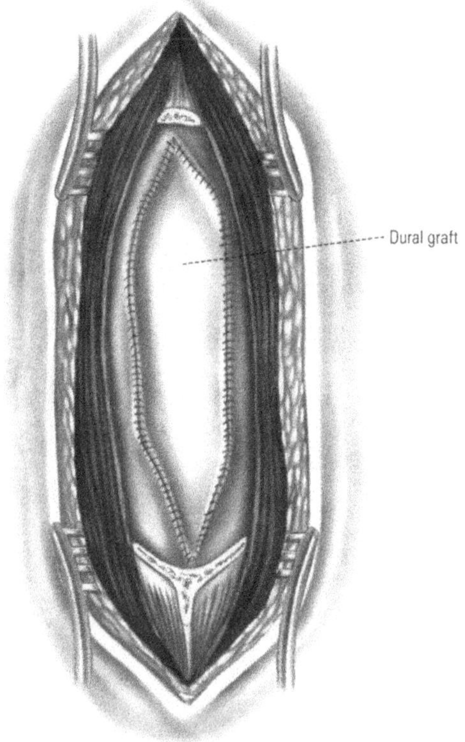

Figure 34-11. A duraplasty is performed by a watertight closure with a dural substitute.

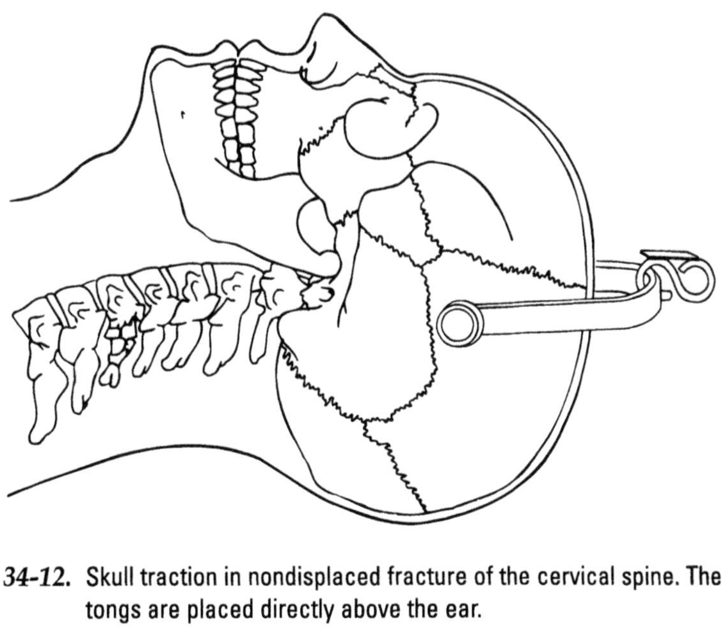

Figure 34-12. Skull traction in nondisplaced fracture of the cervical spine. The tongs are placed directly above the ear.

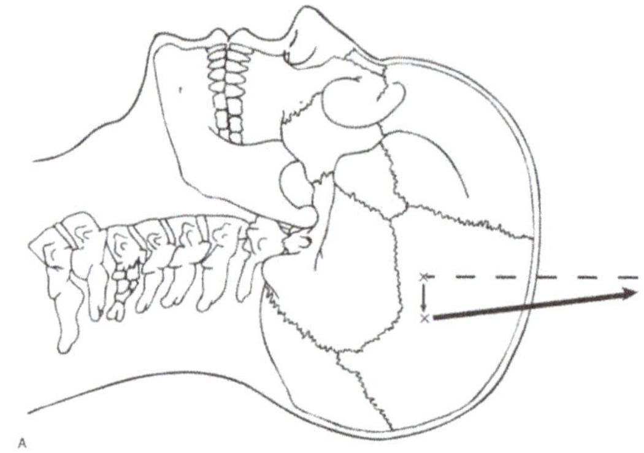

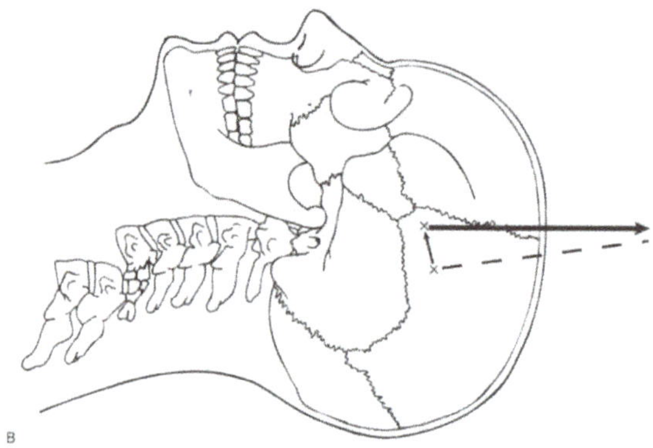

Figure 34-13. A, For a hyperextension injury, the tongs are inserted 2 cm behind the ear. B, For a flexion injury, the tongs are inserted 2 cm in front of the ear.

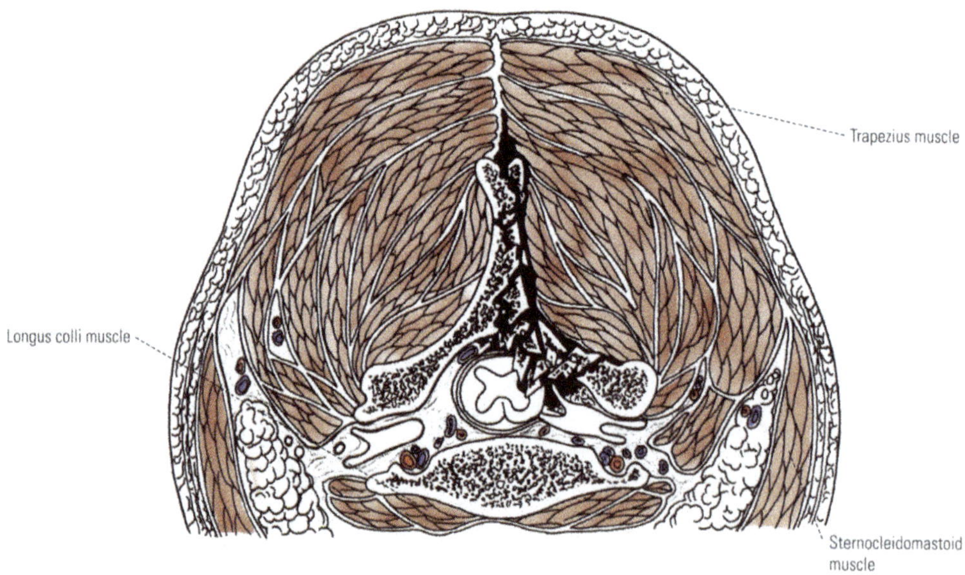

Figure 34-14. Transverse section of the neck at C6 level illustrates the lamina and spinous process fracture of the cervical spine.

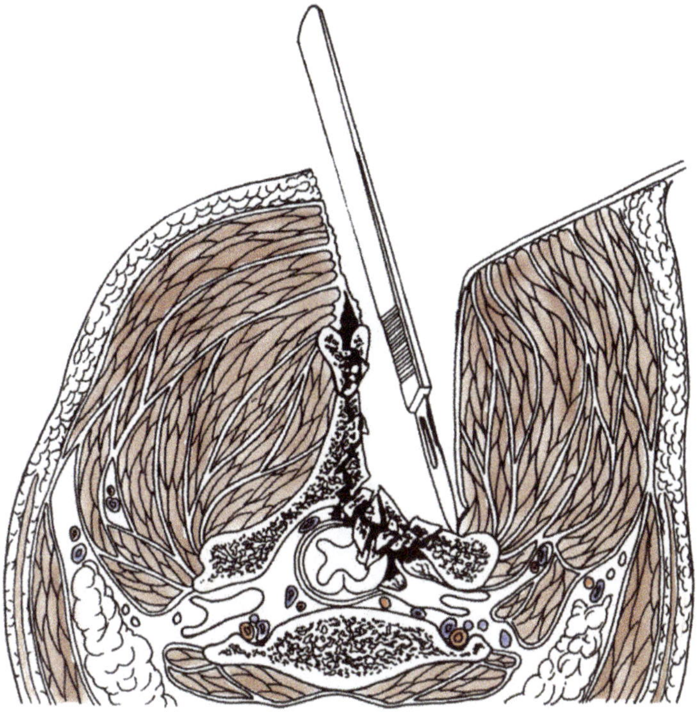

Figure 34-15. Transverse section through the neck at the C6 level. All pressure is directed laterally and dissection is done sharply.

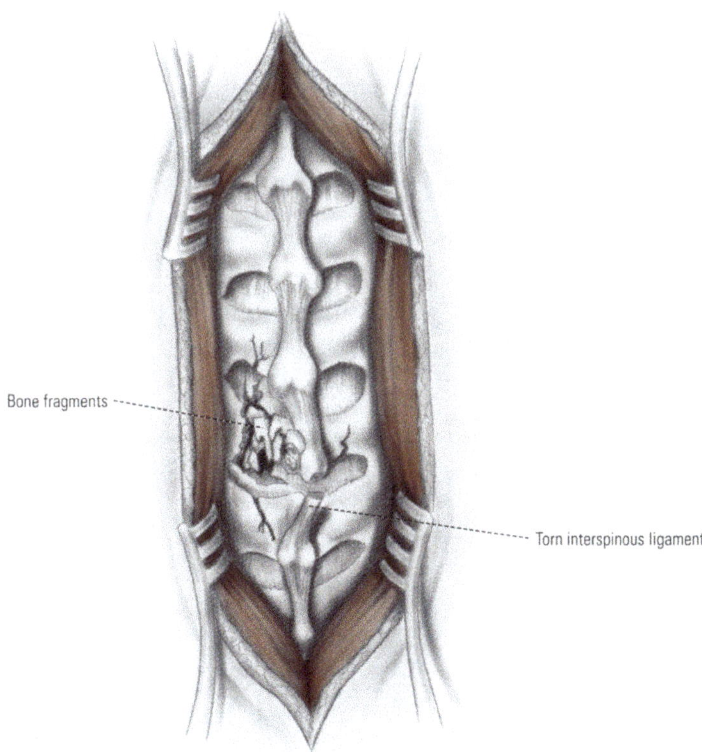

Figure 34-16. Operative view after sharp dissection of the muscle from the spinous processes and laminae.

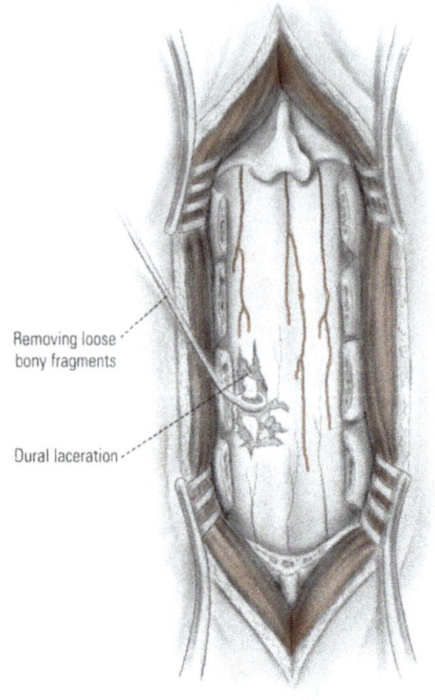

Figure 34-17. Operative view showing removal of the spinous processes and laminae. The dura is partially torn.

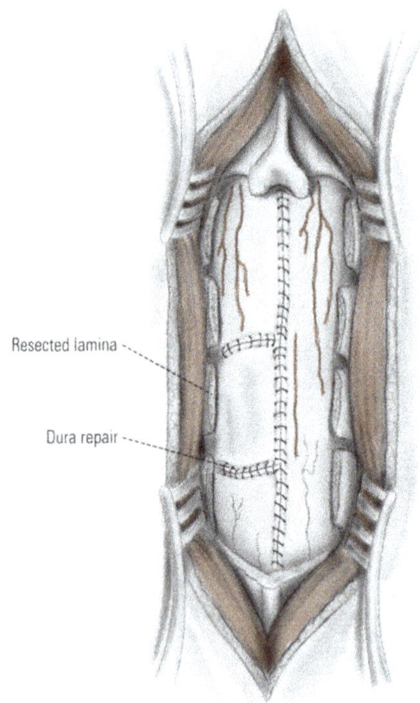

Figure 34-18. Operative view showing a watertight dural closure with a patch graft.

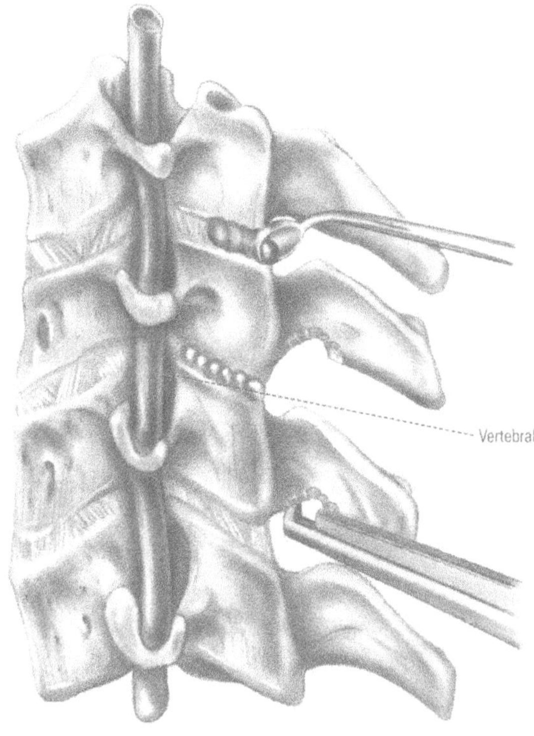

Figure 34-19. Lateral mass plating: preparing the facet. The facet joints are roughened with a curette and packed with pieces of cancellous bone obtained from the inferior spinous process.

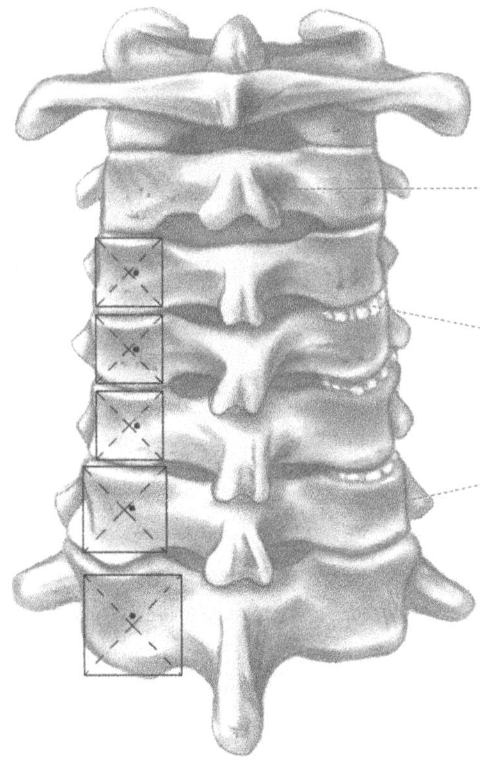

Figure 34-20. Landmarks for center of lateral mass. The center of the lateral mass (x) is the midpoint between the superior and inferior facet rostrocaudally and the lateral edge of the lamina (where the lamina meets the lateral mass) and the lateral edge of the lateral mass. Note the entry point is 1 mm medial to the center. Also note the slightly more lateral and cephalad entry point at C7.

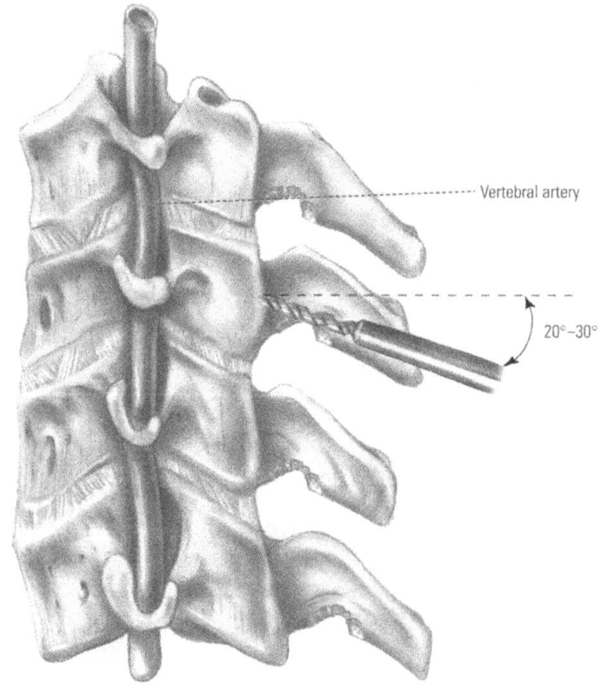

Figure 34-21. Drilling lateral mass. The drill penetrates the lateral mass 13 to 19 mm at approximately a 20° to 30° angle parallel to the facet.

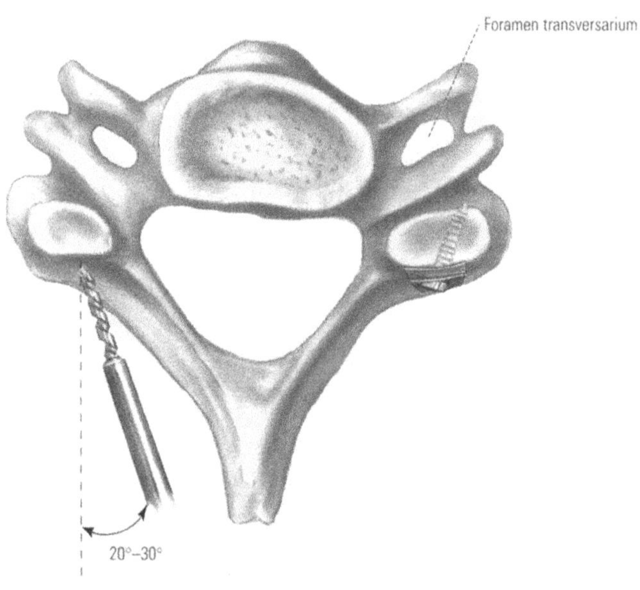

Figure 34-22. Drilling lateral mass continued. The drill is aimed 20° to 30° laterally, almost parallel to the lamina to avoid the vertebral artery.

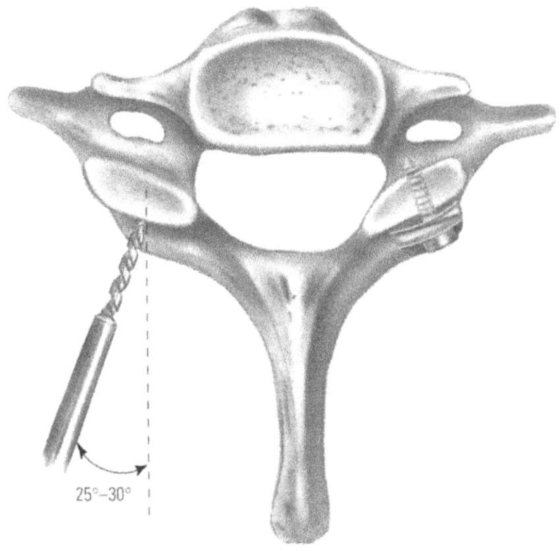

Figure 34-23. Drilling the pedicle of C7. The pedicle of C7 can be entered 1 mm caudal to the facet joint with the drill directed 25° to 30° medially.

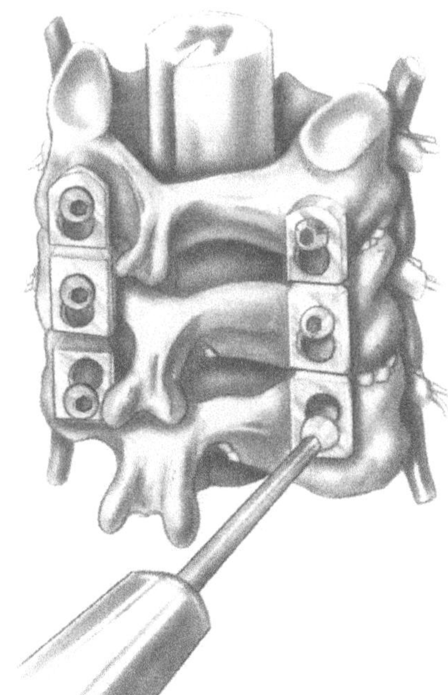

Figure 34-24. Tightening the plate screws. The screws are tightened to a two-finger torque.

Cervical Radiculoneuropathy: Herniated Intervertebral Disk and Spondylosis

Posterior Approach: Keyhole Foraminotomy

Cervical radiculopathy may be caused by a ruptured intervertebral disk, spondylosis, or a combination of these two processes. Soft disk material extrudes when the posterior annulus ruptures after the nucleus pulposus herniates. Figure 35-1 illustrates a typical lateral extruded disk. Laterally, the posterior annulus is weakest and the posterior longitudinal ligament is thinnest. Consequently, most degenerated disks protrude in this area. Because the nerve root is stretched over this area as it enters the intervertebral foramen, even a small amount of extruded disk material can cause the symptoms and signs of radiculopathy.

Progressive wear and tear of the end plates, specifically, of the joints of Luschka laterally, change the vertebral disk and adjacent structures and can cause cervical spondylosis. As a disk degenerates, the intervertebral disk space narrows and osteophytic bars are formed posteriorly and laterally. The result is spurring of the uncovertebral joint. All these changes reduce the size of the spinal canal and intervertebral foramina. Consequently, either myelopathy or radiculopathy can result. It is not unusual for this process to be much more severe on one side than on the other (Fig. 35-2). These changes often occur at the lower cervical levels, primarily at C5-C6 and C6-C7.

Unilateral herniated intervertebral disks can be removed through either an anterior or posterior approach. If the compression is primarily anterior and the patient has myelopathy, an anterior cervical diskectomy or corpectomy should be considered. If the patient has a straightening of the spine or kyphosis, the anterior approach is preferred for both myelopathy and radiculopathy. If, however, the patient's lordosis is normal and radiculopathy is caused only by an uncovertebral osteophyte or lateral ruptured disk, then a keyhole posterior foraminotomy is an excellent alternative. A posterior cervical decompression should be performed if the patient has myelopathy, normal lordosis, and equal anterior and posterior compression or primarily posterior compression (see cervical laminectomy in chapter 34).

Preoperative studies should include magnetic resonance imaging and/or CT-myelography. This chapter illustrates a unilateral semi-hemilaminectomy for removing a soft disk herniation.

The patient is placed in the prone position. The precautions necessary for placing the patient in this position are described in chapter 34. The neck is flexed only slightly, and the head is held in a Mayfield clamp. Venous stasis and tightening of the vertebral muscles result from marked flexion. Intraoperatively, it is more difficult to identify the exact level in the cervical spine from the posterior approach than from the anterior cervical approach. Helpful anatomic landmarks include the bifid C3-C6 spinous processes or the obvious large spinous process of C2 or C7. Using these anatomic landmarks, an incision is made and the location is verified by radiographs once the dissection is closer to the appropriate level.

A 4-cm skin incision is made over the two appropriate spinous processes (Fig. 35-3). The incision proceeds to the ligament nuchae and self-retaining retractors are inserted. The spinous process and laminae of the adjacent vertebra above and below the level of the lesion are stripped subperiosteally only on the symptomatic side. Paravertebral muscles are stripped back as far as the facet joint using sharp curettes.

The lower rim of the superior lamina and the superior rim of the inferior lamina are exposed. Under microscopic visualization and using a thin-lipped rongeur, the inferior half of the lamina of the superior level is removed followed by the superior half of the lateral lamina of the inferior level (Fig. 35-4). With a fine Kerrison rongeur, a foraminotomy is performed laterally, removing some of the medial aspects of the facets. The ligamentum flavum, which is very thin in the cervical region, is removed to expose the dura. If bleeding from epidural veins is present, it is controlled with bipolar coagulation or hemostatic agents and cotton pledgets (Fig. 35-5). Placing pressure on the nerve root or dural sac with cotton pledgets should be avoided.

The nerve root can be quite flattened by protruding disk material. With appropriate instrumentation, usually a number 4 Penfield dissector, the nerve root is separated from the underlying disk and reactive tissue and gently elevated without traction on the dural column. The disk fragment, which is now visible below the nerve root, should be teased out gently with micropituitary forceps (Fig. 35-6). If hard disk material is present instead of soft disk material, a high-speed drill with a diamond tip can be used to remove it after the nerve root is elevated as described previously. Once extruded disk fragments or an osteophyte have been removed, the nerve root will be much less tense and additional dissection, usually with a nerve hook, can be performed to look for other disk material. The nerve hook is used to palpate within the intervertebral foramen to make certain that all disk fragments have been removed.

Anterior Cervical Diskectomy and Fusion

In the early 1960s, Cloward [1] and Robinson and Smith [2] popularized the anterior approach to the cervical spine for the treatment of diskogenic disease. This approach has evolved and provides surgeons with a technique that removes ventral cervical spine disease directly at the site of compression. Performing fusion after a routine diskectomy when no overt structural abnormalities are present remains controversial. The criteria for fusion are evidence of a loss of normal lordosis as determined by preoperative lateral radiographs of the cervical spine and associated axial pain. The diagnostic workup for degenerative disease of the cervical spine includes MR imaging or CT-myelography. Although MR imaging provides excellent information on soft tissue disease, CT is superior for identifying bony pathology.

The patient is placed in a supine position on the operating table on a head rest or donut (Fig. 35-7), and a small sandbag or towel is placed under the left hip. The head is kept straight. General endotracheal anesthesia is used. When myelopathy is present, somatosensory evoked potentials are monitored. Before surgery begins, the patient receives a dose of intravenous antibiotics. Unless the patient is allergic to cephalosporins, one dose of intravenous vancomycin is administered. Additional doses of antibiotics are not given after a routine cervical diskectomy. Although superficial landmarks may not correspond to the exact level of the cervical spine, they serve as rough reference points for selecting the level of the skin incision.

The approach is routinely from the right side unless the patient has undergone a prior approach from the left. Patients with paralyzed vocal cords are approached from the side of paralysis. Although an approach from the right side risks injury to the recurrent laryngeal nerve, an approach from the left side (especially to the lower cervical disk spaces) risks injury to the thoracic duct (Fig. 35-8) [3]. For a one-level anterior cervical diskectomy, as is discussed in this chapter, a transverse incision in a skin crease in the neck at the level of a previously chosen superficial landmark is used. The incision overlies the anterior border of the sternocleidomastoid muscle. The angle of the mandible usually corresponds to the level of the second cervical vertebra, the hyoid bone to the level of C2–C3, and the cricoid cartilage to the level of C4–C5.

The platysma muscle is also sharply incised transversely across the entire width of the skin incision. The platysma muscle is elevated at both the inferior and superior margins of the wound, and blunt dissection proceeds immediately beneath this muscle. The subplatysmal dissection is imperative if more than one vertebral level is being exposed. The cervical fascia is opened vertically just anterior to the sternocleidomastoid muscle. Both sharp and blunt dissection are used to separate the soft tissue plane between the medial aspects of the sternocleidomastoid muscle and the lateral aspect of the laryngeal strap muscles. Next, the carotid sheath is retracted laterally and the trachea and esophagus medially. Once the prevertebral soft tissue has been opened, the longus colli muscles become visible overlying the anterior longitudinal ligament and the vertebral bodies (Fig. 35-9).

With hand retractors, the carotid sheath is held laterally and the esophagus and trachea medially. The prevertebral fascia is opened in the midline. Vertebral bodies and intervertebral disks are easily palpable. The level thought to be appropriate is selected, and without further dissection, a vertebral body post is placed in the middle portion of one of the vertebral bodies or a "bayonetted" spinal needle is placed in the disk space. Lateral radiographs of the cervical spine are obtained.

At this time the autograft from the right hip is obtained. A 3-cm incision starting 2 cm behind the anterior superior iliac spine is carried inferior and parallel to the anterior iliac crest. The incision proceeds down to the fascia lata and iliac crest. The fascia lata is incised from the anterior superior iliac crest, and the muscle is stripped back using a sharp periosteal elevator. With appropriately sized chisels, bone grafts (usually 8 mm wide and 1.2 cm deep) are obtained (Fig. 35-10). The graft must have cortical layers on each end and should be denuded of soft tissue attachments. The graft is wrapped in a saline-soaked sponge and saved. Bone wax is used to control bleeding from the ilium, and the wound is closed in layers.

Having ascertained the appropriate cervical vertebral level by radiography, attention must again be directed to the neck. The hand retractors are inserted as before, and the longus colli muscles are stripped laterally from the anterior surfaces of the two vertebral bodies adjacent to the interspace that will be explored (Fig. 35-11). Self-retaining retractors are then inserted. The teeth of the lateral retracting blade should be inserted into the longus colli muscles and must not be displaced throughout the remainder of the operation. The anterior longitudinal ligament is scraped off the vertebrae (Fig. 35-12).

Vertebral body posts are placed in adjacent vertebral bodies above and below the planned diskectomy site (Fig. 35-13). A window is made into the interspace with a number 11 blade and should be carried laterally as far as the retractor permits. The vertebral bodies are distracted gently using the post spreader.

A diskectomy begins with a rectangular incision in the annulus fibrosus anteriorly (Fig. 35-14). The superficial disk material is resected with cervical curettes and interspace rongeurs. For the deeper portion of the diskectomy, an operating microscope is used. All bony disk material must be removed from the anterior cervical nerve root without disturbing the vertebral artery, which lies lateral to the vertebral bodies between the foramina transversarium (Fig. 35-15*A*). Beginning laterally where the ligament has already been freed, the posterior longitudinal ligament is moved across the entire width of the interspace. Removal of this ligament is an integral part of each anterior cervical fusion (Fig. 35-15*B*). Extruded fragments of disk material or redundant ligaments often are removed during this part of the operation. Each neural foramen is then palpated once again to assure that both nerve roots have been decompressed.

Once the diskectomy and appropriate bony decompression have been completed, fusion can proceed. This section describes the Smith-Robinson fusion [1]. Adjacent vertebral body endplates are drilled along the disk space to promote fusion and to lock the graft into position (Fig. 35-16). The graft can also be countersunk by making a 1- to 2-mm posterior shelf along the superior aspect of the inferior vertebral body. This strategy prevents retromigration of the graft. Along the anteroinferior aspect of the superior vertebral body, a "lip" of approximately 1 mm is left. Just posterior to this lip, more bone is drilled to prevent anterior dislodgment of the graft. To diminish the incidence of nonunion, it is important to refrain from using bone wax along the interspace bone. With minimal distraction (vertebral body post, interspace distractors, or slight manual retraction of the head can be used), an appropriately sized graft is tapped into position. Once the distraction is released, the graft must be snug and immobile within the interspace (Fig. 35-17). At this stage, any planned instrumentation can proceed.

If more than one level is to be fused, a few additional points are worth remembering. All involved interspaces should be exposed at the same time. When the exposed interspaces are not equally accessible, the hardest one should be done first. Each level should be completed before proceeding to the next level and then the bone grafts should be placed at the same time.

Once the diskectomy and fusion are completed, the vertebral posts are removed and bone wax is applied to the bone holes. After the self-retaining retractors have been removed, the patient's carotid pulse is checked and superficial bleeding is controlled with bipolar cauterization. After copious irrigation, the platysma is closed with simple interrupted 3-0 polyglactin sutures. The skin is approximated by running a 4-0 subcuticular stitch. Steristrips are applied to reinforce the suture line, and a sterile dressing is applied. All patients are transferred to their hospital bed in a rigid collar. Anteroposterior and lateral cervical spine radiographs are obtained in the recovery room to ascertain the position of the graft and to serve as a baseline for further comparison.

The patient wears a hard collar for approximately 6 weeks after which lateral radiographs are obtained to document bone fusion. Flexion-extension films are also obtained. If there is satisfactory evidence of union and no pathologic motion is seen on dynamic radiographs, the patient is weaned from the hard collar and begins neck exercises.

Anterior Cervical Plating

Anterior screw plate fixation augments vertebral interbody arthrodesis in the subatlantal (C2–C7) cervical spine. The anterior cervical plate optimizes the environment for bony fusion. The plate resists graft displacement, reduces the incidence of pseudarthrosis, and avoids postoperative bracing such as a halo. Degenerative, neoplastic, infectious, traumatic, and iatrogenic (postsurgical) causes of vertebral column instability with or without concomitant neural compromise are well-suited for treatment with the rigid internal fixation provided by an anterior cervical plate. Whether plating should be routine after one- or two-level diskectomies is controversial. This section describes an anterior cervical plating after diskectomy secondary to trauma.

After the patient is taken to the operating room, a single prophylactic dose of antibiotics is administered intravenously approximately 30 minutes before the skin is incised. In patients with myelopathy, somatosensory evoked potentials (SSEPs) are routinely monitored. Baseline evoked potentials are measured before the patient is intubated or positioned if myelopathy exists. Muscle relaxants are avoided during anesthesia to provide an immediate indication of neural irritation during the procedure. Patients with posttraumatic cervical instability or preexisting myelopathy related to cervical stenosis undergo fiberoptic or awake intubations. If myelopathy is present, patients routinely receive a bolus dose of methylprednisolone followed by drip infusion. Postoperatively, this infusion is discontinued if the patient's neurologic examination is stable.

When the patient is positioned, bony soft tissue prominences are carefully padded to avoid pressure sores or peripheral neuropathy. If an autograft is to be obtained from the iliac crest, the appropriate hip is elevated with a towel roll. The patient is placed in a Caspar head-holder (Aesculap, San Francisco, CA) to support the head and cervical spine (Fig. 35-18). The head is maintained in a neutral position or extended minimally with the assistance of a chin strap. The SSEPs should be observed carefully for any change and intraoperative fluoroscopy should be available to confirm the maintenance of cervical alignment after positioning is complete. Although fluoroscopy is not mandatory, it is useful in selecting an appropriately sized cervical plate and for assessing screw trajectories, final screw position, and alignment of the plate and vertebral column.

Routinely, an incision is made on the right side unless the patient has undergone previous surgery. In that case, the incision is made on the same side as the previous surgery to avoid the possibility of bilateral injury to the recurrent branch of the vagal nerve. Unilateral manifestations can be subtle and otherwise undetected unless evaluated specifically [4]. General orientation along the cervical spine is estimated by external anatomical landmarks (Fig. 35-19). Intraoperative fluoroscopy also ensures precise placement of the skin incision. A transverse incision within a skin crease is cosmetically superior to a longitudinal incision that follows the medial sternocleidomastoid muscle. Consequently, in a routine one-level diskectomy, a transverse incision is used. After the patient has been prepared and draped, the skin incision is sharply made.

The platysma muscle is incised transversely and undermined rostrally and caudally. The underlying sternocleidomastoid muscles and the tracheal esophageal bundle are identified, and the avascular plane between these structures is developed with careful, blunt and sharp dissection. A trajectory medial to the carotid sheath is followed, and the underlying vertebral column is palpated (Fig. 35-20). The medial insertion of the adjacent longus colli muscles is elevated bilaterally from the vertebral column, and self-retaining serrated retractor blades are inserted to expose the anterior vertebral column further. These blades are placed under the longus colli muscles bilaterally. Rostrocaudal exposure can be achieved by adding a blunt blade perpendicular to the first blade (Fig. 35-21). Vertebral body distractor posts can also be added, but they can compromise the integrity of the vertebral body and adversely affect the quality of screw purchase. Once the appropriate level has been identified by either fluoroscopy or lateral radiography, a diskectomy is performed as previously described.

Screw-plate application provides immediate rigid fixation for the cervical spine. However, only an osseous union can ensure long-term stability of the vertebral column. Consequently, the most fundamental principle is that instrumentation cannot substitute for a carefully conceived and meticulously prepared fusion site. Before the screw plate construct is applied, ventral osteophytes should be removed to allow the plate to set flush against the spinal column. The anterior cortical bone layer, however, needs to be maintained because it contributes substantially to the resistance of individual screws to pulling out. After the adjacent end plates are removed, the adjacent vertebral bodies are decorticated. The appropriate bone graft is tapped in line with the anterior margin of the adjacent vertebral bodies to maximize contact with the plate and the entire fusion construct. A small trough along the posteroinferior aspect of one of the vertebral bodies protects against graft retropulsion and epidural compression.

The appropriately sized plate is selected so that it does not overlap the adjacent disk either rostrally or caudally. In fact, the plate should be just short of such overlap (Fig. 35-22). The plate is then placed on top of the bony vertebral column and should not toggle. If it does, either a disk space spreader or vertebral body distractor posts can be used, or axial traction is applied carefully by the anesthesiologist. The plate can be contoured to maximize contact with the vertebral column. Such manipulation, however, fatigues the plate and should be minimized. This section describes the use of a fixed angle screw. Alternatively, variable angle screws can be placed. The advantages and disadvantages of fixed or variable screw fixation devices are beyond the scope of this chapter.

The fixed angle drill guide is selected and seated within the bone screw hole in the plate. Most fixed guides have a predetermined cephalad and medial convergent angle for the upper two screws and a caudal and medial convergent angle for the lower two screws. After the hole is drilled, the outer cortex of the hole is tapped, and appropriately sized screws (they should be as long as possible without penetrating the posterior cortex) are placed (Fig. 35-23). For the final screw torque, two-finger tightness is desired to avoid stripping the screw hole and diminishing the screws' resistance to pull out. When the screws are in place, they are locked into the plate by a locking mechanism that is intrinsic or extrinsic to the plate.

If the tap threads are stripped, options for securing the construct include substituting a larger diameter "rescue" screw or drilling a new screw hole if variable trajectory placement is possible. Alternatively, the entire plate can be moved and a new hole for a fixed trajectory screw drilled, or the initial screws' purchase can be bolstered with methylmethacrylate.

Although not mandatory, fluoroscopy is recommended to confirm appropriate placement of the plate and screw (Fig. 35-24). Violation of the vertebral end plate not only results in suboptimal screw purchase but also risks incorporating a normal motion segment within the fusion construct. The operative site is inspected under both direct visualization and fluoroscopy if available. Specific attention is directed toward the alignment of the vertebral column after fixation, the position of the graft with respect to the epidural space, and the length of the plate and position of the screws with respect to the rostral and caudal disk spaces.

The wound is irrigated with bacitracin-containing saline, and hemostasis is obtained with bipolar cauterization. The self-retraining retractors are removed, and the trachea, esophagus, and carotid are inspected with hand-held retractors for evidence of injury. A persistent carotid pulse above and below the level of the self-retraining retractor is confirmed. The platysma muscle and the dermis are closed in separate layers with interrupted polyglactin sutures, and the skin is reapproximated with a running subcuticular suture and Steristrips.

After screw plate fixation, most patients are considered to be stabilized enough to wear a hard collar when active and a soft collar while sleeping. Immediately after surgery, plain film radiographs are obtained; they are repeated with flexion-extension views 6 weeks after surgery. If there is evidence of graft incorporation and the instrumentation appears stable in the comparative views, the patient is instructed to taper use of the hard collar and to initiate exercises to strengthen the cervical muscles.

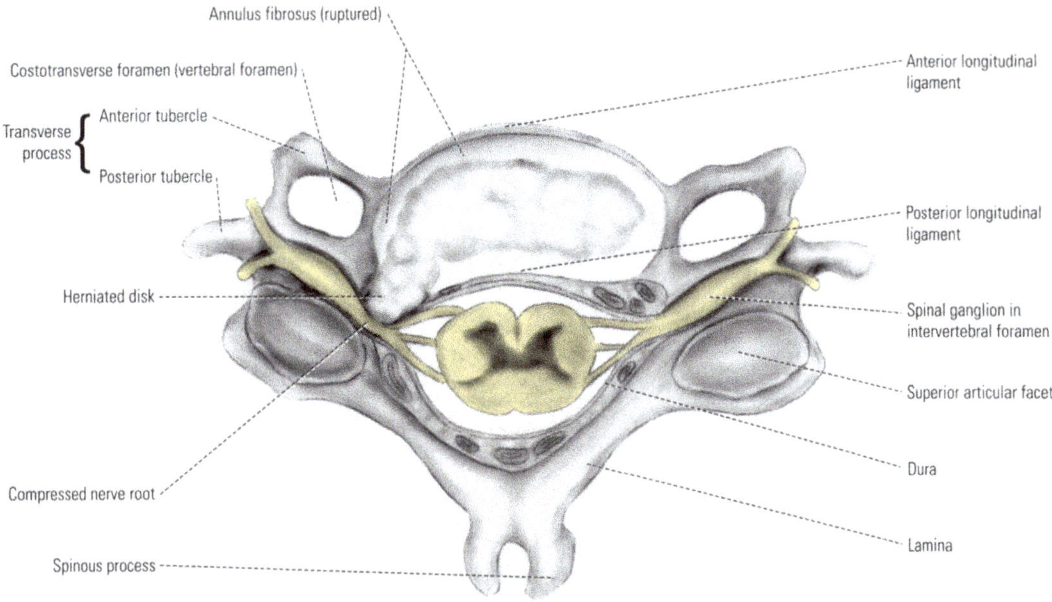

Figure 35-1. Lateral disk herniation showing the relation of the herniation to the lateral extent of the posterior longitudinal ligament.

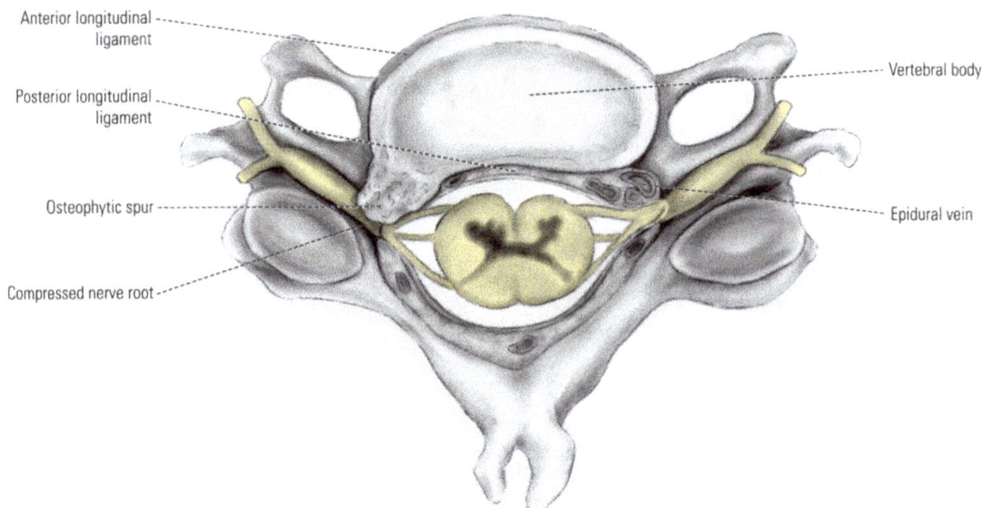

Figure 35-2. Compression of the nerve root by bone spurs on one side only.

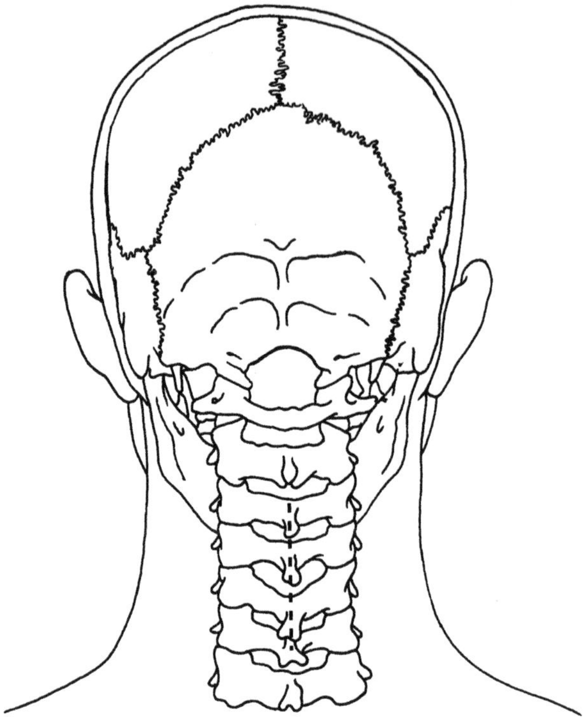

Figure 35-3. A 3- to 4-cm skin incision is made over the two appropriate spinous processes.

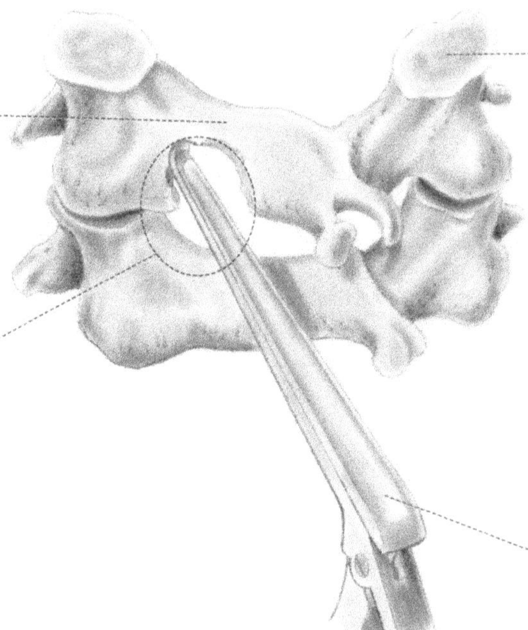

Figure 35-4. The inferior half of the superior lamina and the superior half of the lateral inferior lamina are removed.

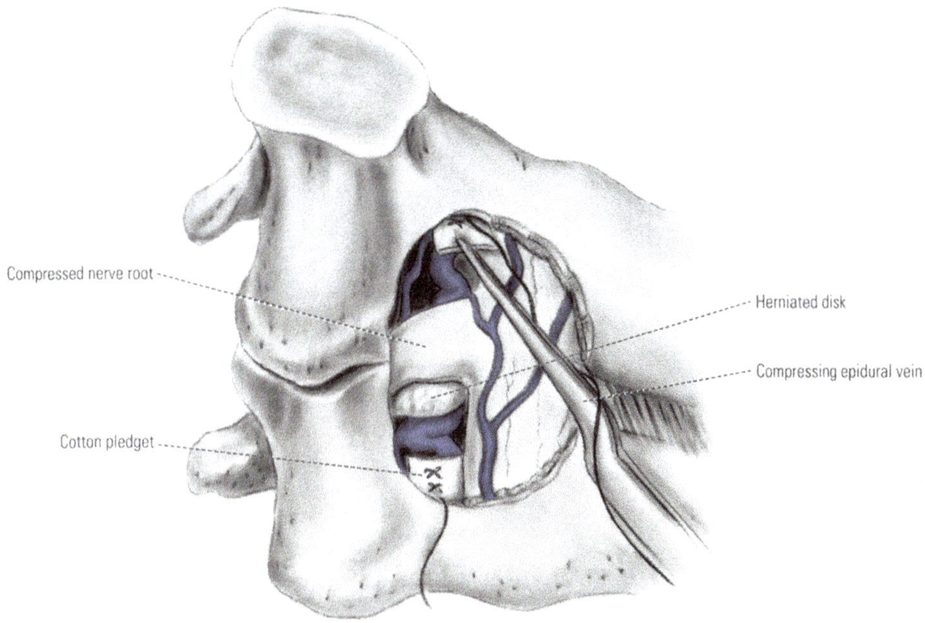

Figure 35-5. Cotton pledgets or bipolar coagulation are used to control bleeding from the epidural veins. The dura covering the spinal cord should not be retracted. The nerve root is displaced by the underlying disk fragment.

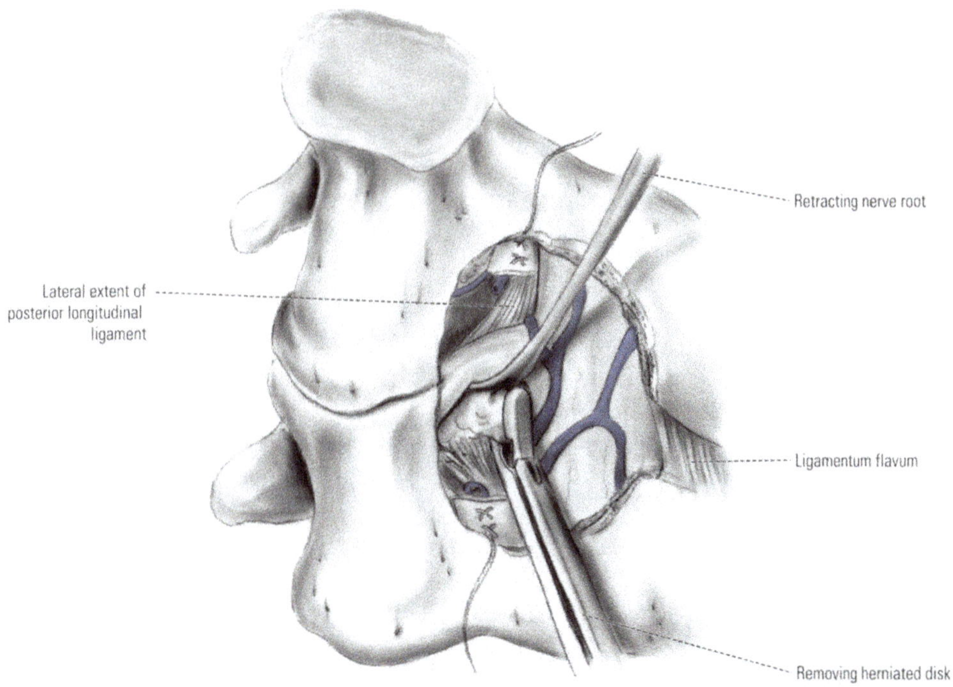

Figure 35-6. The nerve root is gently elevated superiorly and the disk fragment is teased out with micropituitary forceps.

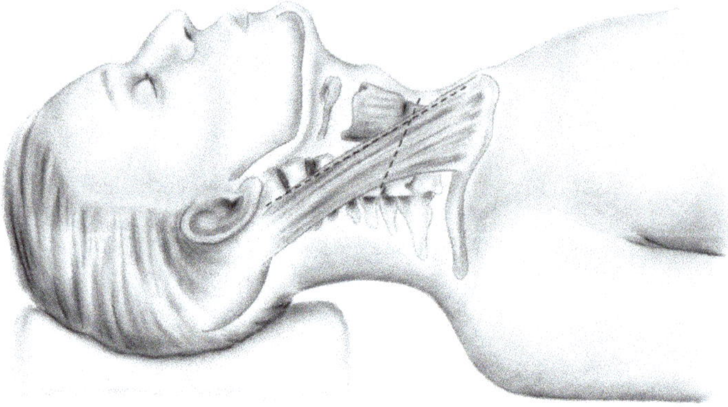

Figure 35-7. A lateral view of the patient after positioning and the planned incision for a single-level diskectomy. The transverse incision is indicated for a multiple-level diskectomy. The incision for the anterior sternocleido-mastoid muscle is shown.

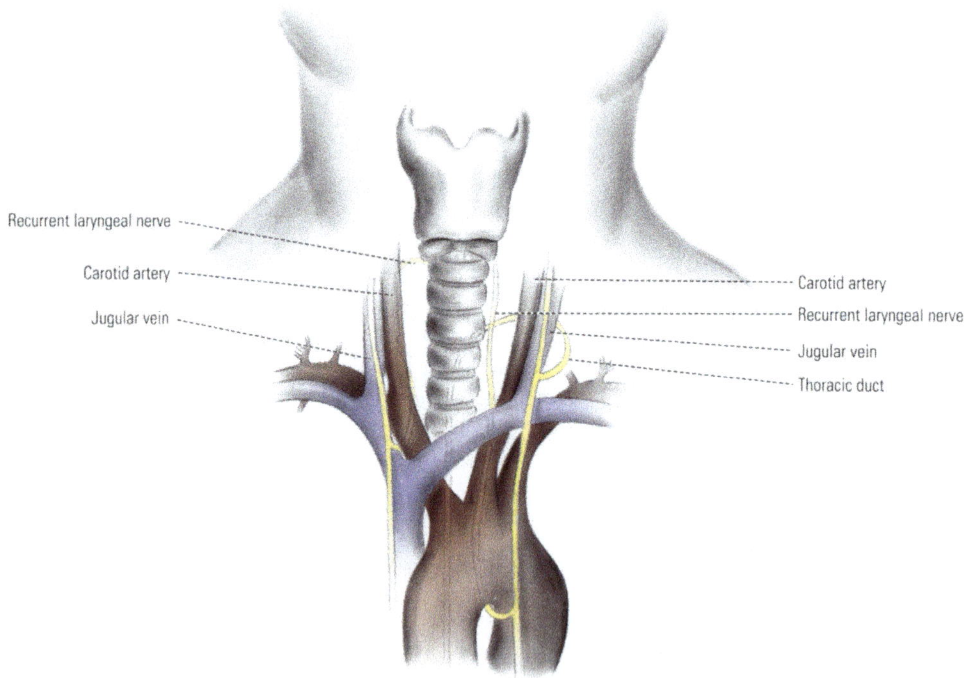

Figure 35-8. The surgical anatomy relevant to an anterior cervical diskectomy. The recurrent laryngeal nerve is more prone to injury on the right side while the thoracic duct is more prone to injury on the left side.

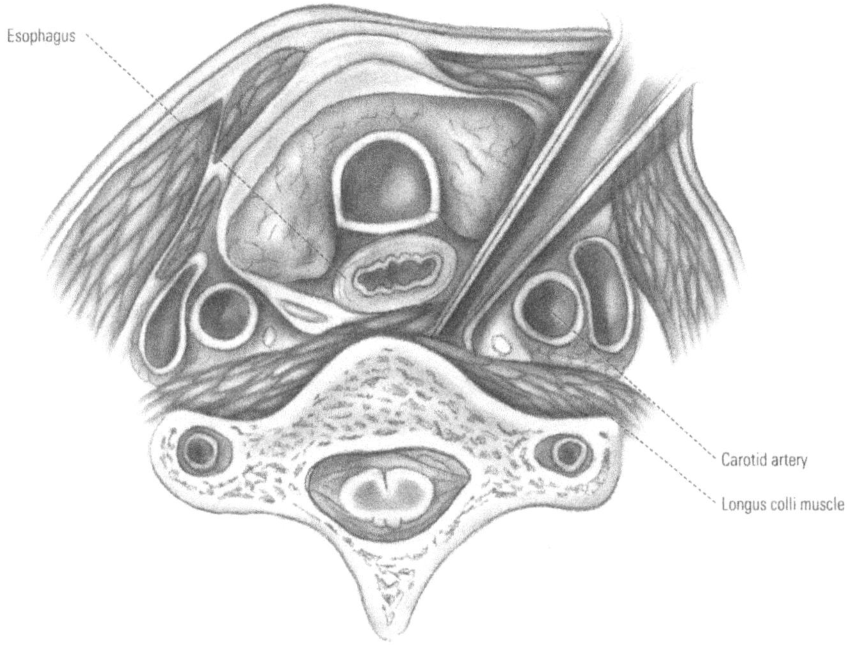

Figure 35-9. Axial section of the neck at C6. The neurovascular structures are retracted laterally and the visceral structures medially. The longus colli muscles need to be stripped laterally so that the retracting blades can be inserted and the vertebra exposed.

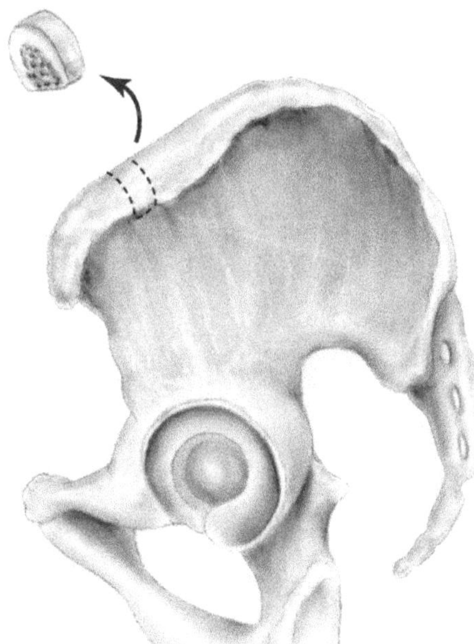

Figure 35-10. Bone graft harvested from the anterolateral ileum should be 2 to 3 cm behind the anterior superior iliac spine to avoid an avulsion fracture. A tricortical bone graft is harvested for a single-level interbody fusion.

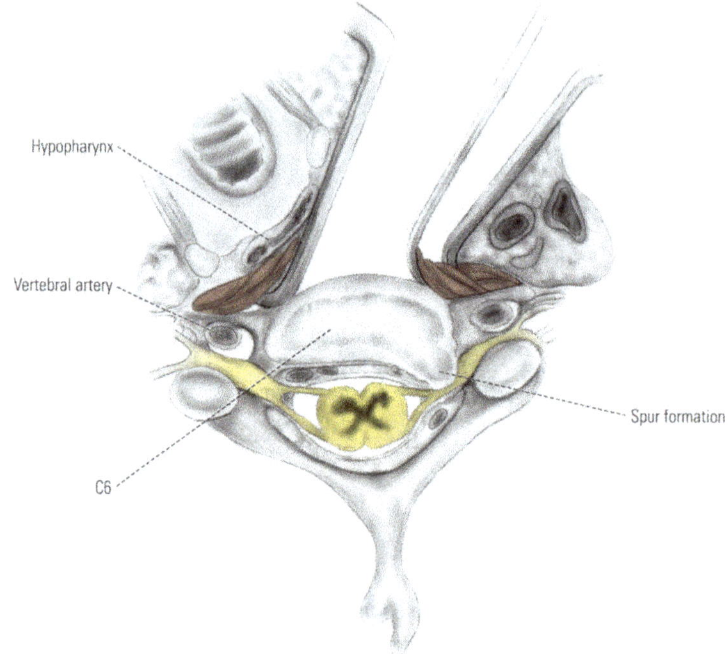

Figure 35-11. Axial section of the neck at C6. The longus colli muscles are stripped laterally to expose the anterior surface of the vertebrae.

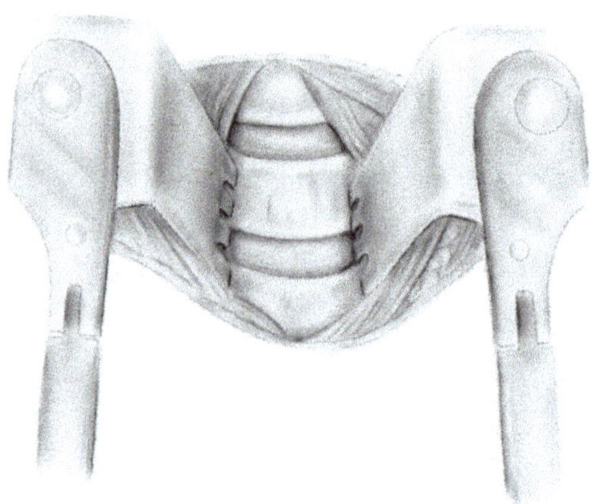

Figure 35-12. Teeth of the lateral retracting plates are inserted under the longus colli muscles and the anterior ligament is scraped off the vertebrae.

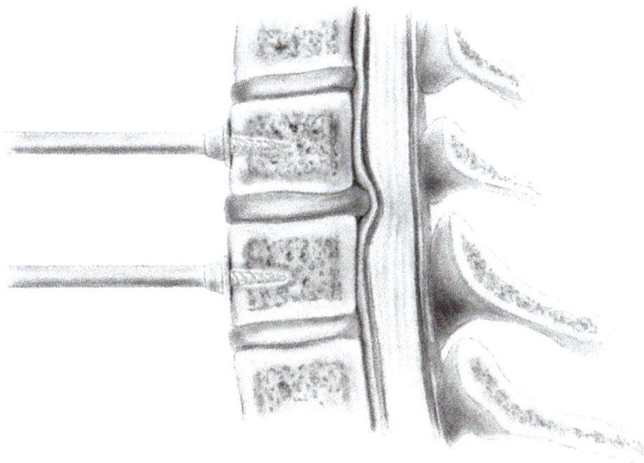

Figure 35-13. Vertebral body posts are placed in the adjacent vertebral bodies above and below the planned diskectomy site.

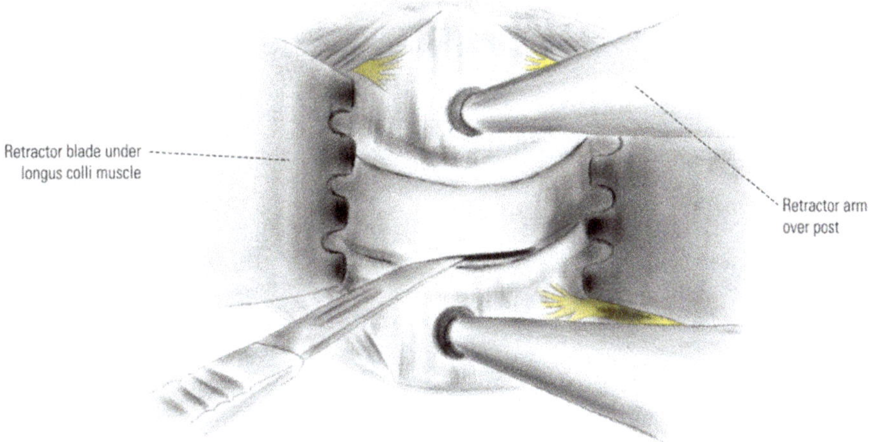

Figure 35-14. The diskectomy begins with a rectangular incision in the annulus fibrosus anteriorly.

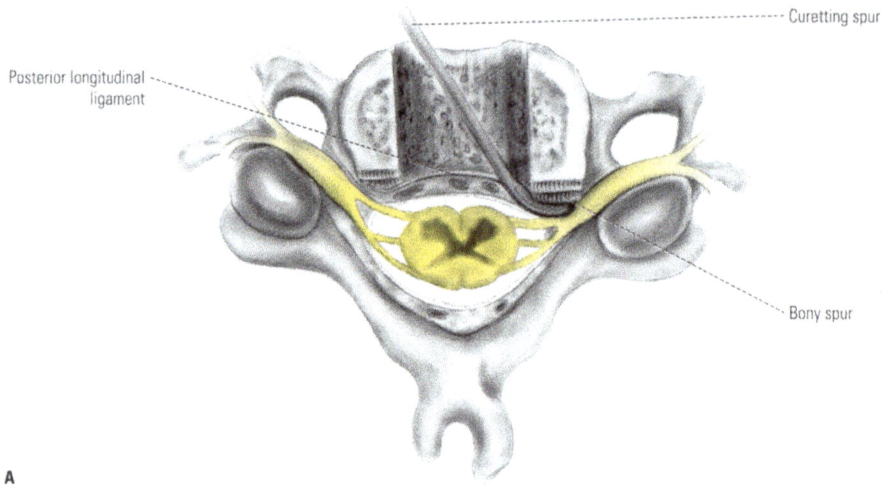

A

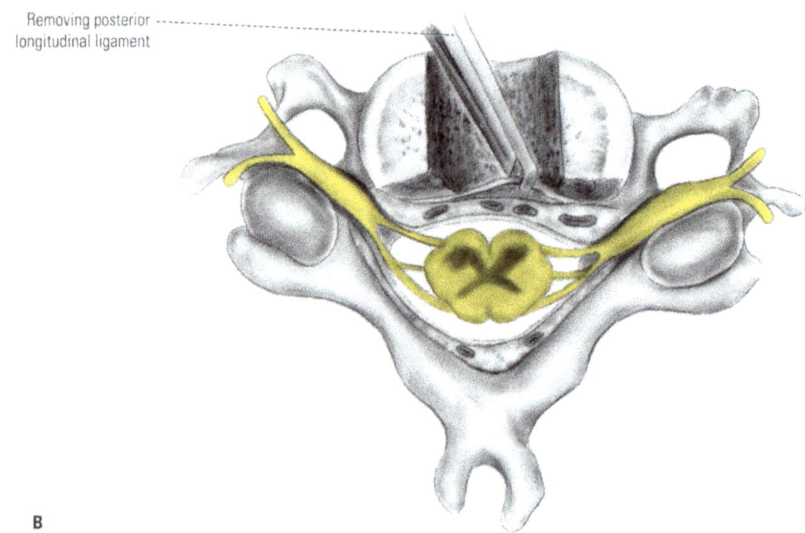

B

Figure 35-15. A, The cross-hatch indicates the portion of bone to be removed, exposing the posterior longitudinal ligament and the nerve root. Curetting is done under direct vision. B, The posterior longitudinal ligament is removed under direct vision after the spurs have been removed.

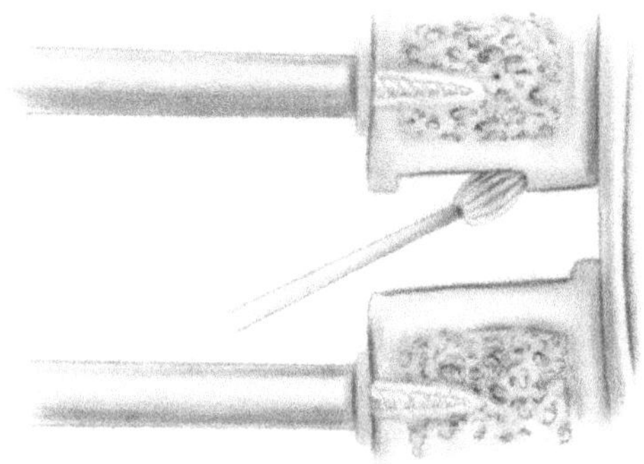

Figure 35-16. Adjacent vertebral body endplates are drilled along the disk space to promote fusion and to lock the graft into position, and a 1-mm posterior and anterior lip is placed to prevent anterior and posterior dislodgment of the graft.

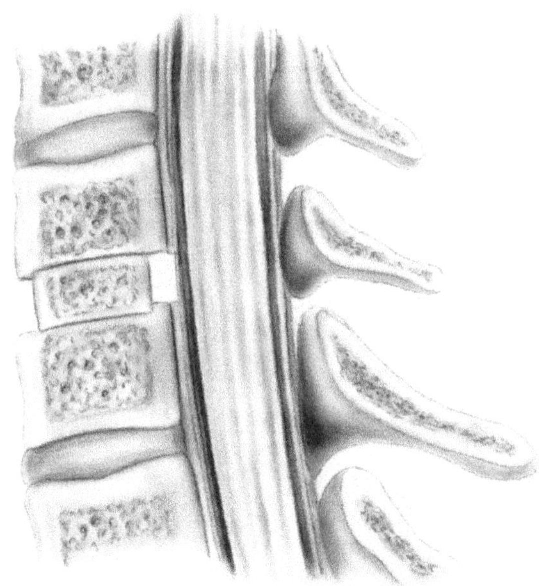

Figure 35-17. The graft is snug and immobile within the interspace.

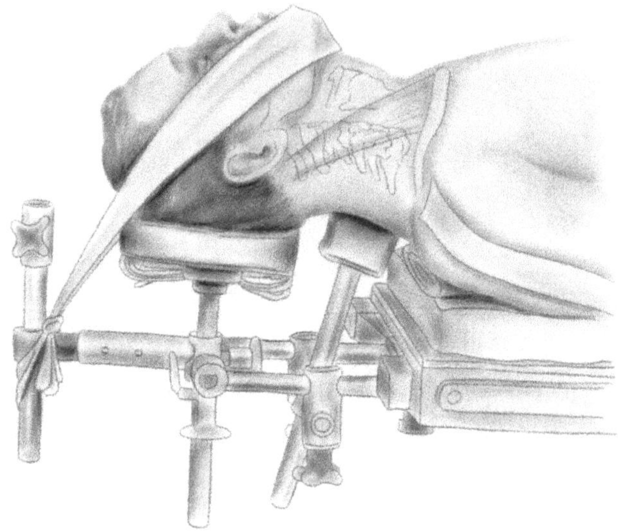

Figure 35-18. The patient is on the Caspar headholder with the cervical spine in a neutral or minimally extended posture to recreate the cervical lordosis. Adhesive tape is used to help hold the shoulders inferiorly.

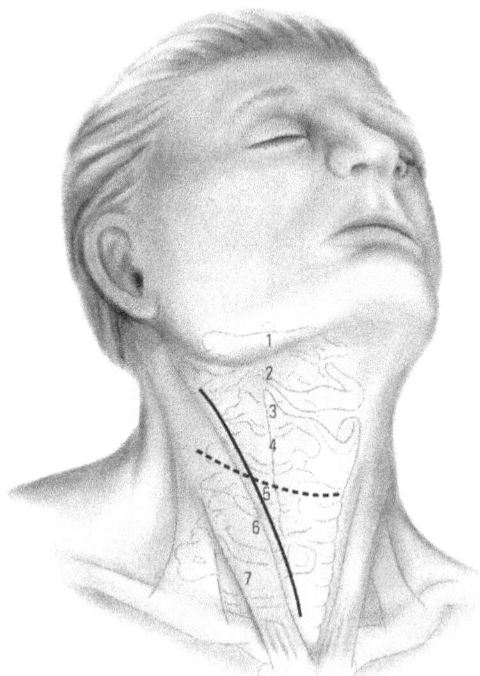

Figure 35-19. Orientation along the cervical spine is estimated by external anatomic landmarks. The top of the thyroid cartilage is at C3–C4 disk space; inferiorly, the thyroid cartilage is at C4–C5. The cricoid ring is at C5–C6 interspace, and the C7–T1 disk space is approximately one-finger breadth above the clavicle.

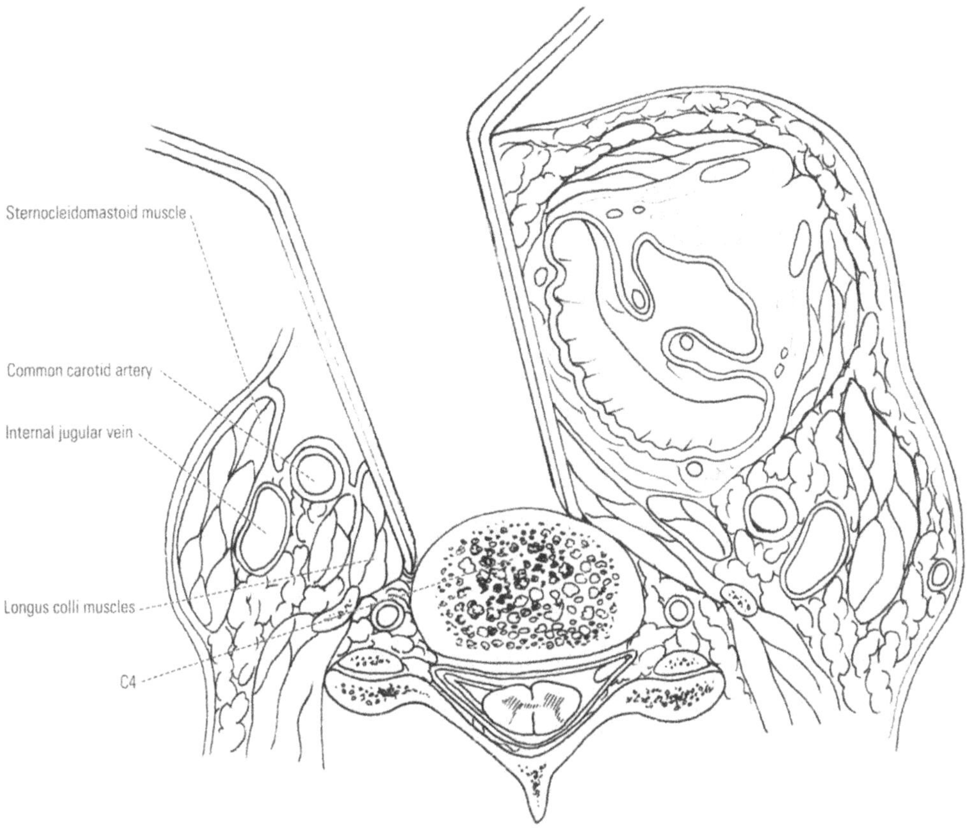

Figure 35-20. The trachea and esophagus are retracted medially and the carotid sheath is retracted laterally.

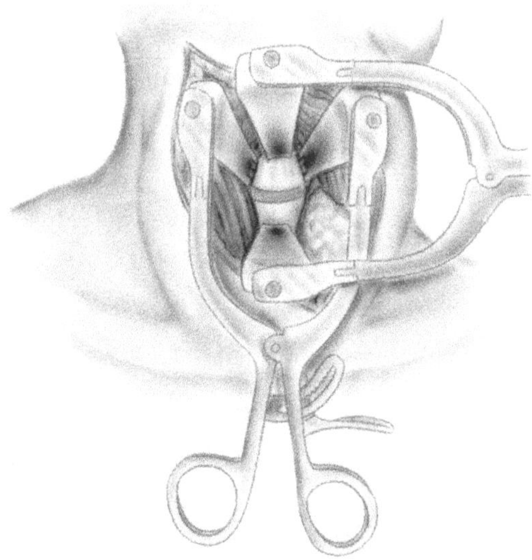

Figure 35-21. Self-retaining retractor blades with teeth are placed under the colli muscle bilaterally. Rostrocaudal exposure can be achieved by placing blunt blade retractors perpendicular to the first retractors.

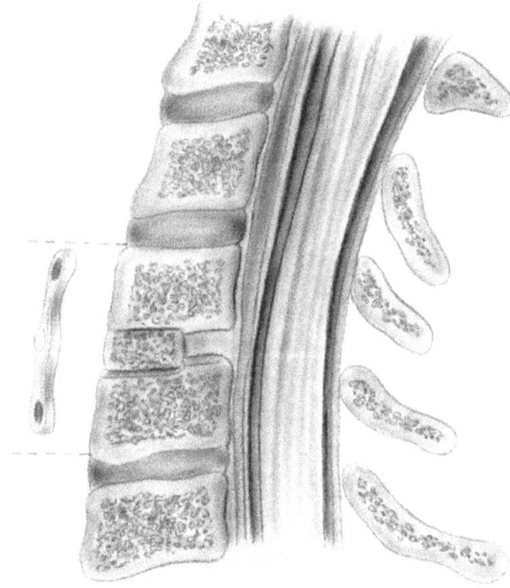

Figure 35-22. The bone graft is tapped in line with the anterior margin of the adjacent vertebral bodies to maximize contact with the plate. A small trough along the posteroinferior aspect of one of the vertebral bodies protects against graft retropulsion. The plates chosen should not overlap the adjacent disk space either rostrally or caudally.

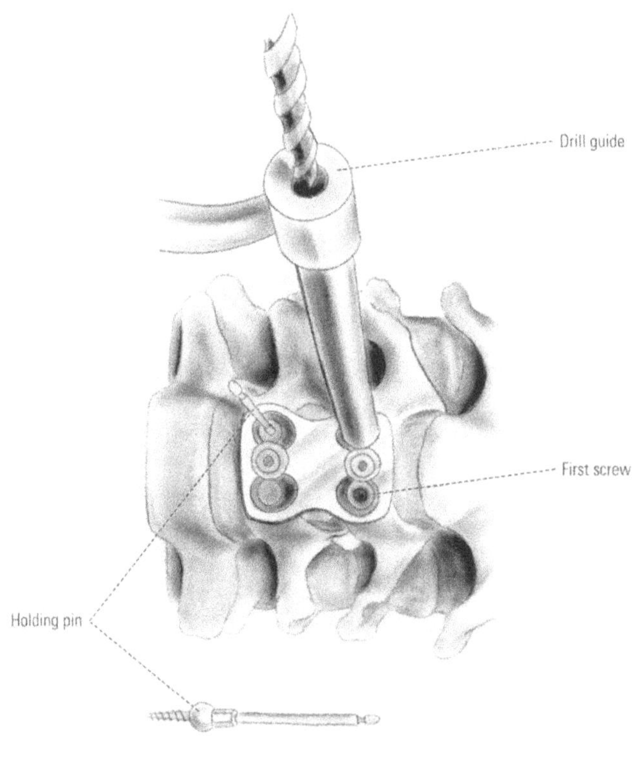

Figure 35-23. After the hole is drilled, the outer cortex of the hole is tapped and an appropriate sized screw is placed. Short, thin, temporary posts may be placed to keep the plate in the desired position.

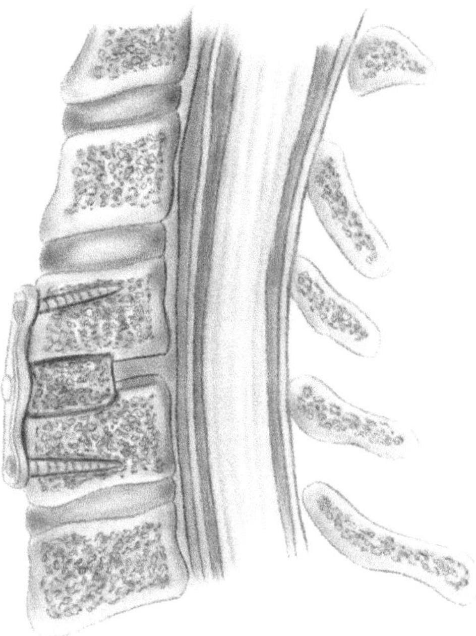

Figure 35-24. Midline location and vertical orientation of the plate can be assessed fluoroscopically by observing the parallel overlay of plate holes and screw trajectory on cross table view.

References

1. Cloward RB: The anterior approach for removal of ruptured cervical disks. *J Neurosurg* 1958, 15:602–617.
2. Robinson RA, Smith GW: Anterolateral cervical disk removal and interbody fusion for cervical disk syndrome. *Bull John Hopkins Hosp* 1995, 96:223–224.
3. Vishteh AG, Baskin JJ, Sonntag VKH: Techniques of cervical diskectomy with and without fusion. *Oper Tech Neurosurg* 1998, 1:84–89.
4. Baskin JJ, Vishteh AG, Dickman CA, Sonntag VKH: Techniques of anterior cervical plating. *Oper Tech Neurosurg* 1998, 1:90–102.

CHAPTER

36

Lumbar Radiculoneuropathy

Herniated Intervertebral Disk: Microdiskectomy

The symptom associated with compression of a nerve root by a herniated lumbar disk is pain down the posterolateral aspect of the lower extremity. The straight leg-raising test (Lasègue's sign) reproducing this pain is a key physical finding. In addition to pain, compression of the lumbosacral nerve roots can produce unilateral radiculopathy characterized by numbness, weakness, and/or loss of deep tendon reflexes. Lumbar intervertebral disks commonly herniate posterolaterally (Fig. 36-1). However, lumbar disks may herniate in the midline causing symptoms and signs in both lower extremities as well as bowel or bladder dysfunction (cauda equina syndrome).

The most common sites for herniated lumbar disks are in the lower two lumbar interspaces (*ie*, L4-5 and L5-S1). Paramedian or lateral herniation of the L5-S1 disk causes compression of the S1 nerve root with resulting hypalgesia along the lateral surface of the foot, weakness in plantar flexion, and depression of the Achilles reflex. Far-lateral herniated disks at L5-S1, however, impinge on the L5 nerve root. Herniation of the disk at L4-L5 is most commonly associated with an L5 radiculopathy (*ie*, decreased sensation over the dorsum of the foot and weakness of dorsiflexion). A relatively large medial herniation at L4-L5 may also compromise the S1 nerve root; conversely, a far-lateral herniation at L4-L5 can compromise the L4 nerve root. The latter presents with pain in the anterior thigh, decreased sensation medial on either side of the calf and foot, weakness of the quadriceps, and depression of the patella reflex. Obviously, the L4 nerve root is more commonly affected by paramedian herniation at the L3-L4 interspace. Figure 36-1 is an anatomic topographic presentation of the common locations of ruptured disks. It illustrates the relationship of the thecal sac and nerve roots to the vertebral bodies and interspaces.

The diagnostic modality of choice is magnetic resonance (MR) imaging. If the patient is unable to undergo MR imaging or the MR image is inconsistent with the patient's clinical presentation, a myelogram-computed tomographic scan can be helpful. Electromyelography is not needed routinely, but it may be helpful in patients whose presentation departs from the classic pattern. A decision to operate is made when conservative treatment fails and the patient has neurologic deficits that correspond to the abnormality seen on imaging studies. Indications for surgery without delay are bladder or bowel dysfunction, progressive neurologic deficits, or intractable pain.

Most unilateral herniated lumbar disks can be removed with the aid of a microscope by hemilaminotomy with minimal bone removal. This section illustrates this operation. Frequently, more bone must be removed from the rostral lamina to gain adequate exposure to the interspace. If two adjacent interspaces are explored, some surgeons prefer a hemilaminectomy. Total laminectomies are indicated for a midline herniated disk when the patient has symptoms in both lower extremities and for lumbar stenosis.

As in all neurologic surgery, it is essential that the surgeon supervise the positioning of the patient on the operating table. After endotracheal anesthesia has been instituted, the patient is placed in the prone position on chest rolls or on a Wilson frame with hips flexed (Fig. 36-2). Supporting sand bags and pillows must not compress the chest or abdomen or the areas indicated in red on Figure 36-3. The epidural veins become markedly enlarged if the return of venous blood to the heart is obstructed or impeded by improper positioning of the patient. This can convert a relatively straightforward surgical procedure into one that is hindered by continuous venous bleeding that obliterates the normal anatomic structures. In an obese patient whose abdomen cannot be kept uncompromised in the prone position, the lateral decubitus position can be considered; some neurosurgeons use it routinely in all patients.

Once the patient is positioned properly, a lateral radiograph with a spinal needle pointing to the appropriate interspace can be helpful in localizing the level. In an L5-S1 herniated disk, a midline vertical skin incision is made from the spinous process of L5 to S1. The fascia is also incised in the midline and the spinous processes on the side of the lesion are stripped of all soft tissue, using a sharp, broad periosteal elevator. Once the lamina is cleared to the facet joint, a Williams or Taylor retractor keeps the soft tissue lateral. If there is any question of localization, repeat radiographs are obtained to verify the L5-S1 level. Usually, however, the anatomy is quite clear because of the nonsegmentation of the sacrum, its hollow note on percussion and the presence of crossing fibers in the muscle fascia.

Having located the appropriate level, the microscope is now placed in the field. The ligamentum flavum, which passes from the posterior surface of the lower lamina to the undersurface of the lamina above, is identified, and the rostral part is exposed by removing the overhanging rim of the superior lamina. The lateral portion of the ligamentum flavum is then incised. As soon as the knife blade goes through the ligament, cotton pledgets are inserted to protect the dura (Fig. 36-4). The incision of the ligament is completed along the superior and inferior bony margins. After the ligament has been removed, the margin of the laminar exposure can be enlarged using Kerrison rongeurs (Fig. 36-5). The ligament is removed laterally, and occasionally it is necessary to remove the medial aspect of the facet joint to obtain a better exposure. Obviously, the amount of facet resected should be limited (Fig. 36-6).

The nerve root is now identified and dissection is begun on its superior aspect to avoid excess stretch. The nerve root is gradually retracted medially to expose the level of the interspace and the ruptured disk (Fig. 36-6). When the nerve root is stretched over the ruptured disk so tightly that it cannot be easily displaced, the patient should be placed in a less flexed position and/or the lateral portion of the disk is removed first. With a downbiting curette under the root, the disk is slowly milked laterally. The nerve root is retracted further medially (Fig. 36-7) and held in position by a nerve root retractor or cotton pledgets. The herniated disk is removed using a number 4 Penfield dissector to free it from the dural sac and the nerve root. The disk material is then teased out with a micropituitary forceps.

If there is no free disk fragment, a window is cut with a number 11 blade into the intact posterior ligament and annulus and the interspace is entered. Epidural veins are often bothersome at this stage, and cotton pledgets can be placed superiorly and inferiorly to tamponade these veins. Cotton pledgets should not exert pressure on the dural sac or nerve root. The interspace is cleaned of degenerated disk material using pituitary forceps and various sized curettes. The sharp curette can be dangerous and must always be used with both hands to avoid inadvertent damage to the neural structures. The cartilaginous plates of both the inferior and superior vertebral surfaces are broken down with a curette and removed with forceps. A reversed angulated curette is very helpful in pushing medial fragments down into the interspace. Pituitary forceps should not be inserted into the interspace deeper than the hinge that controls the movements of the biting cups. A rim of annulus is left anteriorly and laterally to prevent violation of the retroperitoneal vascular and visceral structures. At the L4-L5 interspace, the common iliac artery is especially vulnerable.

Once the interspace has been cleaned to the surgeon's satisfaction, attention is once again directed to the epidural space. Using a Woodson dental instrument, the epidural space is palpated above and below the nerve root well into the neural foramen (Fig. 36-8). This instrument should also be used to palpate medially beneath the dural sac to make certain that a midline mass has not been left behind. Palpation is also performed superiorly and inferiorly after the cotton pledgets have been removed.

If the dura has been violated inadvertently at any point during the procedure, it should be repaired primarily if at all possible. Ignoring dural defects can lead to the formation of psuedomeningoceles or cerebrospinal fluid leakage through the wound. If the dural laceration is in an inaccessible area, the dural opening can be covered with an absorbable gelatin sponge. At this time, the wound is irrigated copiously, inspected for further bleeding (which is controlled by bipolar coagulation), and closed in layers. Closing the muscle layer is unnecessary and might even increase the patient's postoperative pain. The fascia is closed with 2-0 vicryl suture in interrupted layers. Vicryl sutures (3-0) are used for the subcutaneous layer, and a subcuticular running stitch of 4-0 vicryl is used. Steristrips are applied to the skin incision, which is approximately 2 to 3 cm long.

Lateral Recess Stenosis and Central Spinal Stenosis

The classic presentation of lumbar stenosis occurs in patients between the ages of 50 and 70 years who report unilateral or bilateral leg pain upon ambulation. Sitting in the flexed position relieves the symptoms by increasing the sagittal diameter of the spinal canal (Fig. 36-9). Conversely, extension of the lumbar spine either at rest or while walking tends to exacerbate the symptoms. Lateral recess stenosis can produce unilateral symptoms (Fig. 36-10). Bilateral symptoms, which are most common with central stenosis, can be asymmetric or symmetric, although the latter is the most typical presentation. The neurologic examination tends to be unremarkable, but motor, sensory, and reflex changes may be present or induced by exercise.

CT-myelography and MR imaging can help diagnose the stenosis. Flexion-extension films can rule out instability. Surgical decompression of the lumbar neural elements is offered to patients with a history of back and leg pain who have radiographic evidence of lumbar stenosis or lateral recess stenosis and in whom conservative therapy has failed to relieve symptoms.

After general anesthesia is induced, the patient is placed in a frame with hips flexed. A midline incision is made over the stenotic levels. The soft tissues are mobilized laterally by means of subperiosteal dissection. Meticulous hemostasis must be achieved to minimize blood loss. A lateral lumbar spine radiograph helps localize the surgical levels.

A double-action rongeur is used to remove the spinous process insertion into the posterior arch. Kerrison and other rongeurs and curettes of various sizes are used to remove the lamina. At all times care is taken to protect the underlying dura. A drill can also be used to help remove cortical and cancellous bone. While thinning the posterior arch, the surgeon can use the caudal aspect of the arch, which is attached to the ligamentum flavum, as a useful landmark to avoid injuring the dura. The ligament does not protect the underside of the superior aspect of the arch; therefore, bone along the superior aspect of the posterior arch should be removed even more cautiously.

The limit of decompression in the cephalocaudal axis is usually heralded by the appearance of epidural fat, which is absent at the severely stenotic levels. The remainder of the decompression is performed using a surgical microscope. The bed is rolled toward the side to be decompressed, and the microscope is angled to maximize visualization of the contralateral canal (Fig. 36-12*A*).

The dental dissector is used to find the epidural plane (Fig. 36-11). The ligament and bone are removed laterally with a 2- to 3-mm Kerrison punch. The pedicle is visualized and the facet is undercut (Fig. 36-12*B*), thereby decompressing the nerve root along the lateral recess as it courses to and through the foramen (Fig. 36-12*C*).

After decompression is completed on this side, the dental dissector is used to probe the lateral recess, neural foramen, and epidural space for bone, ligamentous fragments, or bulging or herniated disk. Any frank disk herniation is removed. A bulging disk is usually left in place as long as decompression is adequate. The bed and the patient are then rolled to the opposite side and the procedure repeated.

Throughout the procedure, meticulous hemostasis is maintained with bipolar coagulation, hemostatic agents, or both. After the neural elements have been decompressed completely, the microscope is removed from the field. The wound is irrigated with copious amounts of an antibiotic-containing solution. The soft tissue is reapproximated and the wound closed in layers. Steristrips are used to buttress the skin closure, unless an inadvertent dural tear occurs, at which time a nylon skin closure is performed.

Spondylolisthesis: Posterior Fusion Technique

Patients with spondylolisthesis of the lumbar spine usually become symptomatic with lower back pain, radicular pain, or both. Aggressive conservative treatment consists of back exercises, weight control, and posture control. Congenital spondylolisthesis usually occurs at L5-S1 whereas acquired degenerative spondylolisthesis appears at L4-L5. This section discusses the use of pedicle screw fixation for the treatment of L4-L5 spondylolisthesis.

Imaging studies include plain radiography, MR imaging, myelography, and CT to evaluate the extent of decompression needed and the appropriate levels for fixation. Axial CT scans are most helpful for determining the suitability of the pedicles for the placement of screws. In general, the diameter of the lumbar pedicle should be at least 7 mm if pedicle screws are to be placed. In typical adults, the pedicle screws used are usually 6.5 mm in diameter. Fixation follows the rule of two thirds: the diameter of the pedicle screws should be no greater than two thirds the diameter of the pedicle to be instrumented, and the length of the pedicle screw should extend no further than two thirds the length of the vertebral body.

After general anesthesia is administered, the patient is positioned prone on the operating table on chest rolls with knees slightly bent. Pressure points are padded, and the appropriate electrophysiologic monitoring leads are attached. The patient is prepared and draped. If a C-arm is used, it is also draped.

The dissection begins with a dorsal midline incision and proceeds to the bone bilaterally. Self-retaining retractors are placed to retract the soft tissues laterally. Dissection with an electrocautery device or sharp instruments continues laterally over the facets and transverse process. Dissection ventral to the transverse process should be avoided because the nerve roots lying there could be injured. Only the transverse processes that will be fused should be exposed. If a decompression is indicated, it is performed at this point.

The first screw is placed with the guidance of fluoroscopy, anatomic landmarks, or a stereotactic navigational system. The technique described here relies on anatomic landmarks and fluoroscopy for the placement of pedicle screws. The external landmarks are visualized over the dorsal surface of the lumbar spine (Fig. 36-13). A line is drawn so that the axial plane of the transverse process and a sagittal plane through the lateral superior facet intersect at the center of the pedicle. Using a Woodson instrument, Penfield dissector, or both from within the spinal canal, the surgeon can define the superior, inferior, and medial borders of the pedicle, thus gaining tactile information. This maneuver is only an option if a laminectomy has been performed. Radiographic confirmation of the location of the pedicle can be obtained with anteroposterior (AP) and lateral fluoroscopy.

Once the center of the pedicle has been identified, bone is decorticated with a high-speed drill under fluoroscopic guidance. A probe is advanced manually through the cancellous center of the pedicle into the vertebral body (Fig. 36-14). The mediolateral orientation in the axial plane depends on the vertebral level of interest. In general, the trajectory of the pedicle screw is medial and progresses in 5° increments. Thus, the trajectory is 5° medially at L1, 10° at L2, 15° at L3, 20° at L4, and 25° at L5 and S1 (Fig. 36-15). The rostrocaudal orientation through the pedicle is determined by lateral fluoroscopy. The goal is to maintain a trajectory that is parallel to the endplate. The probe is advanced through the pedicle.

An appropriately sized tap is then advanced through the pedicle along the same trajectory as the probe, independently or over the K-wire guide (Fig. 36-16). Once the hole has been tapped, a thin pedicle probe is inserted into the hole to verify that the pedicle wall is intact. An appropriately sized pedicle screw is advanced into the pedicle and vertebral body along the predetermined trajectory (Fig. 36-17). Typically, the screw tip is advanced two thirds of the way through the vertebral body. Once all pedicle screws are placed, their position is evaluated a final time with lateral and AP fluoroscopy.

A malleable endotracheal tube stylet is used as a template for the rod. This step helps to determine both the length and contour of the rod. The rod is cut and bent to match the template. The rod is attached to the pedicle screw with connectors (Fig. 36-18). The surgeon may be able to reduce the deformity partially by using a distractor or compressor or other devices that help reduction. Once the reduction is acceptable, the bolts are tightened provisionally. A torque wrench can be used for the final tightening of the screw. Cross-linking should be added if elements of rotation and instability are present or if more than one level is instrumented. For a single-level fixation, however, there is seldom enough room for such cross-linking.

A bone graft is an integral part of pedicle screw fixation. Instrumentation alone is insufficient to maintain long-term stabilization and provides only interim stabilization while a bony fusion develops.

A graft can be harvested through either the same incision or a separate one made over the posterior iliac crest. The fascia overlying the posterior iliac crest can be incised with an electrocautery device. The incision should extend no more than 8 cm from the posterior-superior iliac spine to avoid injuring the superior cluneal nerves. The cluneal musculature is reflected from the posterior aspects of the iliac crest. Once the musculature has been dissected free, a Taylor retractor can help expose the dorsal surface of the iliac crest. Unicortical strips are obtained by chiseling through the outer dorsal cortex of the iliac crest with a straight, narrow osteotome to create slivers of bone like matchsticks. A gouge can then be used to remove cancellous material. Bone wax is used for hemostasis. The graft area should be irrigated copiously with an antibiotic-saline solution. The overlying fascia is closed primarily. If a separate skin incision is used, the wound is closed in layers. If a laminectomy has been performed, enough bone graft may be available from the lamina and spinous process to avoid the need to harvest bone from the iliac crest.

At this time, adequate lateral exposure of the transverse process is verified. The bony surface of the transverse processes and laminae and spinous processes should be decorticated with pituitary forceps or a drill. Cancellous bone obtained from the iliac crest is packed over the decorticated surface of the transverse processes, laminae and spinous processes. Next, the cortical strips available from the iliac crest are packed over the cancellous graft material (Fig. 36-19). A facet joint fusion also can be performed. The joint capsule is entered with a sharp rongeur. The cartilage is removed and the cancellous bone surface is exposed. The joint is packed tightly with cancellous bone graft obtained from the iliac crest. After the area is irrigated copiously, the wound is closed in layers. Postoperatively, the patient is placed in a thoracolumbosacral orthosis (TLSO) that is worn upright for 1 to 2 months.

Retroperitoneal Approach: Anterior Fusion Techniques

The anterolateral approach to the thoracolumbar spine can be used for trauma, tumors, infection, and degenerative disease. The need for internal fixation is based on the amount of intrinsic instability caused by the primary pathologic condition as well as the potential instability caused by surgical treatment of the primary pathologic condition.

This section describes the treatment of an L1 burst fracture through an anterolateral thoracolumbar approach consisting of an L1 corpectomy, cage placement, and anterolateral plating. Different plate systems are available; this section focuses on the MR imaging-compatible Z-plate system (Medtronic Sofamor-Danek, Memphis, TN).

Once the patient is in the operating room, somatosensory evoked potentials (and/or motor evoked potentials, if available) are monitored before the patient is placed in the lateral decubitus position. An axial roll is placed under the patient's lower axilla and a pillow is placed between the legs. If gross instability is of no concern, the thoracolumbar area is placed perpendicular to the crack of the operating table. By slightly lowering the top and bottom portions of the operating room table, the angle between the rib cage and the iliac crest is opened, thereby providing additional room for exposure (Fig. 36-20). All pressure points are padded. The top arm is padded by using egg crate foam, or it is placed in a cushioned armrest. The body is taped to the bed just below the iliac crest, which must be available should bone graft be harvested. Unless contraindicated, the patient's left side is placed up. The patient is intubated with a double-lumen endotracheal tube to facilitate collapse of the lung ipsilateral to the side of the approach to obtain better exposure.

The procedure consists of five phases: 1) exposure; 2) resection of the pathology and decompression of the thecal sac; 3) realignment, where applicable; 4) reconstruction and internal fixation; and 5) closure. A lesion at the thoracolumbar junction (T11-L1) is usually approached through the thoracic abdominal approach and the diaphragm is taken down. The fluoroscope may be positioned at the onset of surgery or later as needed. The initial exposure is usually performed by a thoracic or general surgeon.

Once the lateral vertebral bodies are exposed, the segmental vessels of the aorta are sutured, ligated, and divided. The aorta can be mobilized medially and more anterior to the vertebral bodies. In the thoracic spine, the adjacent rib heads must be resected and the neural foramina identified to permit plating. Consequently, the rib head of T12 is resected in this case.

Figure 36-21 shows a burst fracture of L1 to be treated with a corpectomy and plating. Typically, the corpectomy begins with resection of the middle portion of the vertebral body with rongeurs, curettes, or a power drill to create a gutter. Decompression is performed by turning the patient slightly from the surgeon who stands on the abdominal side. Under microscopic visualization, bone and disk material near the thecal sac are removed with small curettes, which are used to pull or wedge the fracture fragments or disk material away from the spinal canal and into the corpectomy gutter created earlier. Alternatively, once the thecal sac has been identified, a diamond bur can be used to hollow out the pathologic bone from the inside before curettage of the outer shell (Fig. 36-22).

Once the thecal sac is decompressed, the operating microscope is removed and a spacer is placed into the site of the corpectomy. Multiple spacers are available. In this example, a titanium cage packed with autograft bone obtained from the corpectomy site and/or any resected rib is used. Once the cage is filled, rings and manhole covers are placed on both ends to prevent the cage from subsiding into the adjacent vertebral body.

The lengths of the bolts and screws are estimated by measuring the width of the adjacent superior and inferior vertebral bodies on axial CT or MR imaging. The bolt should be the exact length of the width of the appropriate vertebral body. The screw should be 5 mm longer than its corresponding vertebral body bolt.

Before the cage is inserted, the bolts are placed into both adjacent vertebral bodies. In the lumbar spine, the bolts are positioned at a point 8 mm from the spinal canal and 8 mm from the disk space (Fig. 36-23). In the lower thoracic spine, the bolt is placed 4 mm from the spinal canal and 4 mm from the disk space. An awl guide is used to guide the awl along the appropriate angle, which is 10° away from the spinal canal (Fig. 36-24). A self-tapping bolt is inserted (Fig. 36-25). After the second bolt is placed in the other vertebral body, the bolt distractors are used to achieve reduction. Then, the appropriately sized cage filled with autologous bone is tamped into place in the middle of the corpectomy site (Fig. 36-26). Care is exerted to avoid impinging on the thecal sac.

Next, an appropriate plate is chosen. It should not overlap with the superior and inferior disk spaces (Fig. 36-27). The plate is placed and the bolt nuts initially are tightened to finger torque. Eventually, however, the bolts are tightened to approximately 80 to 100 inch-pounds. Before the bolt nuts are placed, a washer, which has an extension that helps lock the screw into place, is placed on the bolt. Compression can also be performed while the bolt nuts are being tightened (Fig. 36-28). For the anteriorly placed screws, an awl through a guide is angled 10° toward the spinal canal to create a screw hole (Fig. 36-29). Two screws, each 5 mm longer than its adjacent bolt, are now put in position through the washer and plate (Fig. 36-30). After the last screw is positioned, anteroposterior and lateral fluoroscopy is performed to assure bicortical purchase of both the bolts and the screws.

After copious irrigation, the wound is closed in layers. Routinely, a chest tube is kept in place 1 to 2 days. After the chest tube is removed, supine and upright lateral radiographs are obtained with the patient in a TLSO. If no abnormal motion is apparent, the patient can ambulate liberally in his or her brace and is usually sent home on the third or fourth postoperative day. Typically, patients wear the brace for 6 to 8 weeks.

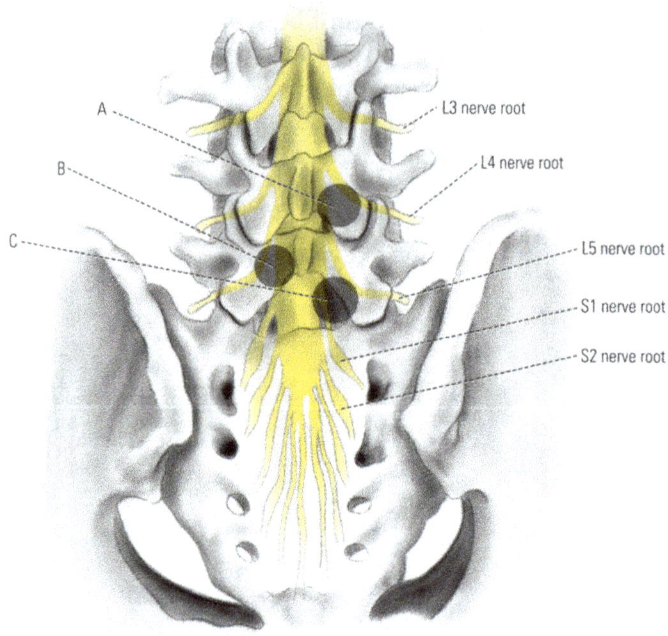

Figure 36-1. Relationship of the thecal sac and nerve roots to the intervertebral disk spaces and foramina. At *A*, a herniated disk (at L4-L5 interspace) can compress the L4 nerve root laterally and the L5 nerve root medially. At *B*, a lateral herniated disk can compress the L5 nerve root. At *C*, a herniated nucleus pulposus at the L5-S1 interspace can compress the L5, S1, and S2 nerve roots.

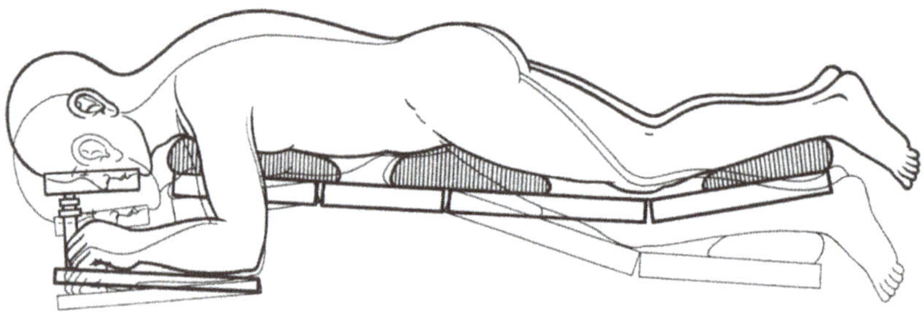

Figure 36-2. Operative position. The patient is placed on the Wilson frame. Elbows and knees are padded (compare with Fig. 36-3).

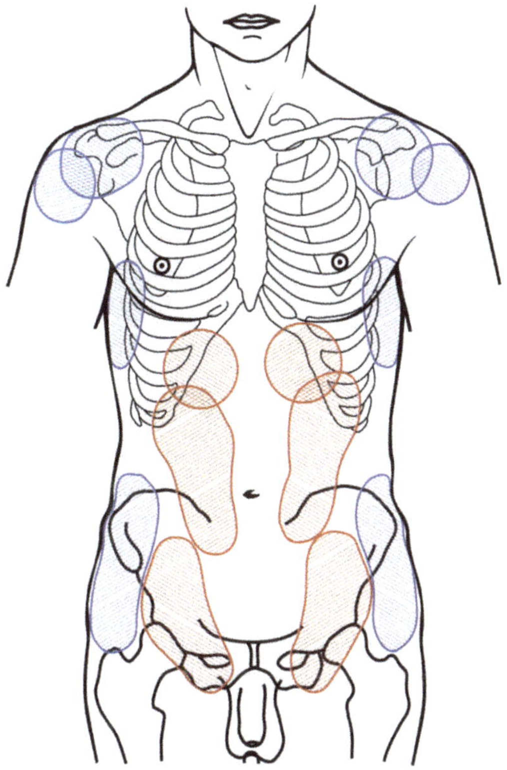

Figure 36-3. Anterior surface of body showing pressure points to use (*blue*) and to avoid (*red*) in the prone position. Compression over red areas can obstruct venous pathways and force distension of epidural veins.

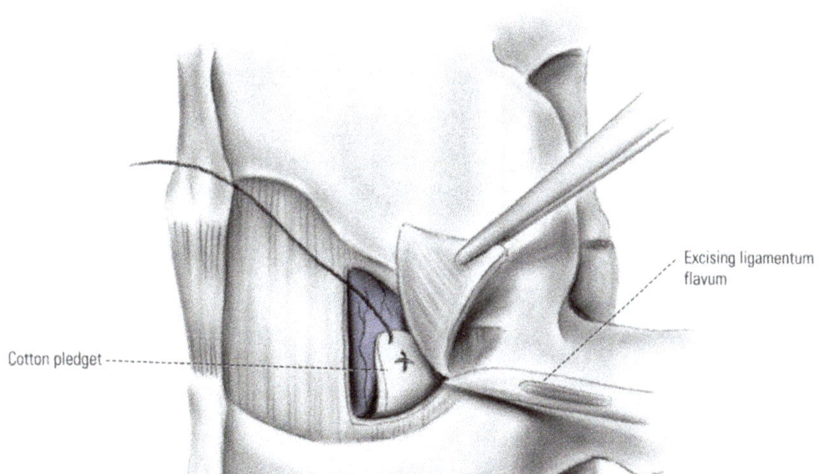

Figure 36-4. Excision of ligamentum flavum. The incision of the ligamentum flavum is begun medially. A cotton pledget protects the dura.

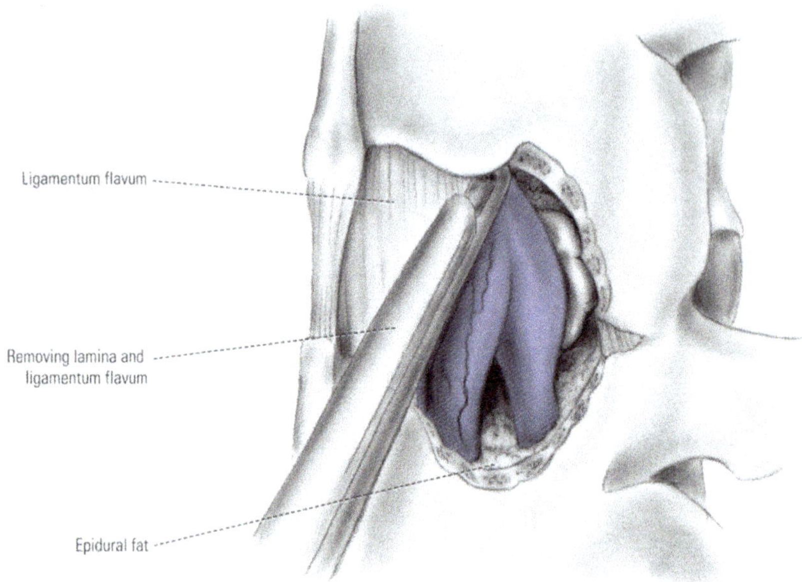

Figure 36-5. The interlaminar exposure is enlarged by removing a small portion of the superior and inferior lamina.

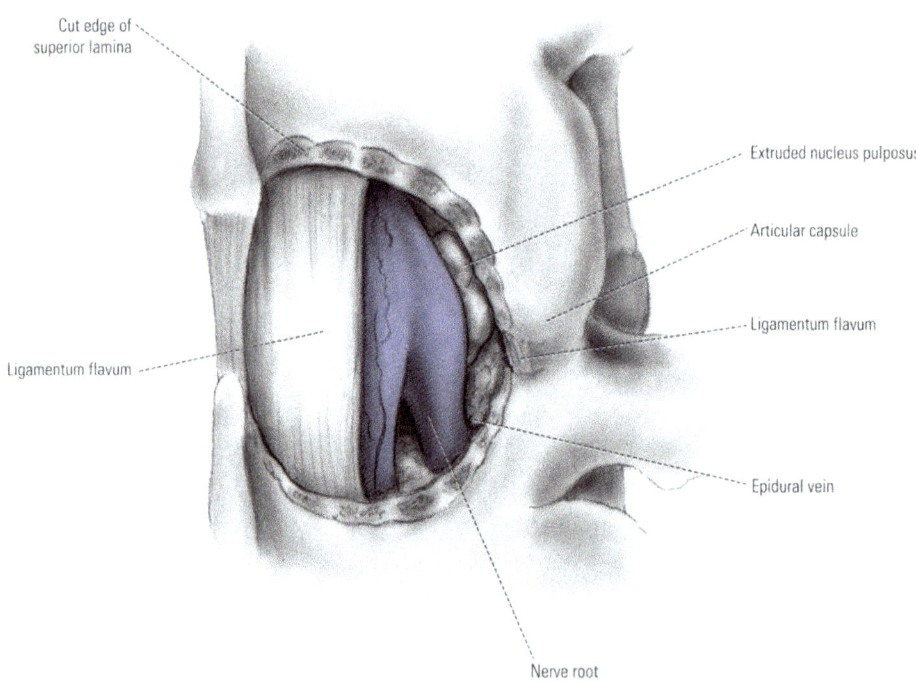

Figure 36-6. Exposure after the bone and ligamentum flavum have been removed. The ligamentum flavum is left intact close to the articular capsule and medially.

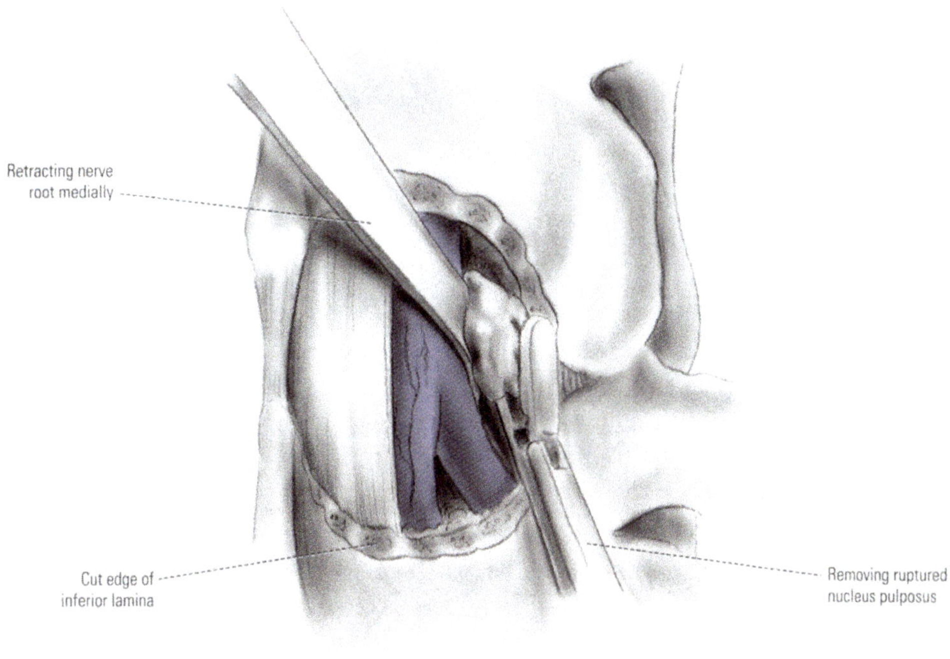

Figure 36-7. The disk is removed with pituitary forceps. The exiting nerve root is gently retracted medially; cotton pledgets placed superior and inferior to the disk space can aid retraction and hemostasis.

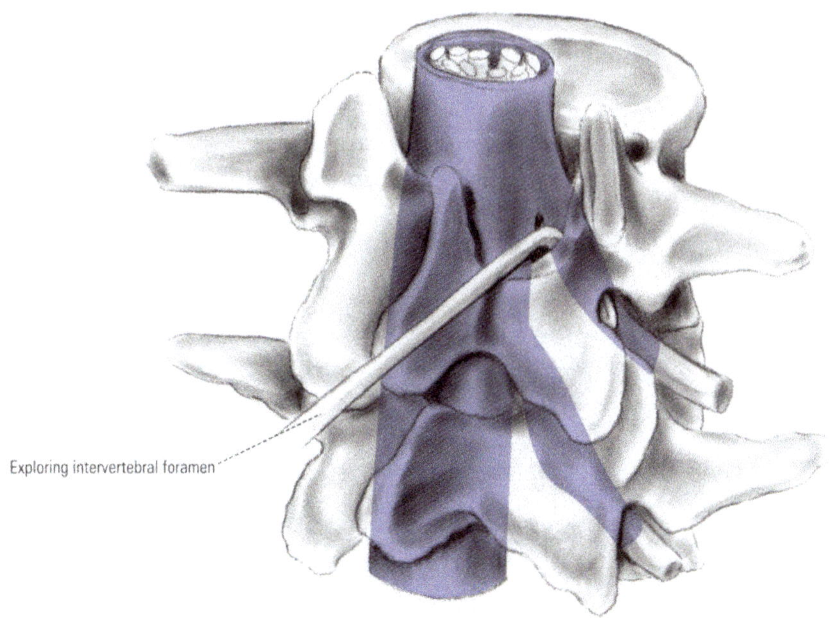

Figure 36-8. The intervertebral foramen is explored after the disk is removed. The probe is guided dorsal to the nerve root through the intervertebral foramen.

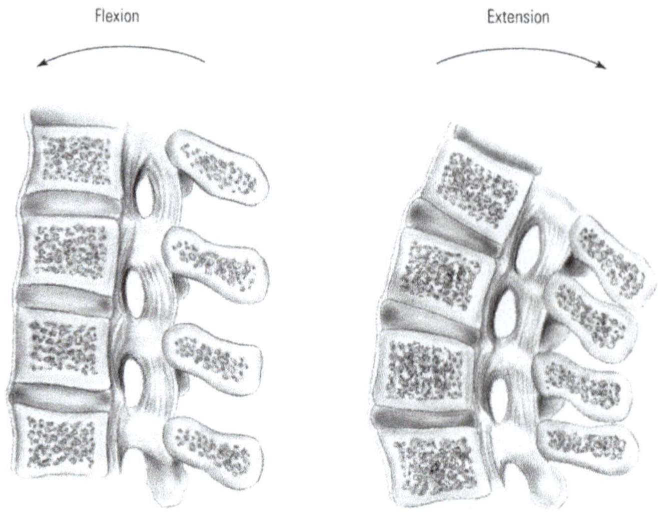

Figure 36-9. When the patient flexes the spinal canal central lumbar stenosis is partially relieved.

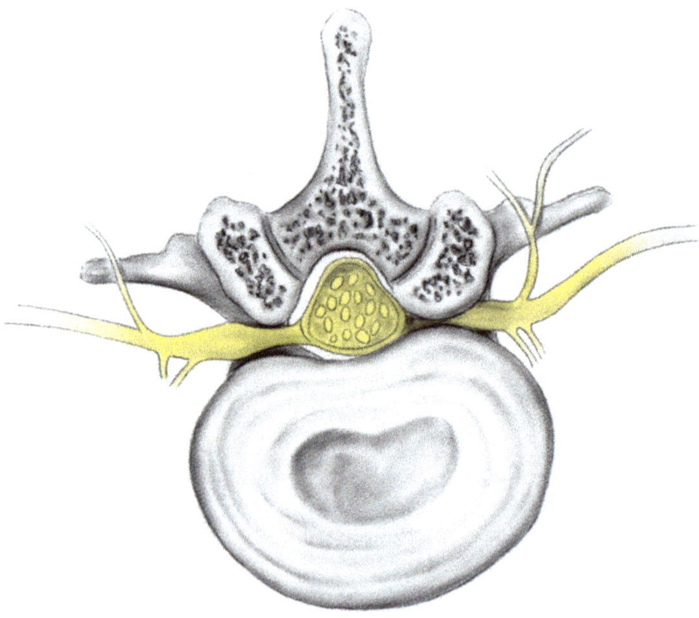

Figure 36-10. Lumbar stenosis (lateral recess stenosis) with the left foramen compressed more than the right.

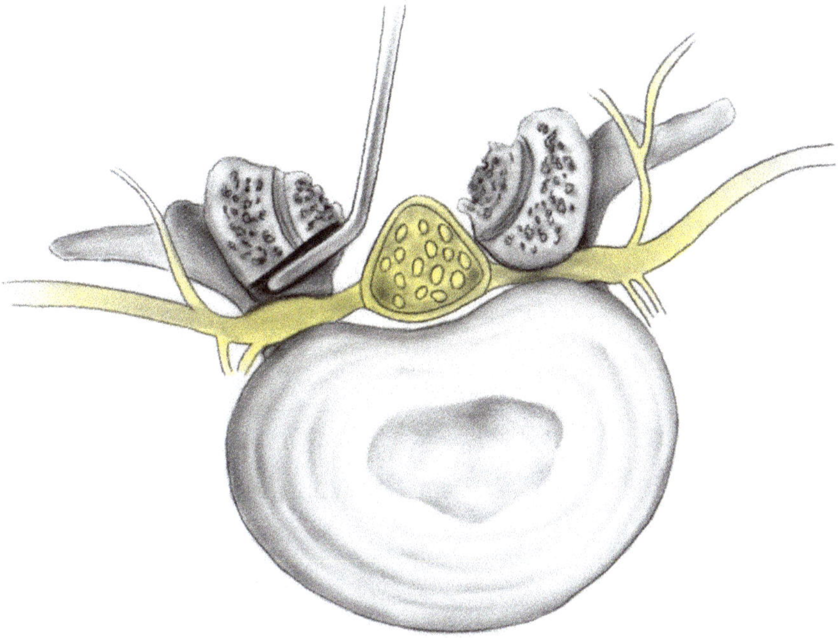

Figure 36-11. Evaluating decompression of the dura with a dental tool.

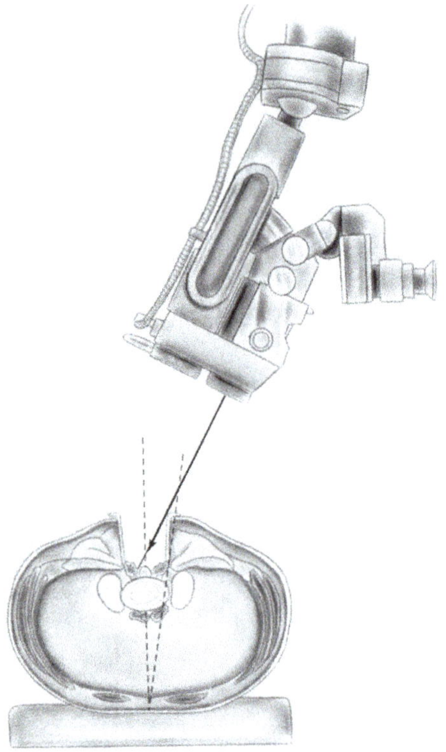

A

Figure 36-12. A, The facets are preserved by angling the patient away from the surgeon, using the operating microscope. B, Kerrison rongeur undercutting lateral recess. C, The nerve roots are decompressed along their path through the lateral recess and the neural foramen while the facets are preserved.

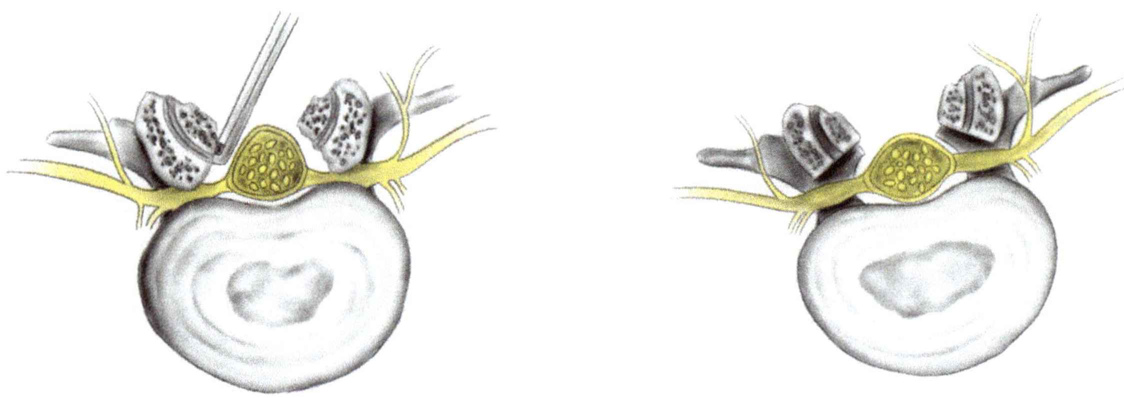

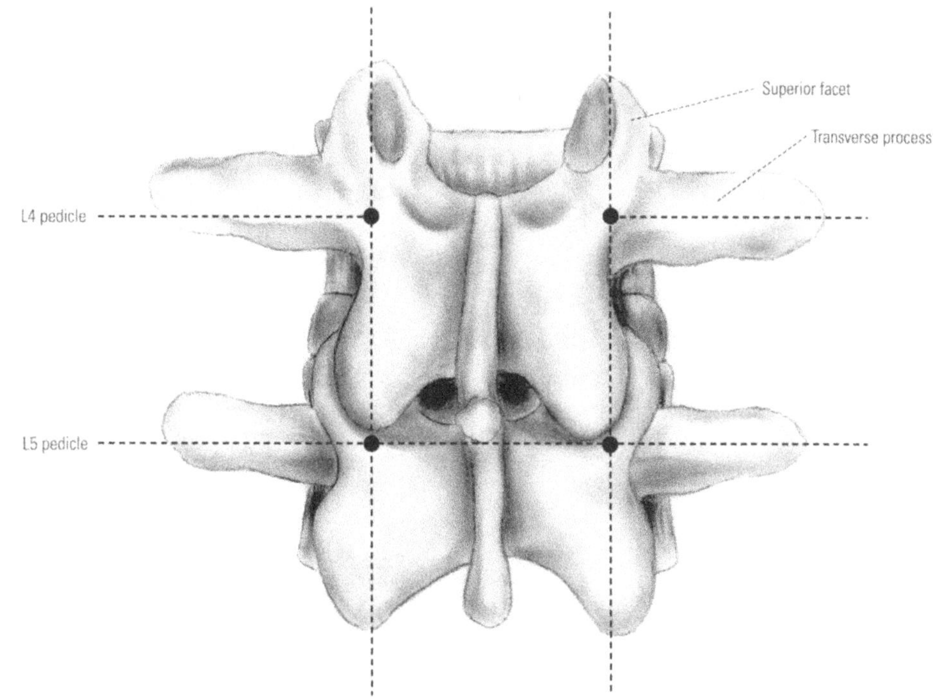

Figure 36-13. Lines are drawn to indicate where the axial plane of the transverse process and the sagittal plane through the lateral superior facet intersect at the center of the pedicle.

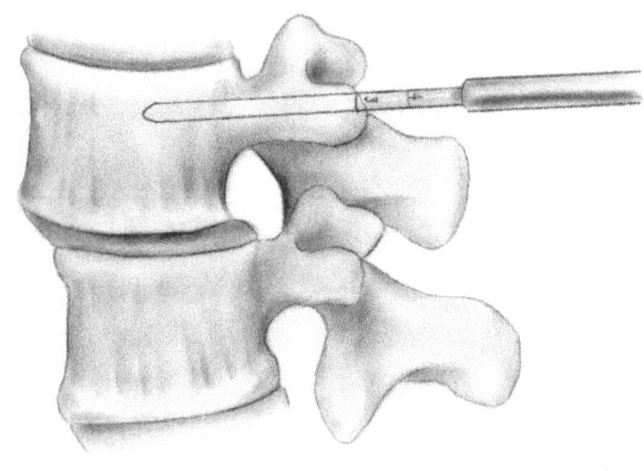

Figure 36-14. A probe is advanced manually through the cancellous center of the pedicle into the vertebral body.

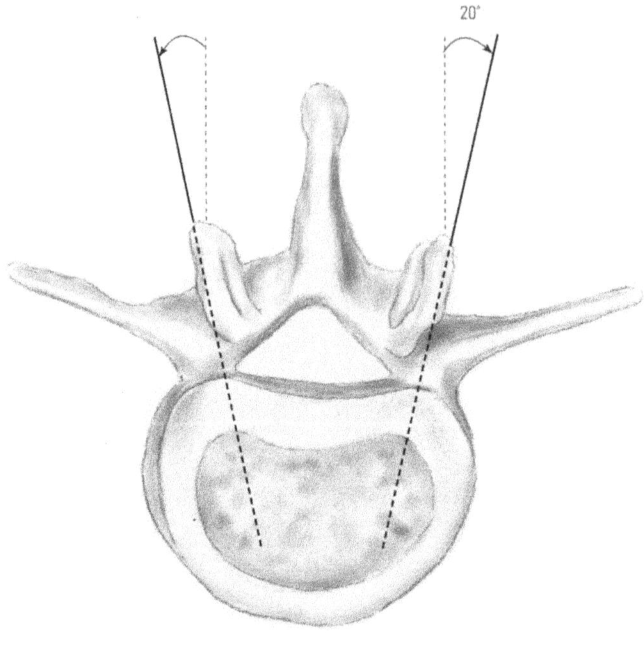

Figure 36-15. The trajectory is aimed 20° medially into the body of L4.

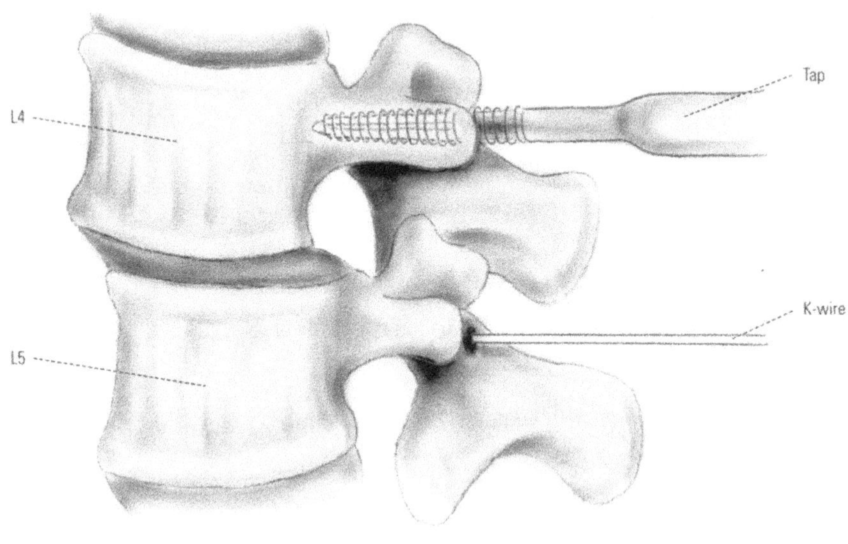

Figure 36-16. An appropriately sized tap is advanced independently or over the K-wire in the pedicle hole.

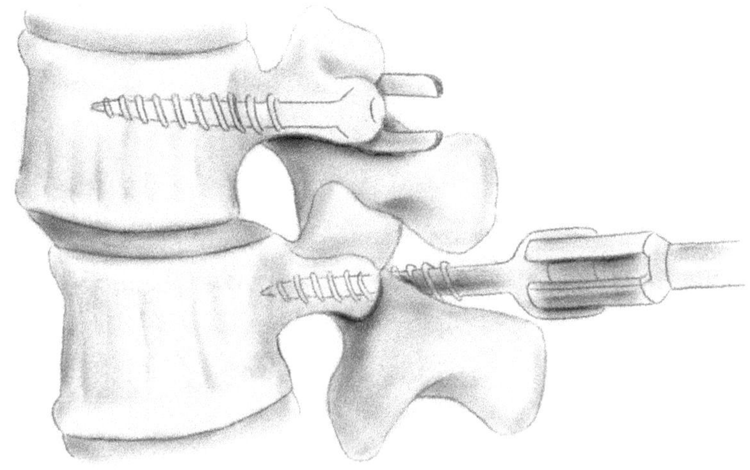

Figure 36-17. An appropriately sized pedicle screw is advanced into the pedicle and vertebral body along the predetermined trajectory.

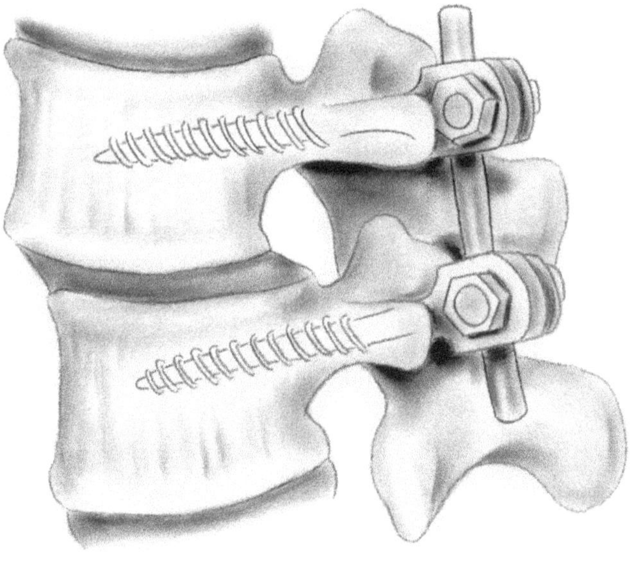

Figure 36-18. The screws are connected to the rod. Cross-linking can be added if rotational instability is present or if more than one level is instrumented.

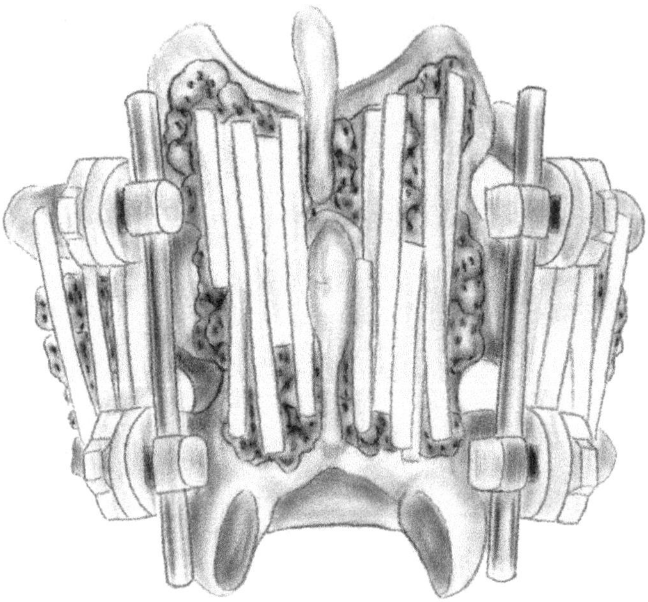

Figure 36-19. Cancellous bone and cortical bone strips are placed laterally over the transverse process, which has been decorticated.

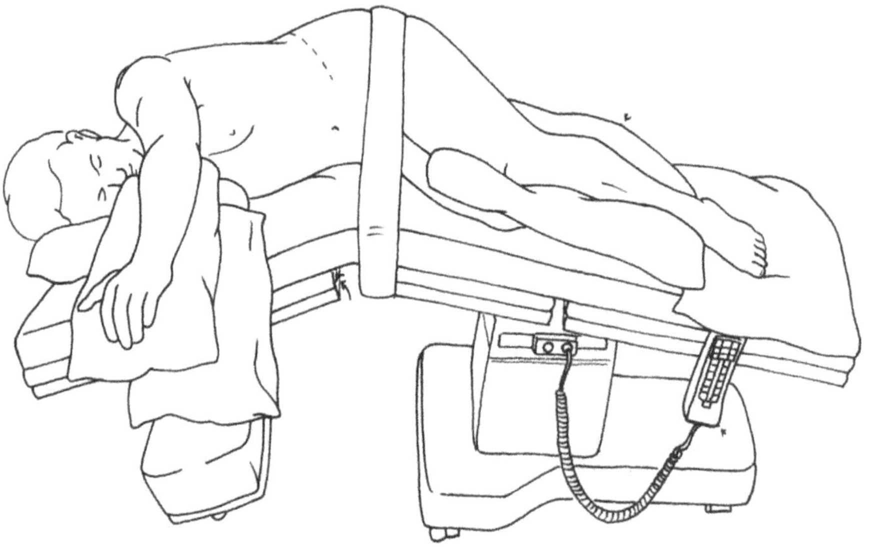

Figure 36-20. The patient is in a lateral decubitus position with the thoracolumbar area perpendicular to the crack of the operating table. The top and bottom of the operating table are slightly lower to increase the exposure between the rib cage and the iliac crest.

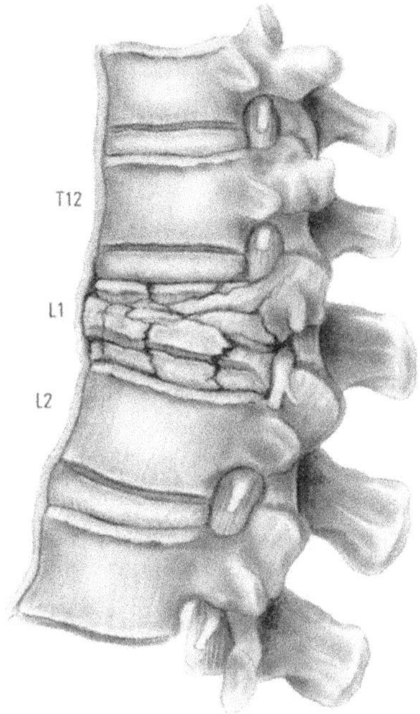

Figure 36-21. A lateral view of the thoracolumbar junction showing an L1 burst fracture (T11 and T12 ribs are not drawn).

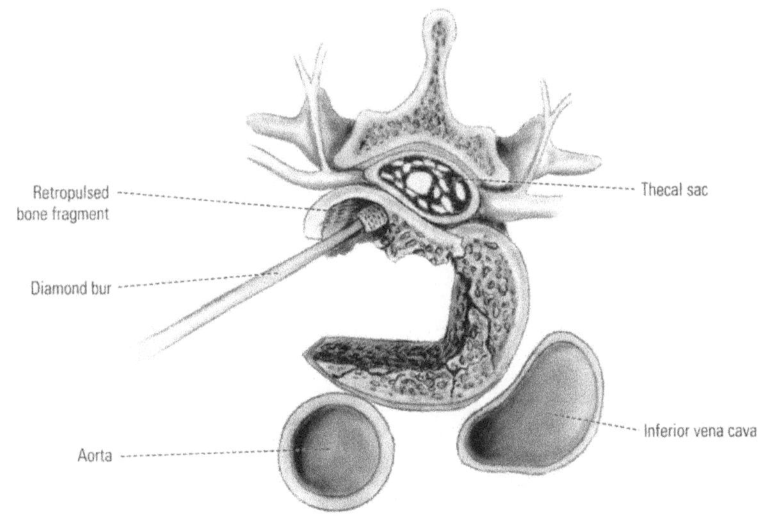

Figure 36-22. Diamond drill bur is used to hollow out compressive bone fragments. A curette can also be used to wedge the thinned bone shell out of the spinal canal.

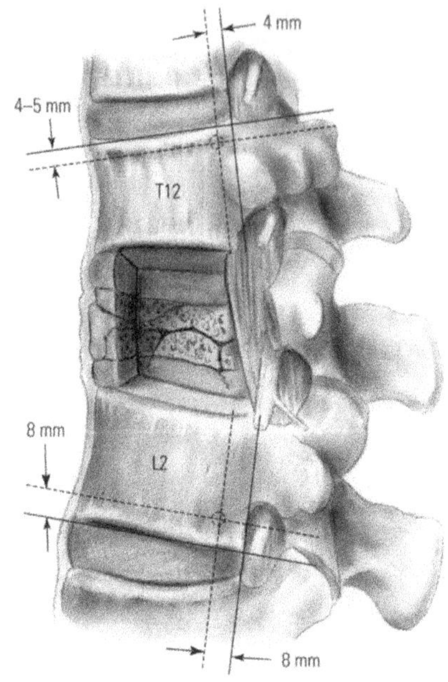

Figure 36-23. A distance of 8 mm from the spinal canal and 8 mm from the disk space are coordinates for placement of the bolts.

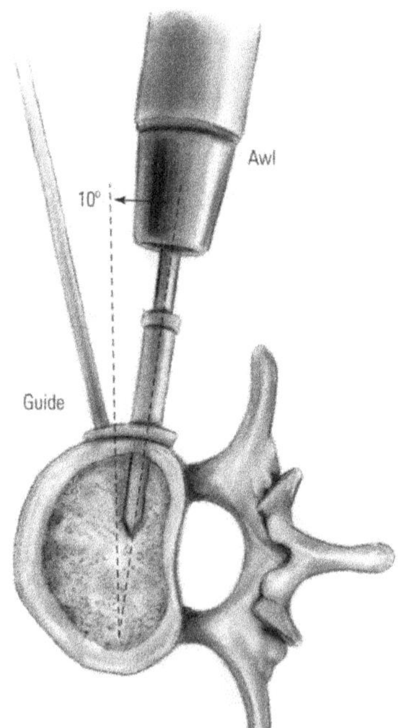

Figure 36-24. Axial section showing a bone awl guide used to guide the awl through the vertebral body to create the bolt hole. The awl is directed 10° away from the thecal sac.

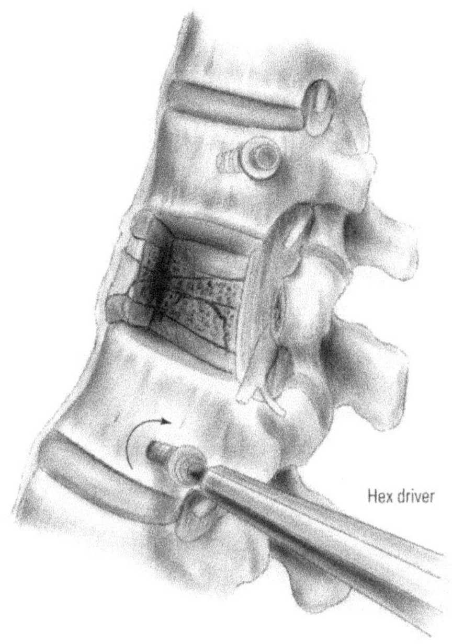

Figure 36-25. The bolt is put in place with a hex driver.

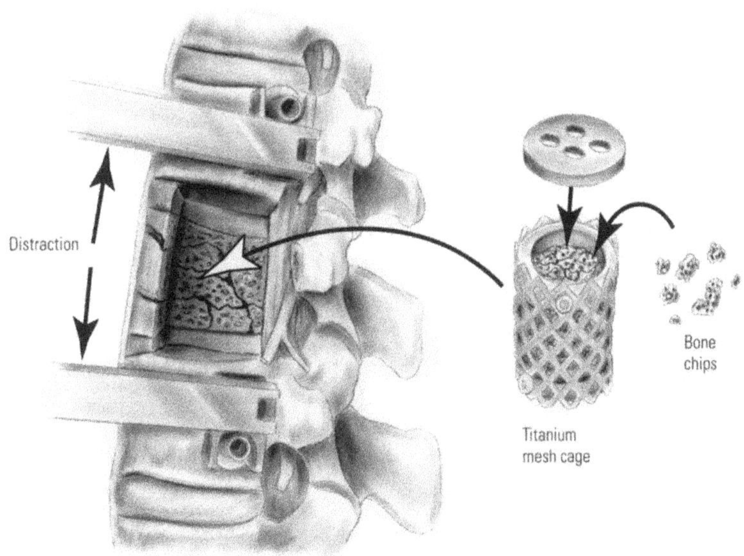

Figure 36-26. A distractor is used to reduce the deformity and to prepare the corpectomy site for the placement of the Harm's cage packed with bone chips.

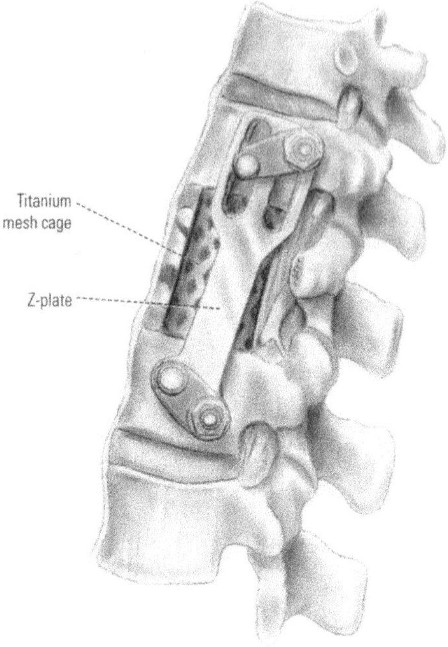

Figure 36-27. An appropriately sized plate is positioned. Bolt nuts are initially placed to finger tightness and eventually tightened to 80 to 100 inch–pounds on the bolt and washer.

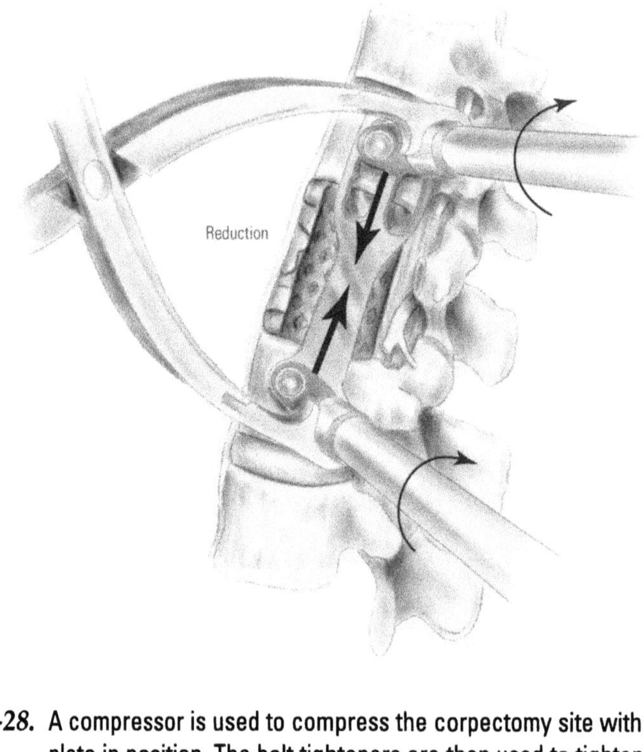

Figure 36-28. A compressor is used to compress the corpectomy site with the plate in position. The bolt tighteners are then used to tighten the bolt nuts while compression is applied.

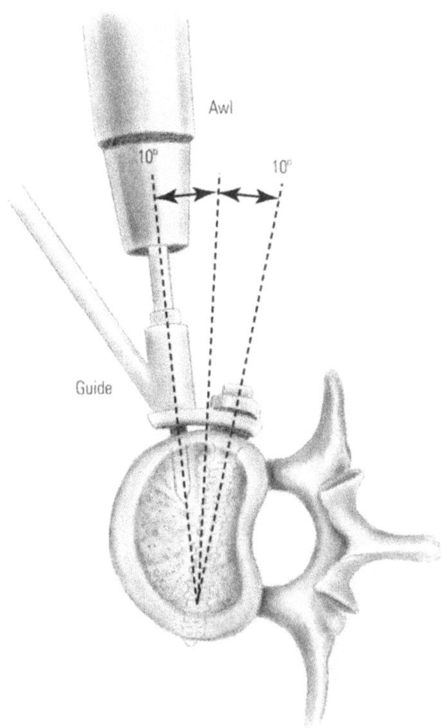

Figure 36-29. Axial section showing an awl guide being used to create a screw guide hole. The screw is directed approximately 10° toward the thecal sac.

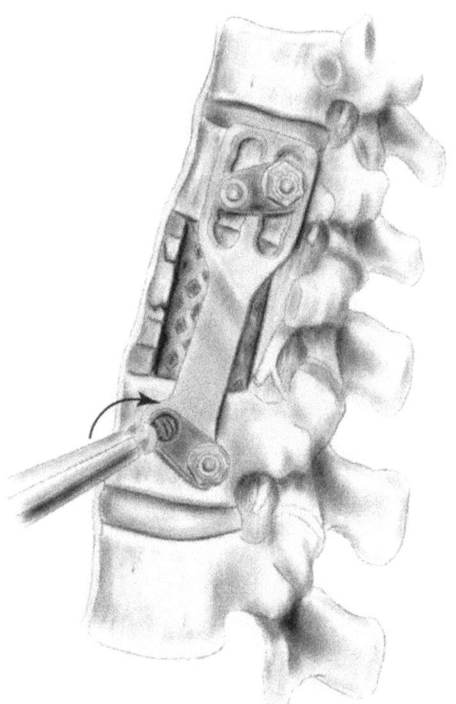

Figure 36-30. The Z-plate screw is tightened with a hex driver over the plate and washer.

CHAPTER

37

Intramedullary Spinal Cord Tumor: Ependymoma

Ependymomas are the most common intramedullary spinal cord tumors in adults. They occur throughout life but are most frequently seen in the middle adult years. Men and women are affected equally. Magnetic resonance imaging with enhancement nicely demonstrates the size and location of an intramedullary tumor. In this particular case, an intramedullary ependymoma of the cervical cord is described.

The patient is placed in the prone position with the neck neutral or slightly flexed. The laminectomy usually extends one level rostral and one level caudal to the extent of the tumor (Fig. 37-1). After the dura is exposed and secured laterally with stay sutures, the normal spinal cord is seen at both poles of the exposure. The spinal cord is visibly swollen secondary to the intramedullary tumor. The arachnoid is also opened in the midline and can be retracted laterally with the dura.

The myelotomy is usually made in the midline or where the spinal cord appears thinnest secondary to the tumor, which is often just off midline. The myelotomy should extend over the entire length of the spinal cord enlargement (Fig. 37-2). After initial dissection of the surface of the tumor with a micro-Penfield dissector, 6-0 stay sutures are placed in the edges of the pia at the site of the myelotomy and the cord itself can be gently retracted laterally to both sides.

Intramedullary ependymomas are usually well-defined, grayish, and somewhat granular tumors. They can be associated with caudal and rostral cysts which help define the tumor capsule. Dissection begins at one of the poles with bipolar coagulation and microscissors. The tumor capsule is separated from the gliotic surface of the spinal cord. Bipolar coagulation forceps are used as feeding vessels are encountered. Figure 37-3 illustrates dissection of the tumor with stay sutures in place in the pia. Dissection proceeds from one pole to the opposite pole while the tumor is lifted away from the spinal cord. Gentle retraction should always be applied to the tumor but never to the spinal cord. The tumor is held up to facilitate vision rather than to remove it. If an area is encountered where the tumor margin cannot be defined, the lesion must be transected even though some tumor tissue will be left behind. Later, this area can be reexplored and further obvious tumor tissue removed. Alternatively, ultrasonic aspiration can be used to help debulk and remove the tumor.

After the mass is removed, the tumor cavity is irrigated with a copious amount of warm saline (Fig. 37-4). The stay sutures in the pia and dura are cut and a watertight closure is obtained. Systemic steroids are given before surgery begins and are continued 1 to 2 days after surgery.

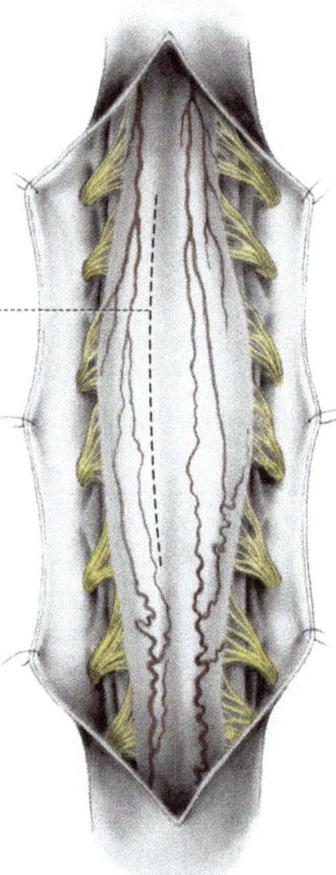

Figure 37-1. A midline or paramidline incision is made over the avascular dorsal surface of the spinal cord. Fusiform enlargement of the spinal cord is noted. The laminectomy is performed one level above and one level below the area of the tumor.

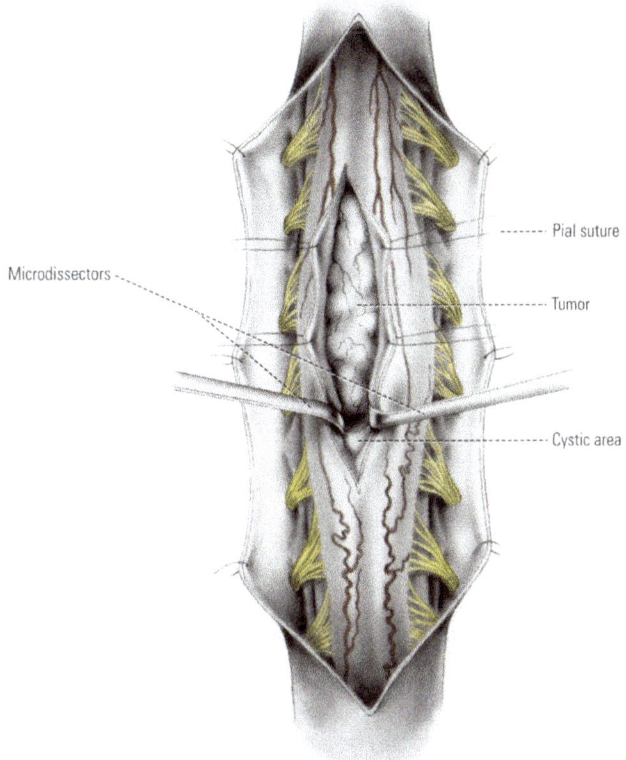

Figure 37-2. An incision of adequate length allows the tumor to be exposed by gentle retraction on the pia with 6-0 stay sutures.

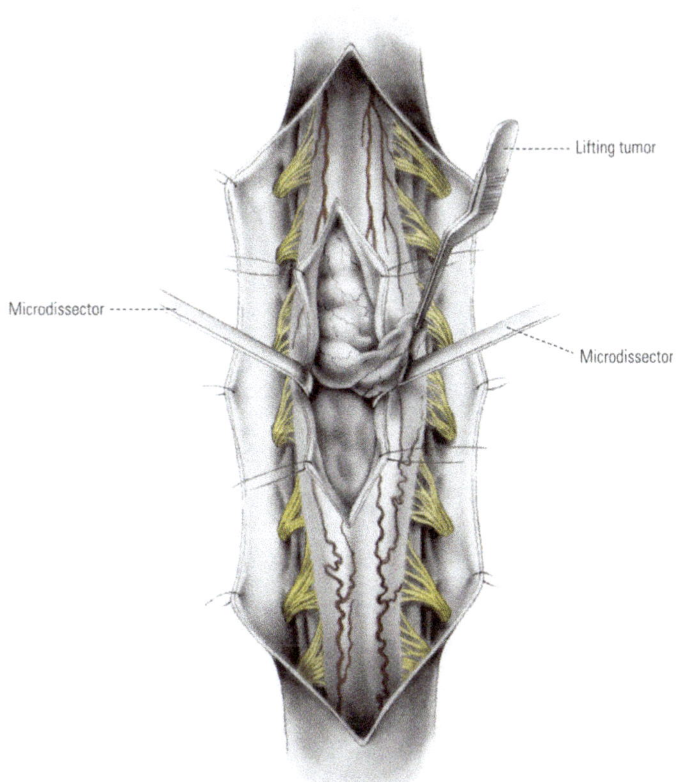

Figure 37-3. Gentle upward retraction of the tumor can facilitate careful dissection of the tumor from the spinal cord.

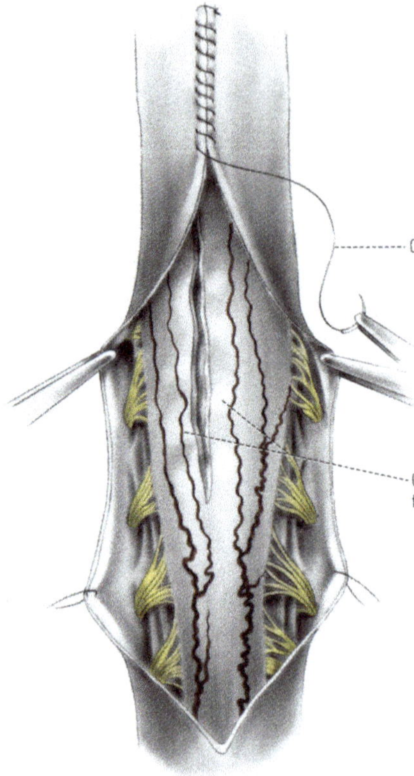

Figure 37-4. The dura is closed in a watertight fashion.

CHAPTER

38

Cauda Equina: Conus Medullaris Ependymoma

Tumors of the cauda equina–conus medullaris region are often well-defined, small masses attached to the filum terminale. These lesions are dissected from the nerve roots and the tip of the spinal cord relatively easily. A portion of uninvolved filum terminale is usually present between the tumor and spinal cord. The afferent and efferent segments of the filum must be amputated to remove the tumor. Small and moderate-sized tumors do not require internal decompression. Recurrences after successful en bloc resections are rare.

These tumors can envelop the nerve roots and conus so that the origin of the lesion is questionable and its total removal impossible. Large filum terminale ependymomas also can be difficult to resect completely. In such cases, the goal of surgery becomes decompression of the nervous elements surrounded by the tumor. The blood supply to the conus must be preserved. Large vessels often accompany sacral nerve roots rostrally to supply not only the tumor but the conus as well.

Ependymomas in this region can cause both upper and lower motor neuron–types of neurologic deficits. Initially, a tumor can cause symptoms and signs referable to only one or two nerve roots and may be interpreted as radiculopathy secondary to a herniated nucleus pulposus. Consequently, when patients are evaluated for radiculopathy, it is a good rule for magnetic resonance (MR) imaging studies to include the area of the conus. MR imaging with and without enhancement is the best preoperative diagnostic study both to localize the tumor and to delineate its relationship to the conus and filum.

The operation described in this chapter is for a typical well-defined myxopapillary ependymoma that arises from the filum terminale. The operating microscope and microsurgical instrumentation greatly facilitate the resection of these lesions. The patient is placed in the prone position on the operating room table. The lesion is exposed through a midline incision, and the laminectomy is extended one level rostral and one level caudal to the tumor. Figure 38-1 illustrates the exposure after the dura and arachnoid have been opened. The filum terminale is identified in the midline by gently separating nerve roots below the tip of the conus. Compared to the rootlets, the filum terminale is fibrous and firm because the pia of the conus continues to encase it. The filum terminale is clipped at its origin (Fig. 38-2) and divided. Beginning dissection at this end of the mass precludes placing traction on the conus and injuring it. The nerve roots are dissected free of the tumor and the tumor is gradually removed (Fig. 38-3). The dura is closed in a watertight fashion, and the wound is closed in layers.

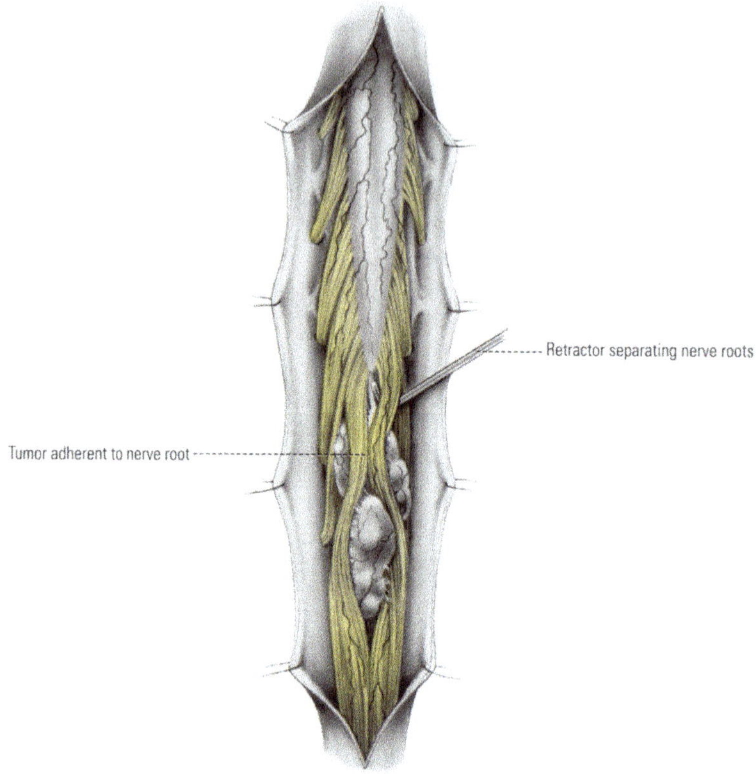

Figure 38-1. The exposure should extend at least one level caudal and one level rostral to the site of the tumor. Exposure of the tumor begins rostrally with identification of the conus medullaris and filum terminale. Nerve roots must be separated to identify the origin of the filum.

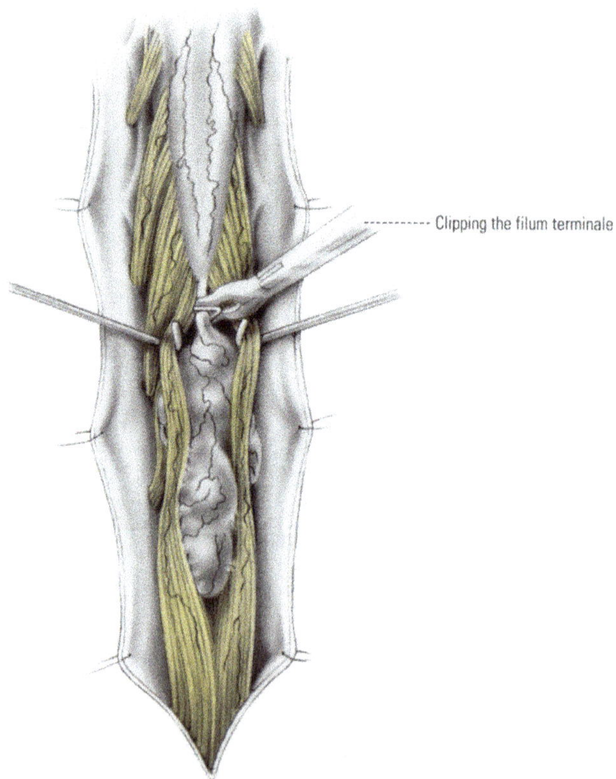

Figure 38-2. The filum terminale is clipped at its origin just distal to the conus medullaris before the tumor is dissected from the surrounding nerve roots.

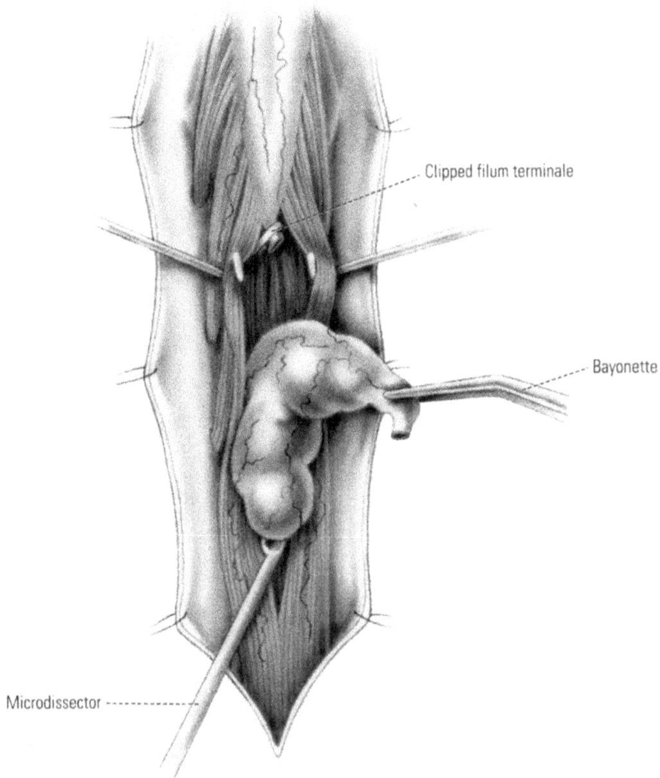

Figure 38-3. Tumor removal begins rostrally and proceeds caudally to prevent injury to the conus medullaris. The nerve roots are gently dissected from the tumor.

CHAPTER

39

Intra- and Extramedullary Tumor: Thoracic Meningioma

Meningiomas of the spinal canal account for approximately 25% of intradural spinal cord tumors in adults. They can arise in any age group but most occur between the fifth and seventh decades of life. Approximately 80% occur in women and approximately 80% are located in the thoracic region. Magnetic resonance imaging is the best diagnostic study; it not only demonstrates the level of the tumor but also its relationship to the spinal cord. Classically, these tumors are located anterolaterally in the intradural space. Most are entirely intradural, but about 10% are both intradural and extradural or entirely extradural. Meningiomas are often covered by a shell-like envelope of spinal cord giving the initial appearance of an intrinsic tumor. Complete surgical removal is the treatment of choice for spinal meningiomas. A meningioma in the upper thoracic area is discussed.

The patient is placed prone on the operating table. Typically, a complete laminectomy provides adequate exposure and should be extended one level rostral and one level caudal the level of the tumor. After the dura is opened in the midline, the spinal cord is exposed (Fig. 39-1); the focal enlargement can be mistaken for intrinsic tumor. Under the operating microscope, however, the tumor can be seen in the anterolateral gutter of the spinal canal after gentle dissection of the arachnoid and section of the dentate ligaments, if necessary. Exposure can be increased by using the dentate ligaments to rotate the spinal cord gently away from the tumor or by internally decompressing the tumor.

With microdissectors, the tumor is dissected away from the spinal cord. Bleeding is controlled with bipolar coagulation (Fig. 39-2). Dissection continues around the encapsulated tumor to determine its origin (Fig. 39-3). Usually there is a dural attachment along the anterolateral portion of the spinal canal. To visualize the tumor better, it is often helpful to depress the paraspinal muscle mass with table-mounted retractors and to turn the patient away from the surgeon. Occasionally, a costotransversectomy or lateral extracavitary approach can be used for tumors in more ventral locations. The arachnoid over the exposed portion of the tumor is incised and reflected so that dissection can proceed directly on its surface. The rostral and caudal tumor poles should be identified. Small pledgets can be placed in the lateral gutters on either side of the tumor to minimize blood spilling into the subarachnoid space. The exposed surface of the tumor can be cauterized to diminish its vascularity and to shrink its mass.

If the lesion has a firm, lateral attachment, the dura is excised with the tumor and then must be repaired with a periosteal or fascial graft or pseudodura. If the dura of the anterolateral region is excised, bleeding from epidural veins and tumor-feeding vessels can be controlled by exerting pressure laterally or anteriorly from inside the dura and/or by bipolar coagulation. Large tumors can be bisected and debulked through the central trough. The tumor segment facing the spinal cord is then delivered into the cavity with gentle traction. The site of the tumor's attachment to the dura is coagulated extensively. All bleeding is controlled with bipolar coagulation, and blood and debris are irrigated from the subarachnoid space with a warm saline solution. Arachnoid adhesions that hold the spinal cord in a deformed position are divided to decrease the risk of tethering. A water-tight dural closure is accomplished. Subsequently, the wound is closed in layers.

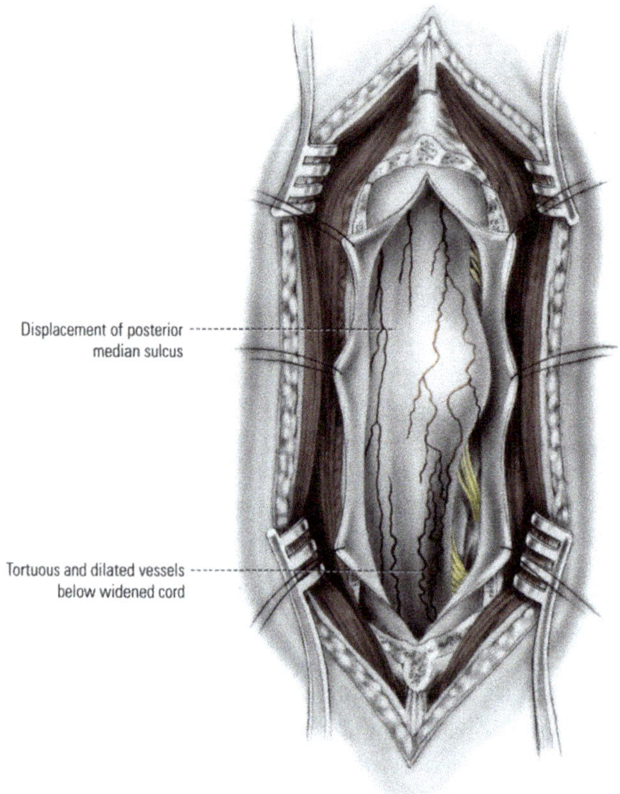

Figure 39-1. **Intradural extramedullary tumor in an anterolateral location. The spinal cord forms a shell-like cover over the meningioma.**

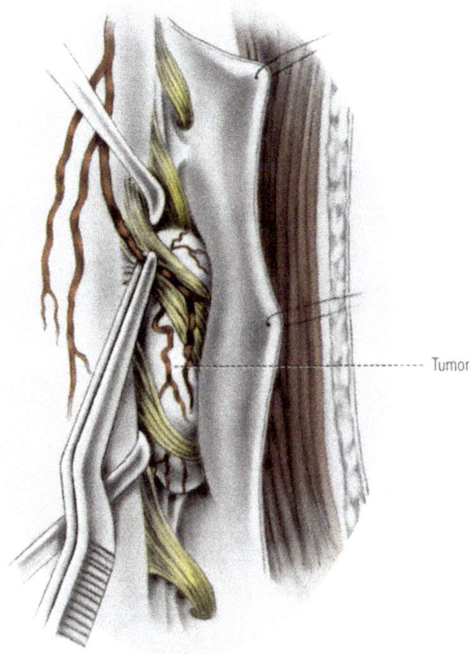

Figure 39-2. Bipolar cauterization is used to coagulate the blood vessels and the capsule of the tumor.

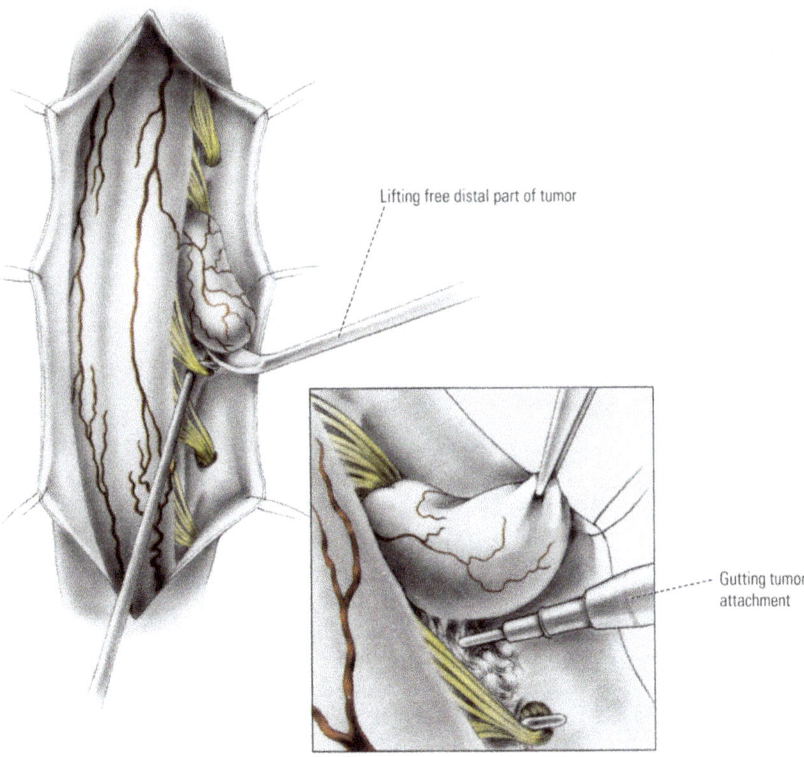

Figure 39-3. Traction of the tumor is always away from the spinal cord. Small tumors can be removed in one piece, but large tumors need to be removed piecemeal.

CHAPTER

40

Intra- and Extradural Tumor: Dumbbell Schwannoma

Schwannomas and neurofibromas together comprise one third of primary spinal cord tumors and show a predilection for the thoracic spine over the lumbar and cervical spine. Characteristically, these tumors originate from the sensory nerve root intrathecally. The tumor then may extend along the nerve peripherally through the intravertebral neural foramina. The extradural portion of the well-encapsuled tumor may reach an extreme size. A standard radiograph of the spine may show erosion or complete absence of the pedicles and lamina as well as vertebral scalloping.

Irrespective of the level of the spine that is involved, the patient is placed in the prone position. Depending on the size of the intraspinal component of the tumor, a total laminectomy or hemilaminectomy is performed. Figure 40-1 illustrates the exposure after a laminectomy and facetectomy have been completed to expose a tumor with a large intradural component. It is important to expose fully the intraspinal foramina and extraspinal extension; this usually requires a facetectomy on the side of the tumor.

Depending on the size of the tumor, the dura is usually incised in the midline or toward the side of the tumor. The arachnoid is then sharply dissected over the tumor. The smooth, encapsulated tumor is traced to its dural exit. The tumor is usually constricted at this point, giving it a dumbbell configuration. The dura is incised perpendicular to the original vertical incision over the exiting nerve root (Fig. 40-2).

The subdural portion of the tumor is gently dissected away from the adherent nerve roots and arachnoid adhesions, and between the tumor capsule and spinal cord. Any retraction or dissection always must be directed away from the spinal cord. If the tumor is too large to permit dissection of its border, the capsule is opened and the tumor is gutted using microcurettes or ultrasonic aspiration. Once the intradural portion of the tumor has been removed, the foraminal portion of the tumor is followed to its extradural component. The remaining spinal cord is somewhat deformed and the nerve root elongated (Fig. 40-3). The extradural portion of the schwannoma is dissected free of its surrounding tissues. The tumor usually has a definitive capsule, which is dissected free from the surrounding soft tissue. In the cervical area, where the vertebral artery is often displaced by the tumor, extra care must be exerted during dissection. The tumor is dissected and can be elevated (Fig. 40-4) to help identify its distal boundaries and the normal nerve root extending from it. It is not unusual for a portion of the nerve root to be dissected free from the schwannoma. If such dissection is impossible, it is advisable to coagulate the nerve root and transect it.

At all levels, it is important to preserve the radicular arteries arising from the posterior branches of the intercostal arteries. Their preservation is especially important in the lower thoracic and upper lumbar levels where these arteries can serve as the origin for the artery of Adamkiewicz.

The dural defect is closed in a T-fashion or using pseudodura or a fascial graft (Fig. 40-5). The dural closure should be watertight. The wound is then closed in routine fashion.

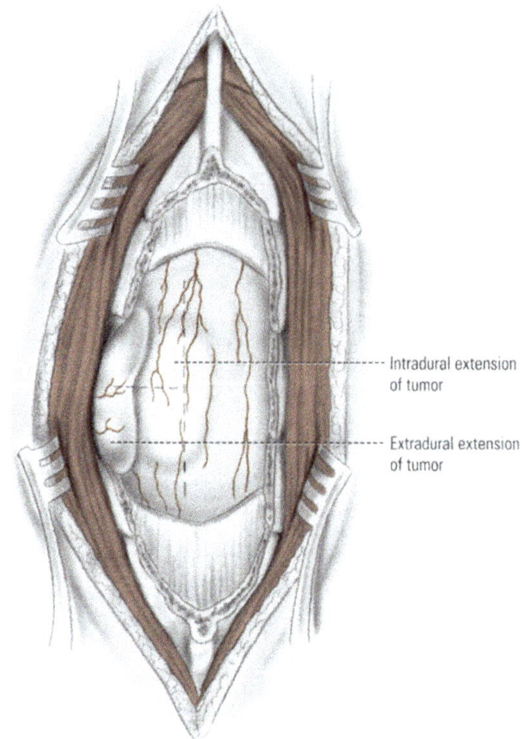

Figure 40-1. Exposure of an intra- and extradural tumor (dumbbell neurofibroma of a thoracic nerve root). The tumor is exposed so that the superior and inferior borders are clearly visible. The dura is tense and bulging from the intradural portion of the tumor.

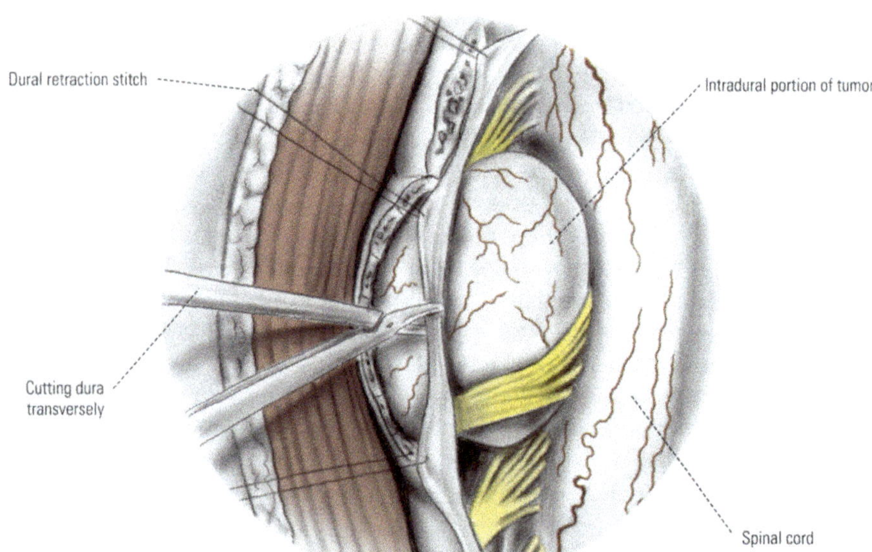

Figure 40-2. The nerve roots and spinal cord are displaced by the tumor. The dura is first incised longitudinally. A second incision is made perpendicular to the first one over the lateral aspects of the tumor.

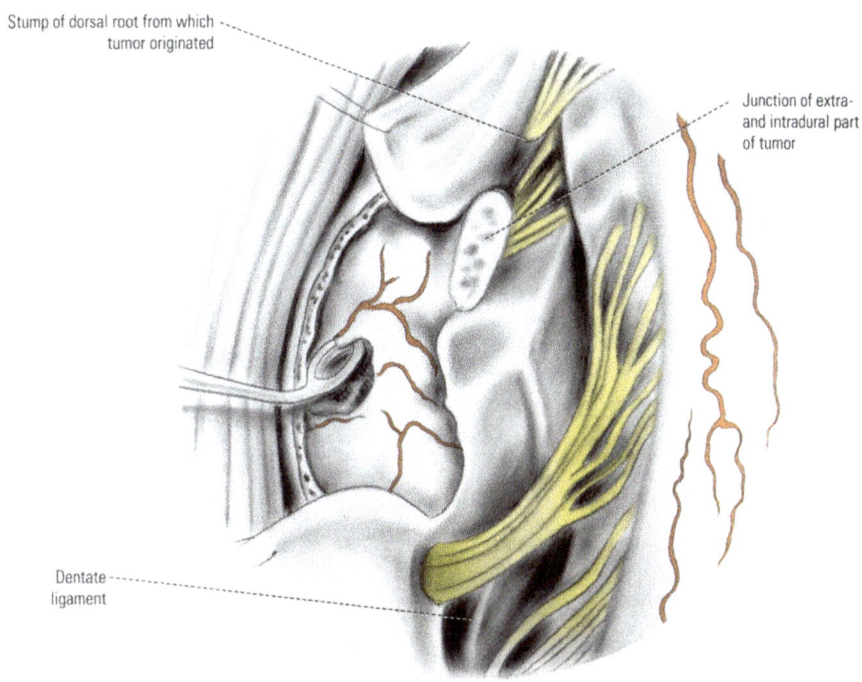

Figure 40-3. The size of the tumor can be decreased by opening the capsule and removing the internal portion. Note the deformity of the spinal cord after intradural tumor has been removed.

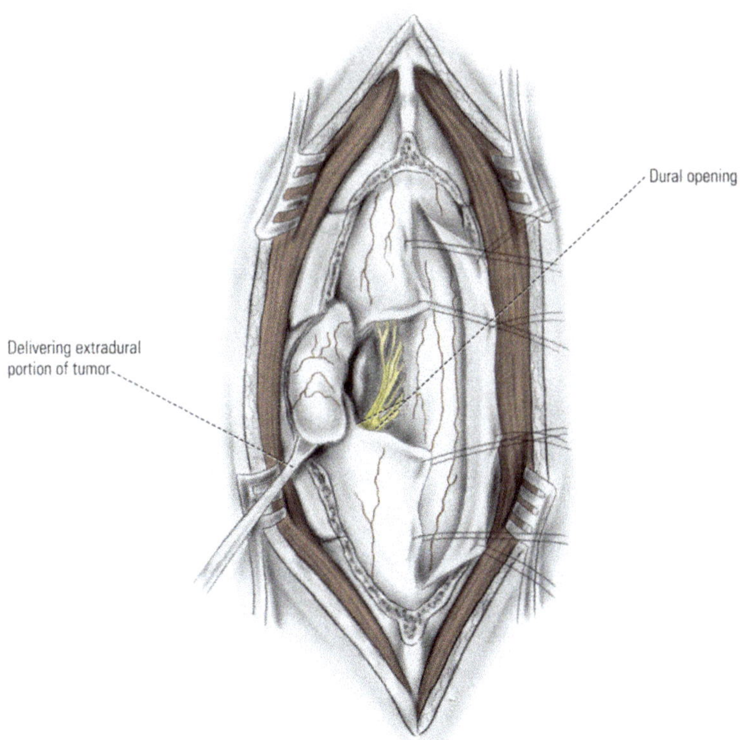

Figure 40-4. Excision of the extradural tumor from its surrounding tissue.

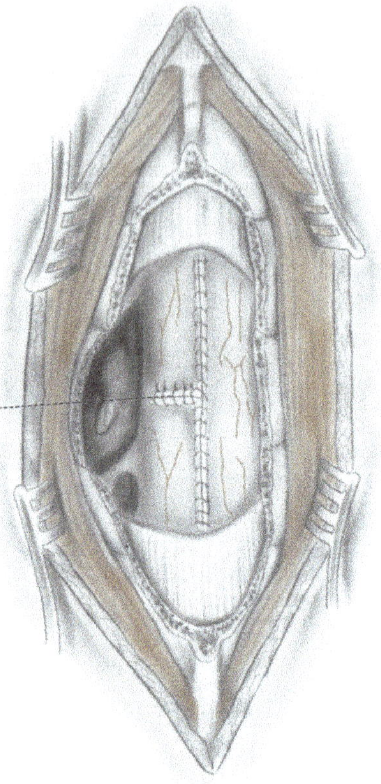

Figure 40-5. The dura is closed primarily in a T-fashion.

CHAPTER

41

Carotid Endarterectomy

Indications for carotid endarterectomy are generally well established: moderate to severe carotid stenosis with ipsilateral transient ischemic attacks or amaurosis fugax, ipsilateral mild or moderate stroke with good recovery or high-grade asymptomatic disease in relatively young and healthy patients. We prefer to do the operation under general anesthesia and use electroencephalographic (EEG) monitoring to determine when to shunt, although many surgeons prefer regional and/or local anesthesia and either no monitoring or routine use of an intraoperative shunt. The skin incision is made along the lower anterior border of the sternocleidomastoid muscle with the upper part of the incision gently curving backwards toward the mastoid at a point about two finger breadths below the angle of the jaw, to avoid injury to the mandibular branch of the facial nerve (Fig. 41-1). The incision is carried sharply through the platysma, carefully avoiding injury to the great auricular nerve, which runs just deep to the platysma in the superior-most aspect of the incision. Dissection is then continued along the anterior aspect of the sternocleidomastoid muscle until the internal jugular vein is identified. In this plane, the descending branch of the hypoglossus nerve (ansa cervicalis) is identified. The dissection plane is between the internal jugular vein laterally and the ansa medially (Fig. 41-2). The common carotid artery (CCA) is then identified inferiorly and a tape is passed around for its control at this point. The surgeon must be careful to dissect in the plane between the CCA and the vagus nerve, which runs posterior to the artery and avoid injury to the nerve. The plane of dissection is then continued superiorly to the carotid bifurcation where the common facial vein is commonly encountered. This vein should be carefully ligated and divided between ligatures. The exposure is then carried superiorly to dissect free the origin of the internal carotid artery (ICA), the external carotid artery (ECA), and the superior thyroid artery, which most frequently arises from the ECA right at the level of the bifurcation. As the surgeon progresses distally, the dissection must stay lateral to the hypoglossus nerve, which can be easily mobilized medially by gradually coagulating and dividing the small veins and arterial muscular branches that hold it in a lateral position (Fig. 41-3). The dissection of the ICA should be carried out well distal to the plaque, the end of which can usually be carefully palpated. Tapes are then passed around the distal ICA, the ECA, and the superior thyroid artery (Fig. 41-3). After applying either atraumatic vascular clamps or aneurysm clips first on the ICA, then on the CCA and finally on the ECA and superior thyroid artery, the surgeon makes an arteriotomy starting just below the bifurcation as in Figure 41-4. We prefer to carry the arteriotomy only to the level of the plaque and then dissect with a Penfield 4 the plane between the plaque and the wall of the artery (Fig. 41-5). This plane is then carried distally to the end of the plaque using Pott's scissors as in Figure 41-6. The surgeon then cuts across the plaque after passing a right-angle instrument under its proximal end as in Figure 41-7. If necessary to get proximal to the beginning of the thick plaque, the surgeon can extend the incision in the CCA as far as necessary. The plaque is then carefully separated from the wall of the artery, first at the origin of the ECA working particularly carefully behind the birfurcation, as in Figure 41-8. The plaque is then removed from the ECA, carefully dissecting as distally as possible in the plane between the plaque and the ECA. Only then is the surgeon ready to deal with the most difficult part of the operation, which is to carefully remove the plaque from the ICA. The plaque must be removed completely until the point that it tapers imperceptibly into the normal intima of the artery distally. Frequently, bits of plaque and loose intima have to be carefully removed under irrigation until the surgeon is satisfied that the lumen of the ICA is perfectly clean. At times, the plaque does not come away perfectly and a "shelf" of intima is left distally. Exquisite judgment is necessary here, but frequently the surgeon is left with no choice but to "tack" down the intima with horizontal mattress sutures. In most cases, the plaque comes off completely, leaving a smooth intimal edge as in Figure 41-9. The surgeon is then ready to close the arteriotomy, which we prefer to do with a running suture of either 5-0 or 6-0 prolene, depending on the size of the lumen (6-0 is used when the lumen is relatively narrow) (Fig. 41-10). We prefer to use a doubly armed suture as a horizontal mattress suture starting from the lumen and going out to each side of the apex of the arteriotomy with each needle at a time as indicated in Figure 41-9. Figure 41-11 indicates the finished suture line. It is important to allow backflow temporarily, first from the ICA and then from the ECA to wash out air and debris. The clamps are then removed sequentially, first from the ECA, then from the CCA, and finally from the ICA.

We use an internal shunt only when the EEG changes significantly or in patients who have had a recent stroke or are known to have contralateral carotid occlusion with poor intracranial collateral circulation. We prefer to use a straight shunting tube with tapered edges as indicated in Figure 41-12. When the EEG changes immediately and dramatically, we cut right through the plaque being careful to extend the arteriotomy beyond the end of the plaque and then insert the shunt through the plaque. After the shunt is inserted in the ICA first and then in the CCA, tourniquets are tightened, as indicated in Figure 41-12, to prevent bleeding. The plaque can then be dissected carefully and completely, but the dissection, in the presence of the shunt, is a bit more difficult. For this reason, when the EEG changes are not dramatic, we prefer to remove the plaque completely, in the usual manner, then insert the shunt. The removal of the plaque should take no longer than 5 or 6 minutes and ischemia of this duration is generally well tolerated. In cases where the lumen is relatively narrow or in cases of re-do endarterectomy, we prefer to use a vein patch. We generally obtain the patch from the saphenous vein in the leg. Other surgeons prefer to use synthetic material for patching.

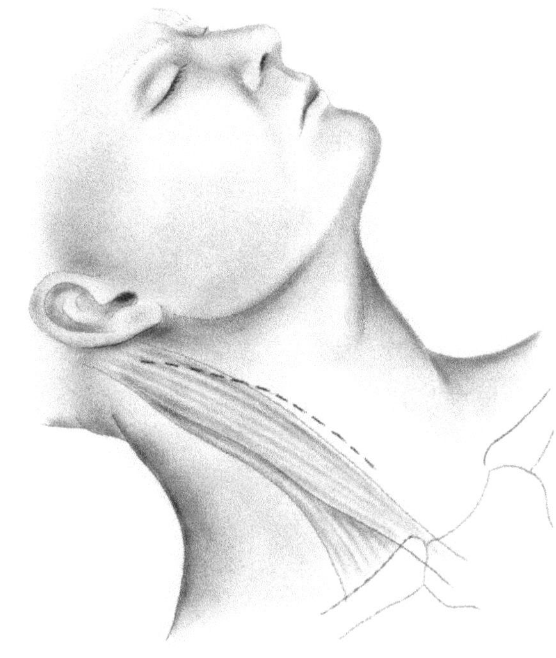

Figure 41-1. Skin incision and initial exposure. Note that the upper end of the incision curves over the sternocleidomastoid muscle toward the mastoid process. (*Adapted from* Ojemann *et al.* [1].)

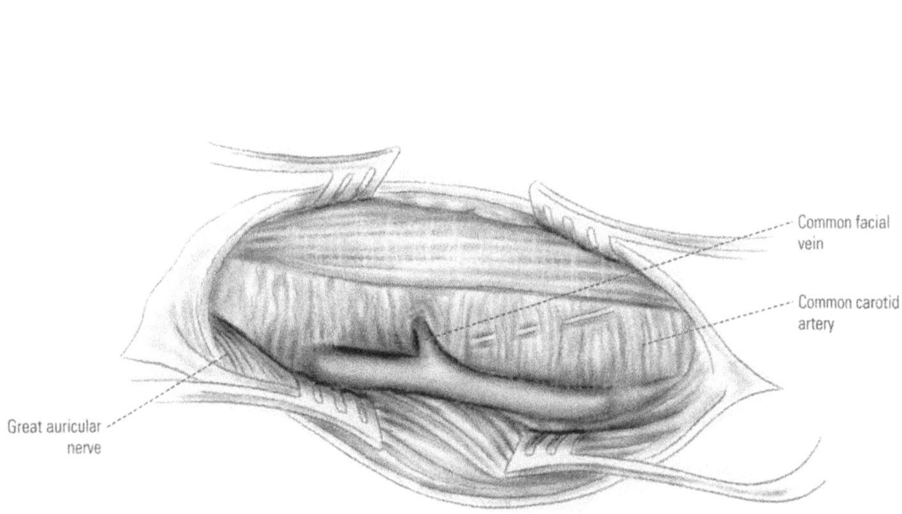

Figure 41-2. The proximal common carotid artery is exposed and a tape passed around it. The common facial vein is ligated and divided. (*Adapted from* Ojemann *et al.* [1].)

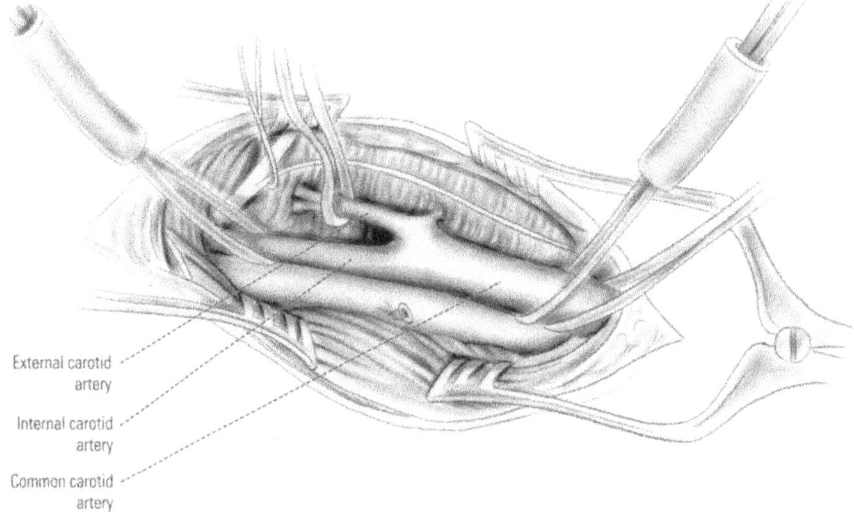

Figure 41-3. Vascular tapes have been placed. The common carotid artery is occluded with a Fogarty clamp and the other arteries with temporary aneurysm clips. (*Adapted from* Ojemann *et al.* [1].)

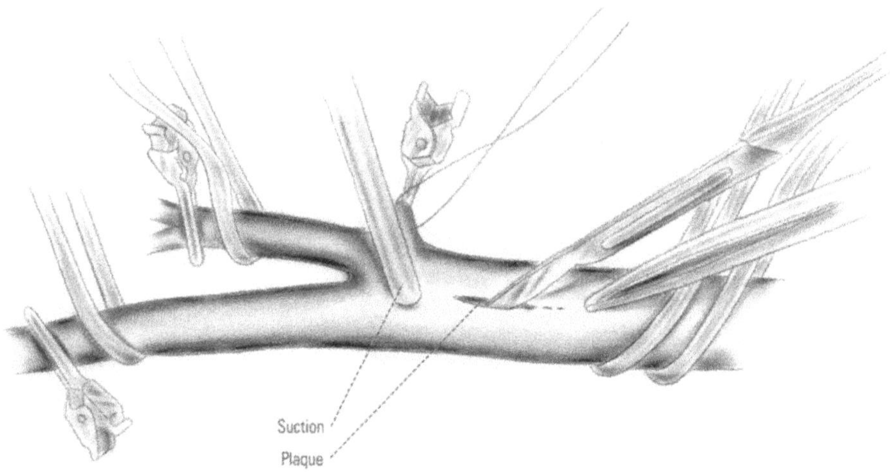

Figure 41-4. Some surgeons use a marking pen to outline arteriotomy incision, which starts on the distal common carotid artery. It is carried down but not through the atheromatous plaque. Suction is ready, and a forceps steadies the vessel. (*Adapted from* Ojemann *et al.* [1].)

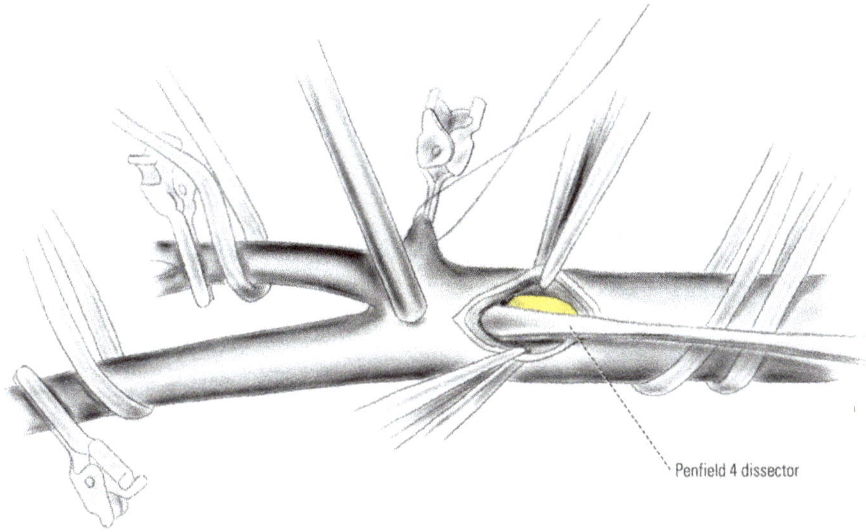

Figure 41-5. Plaque being separated from the anterior wall of the artery by Penfield 4 dissector. (*Adapted from* Ojemann *et al.* [1].)

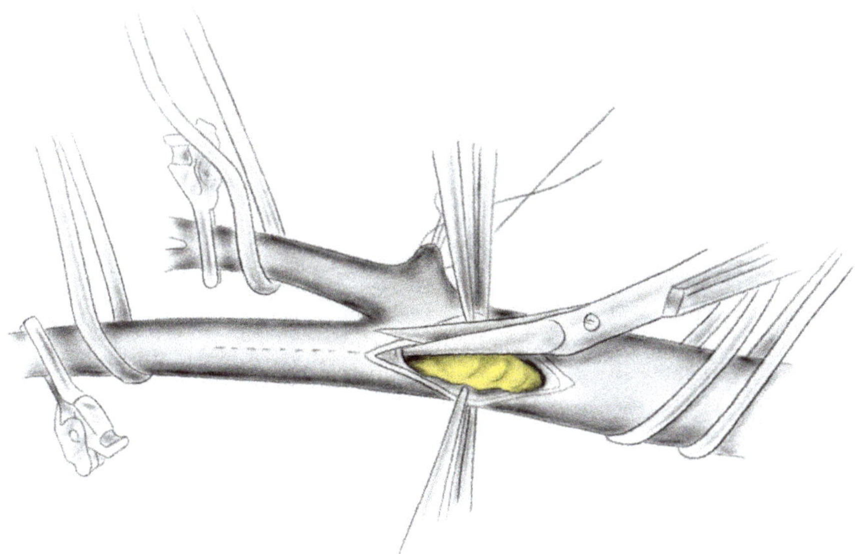

Figure 41-6. The arteriotomy is extended distally using a Potts scissors. (*Adapted from* Ojemann *et al.* [1].)

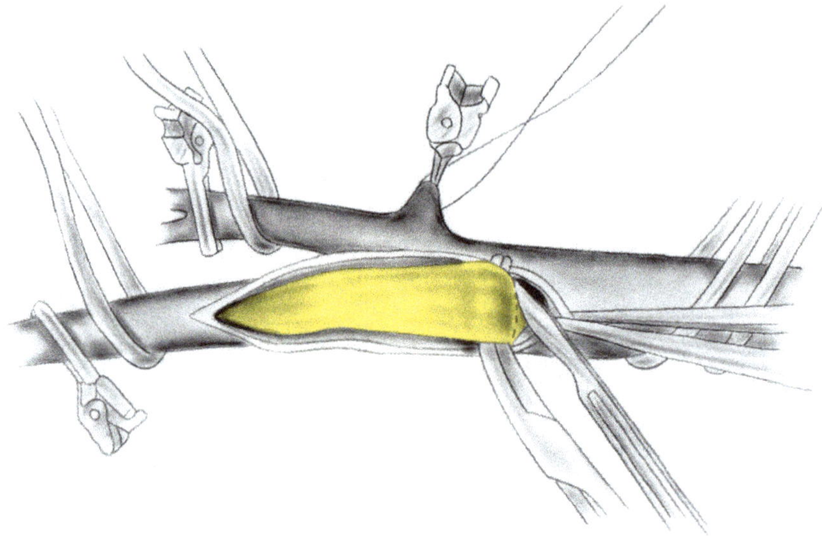

Figure 41-7. A right-angled clamp has been placed around the atheromatous plaque at the proximal end of the arteriotomy. The plaque is being cut off sharply with a number 15 knife blade. (*Adapted from* Ojemann *et al.* [1].)

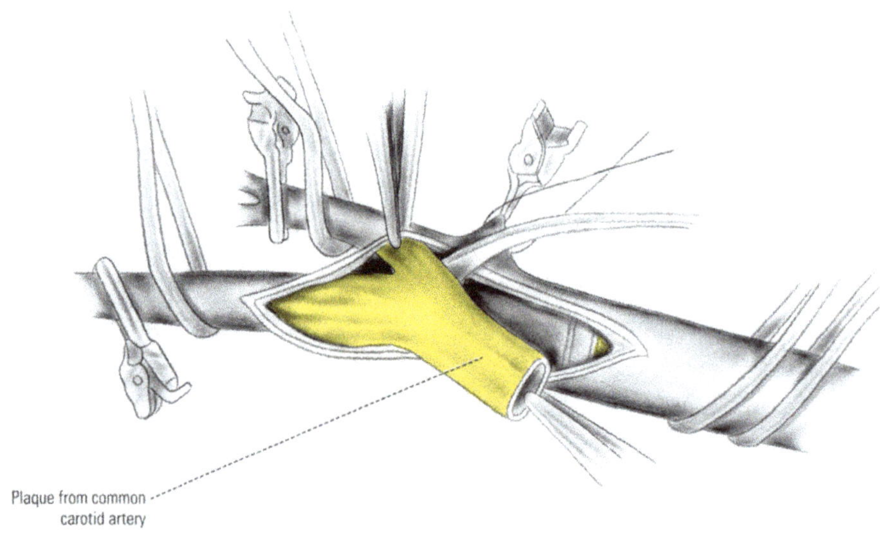

Figure 41-8. The plaque has been separated from the outer wall of the common carotid artery and is now being removed from the origin of the external carotid artery. (*Adapted from* Ojemann *et al.* [1].)

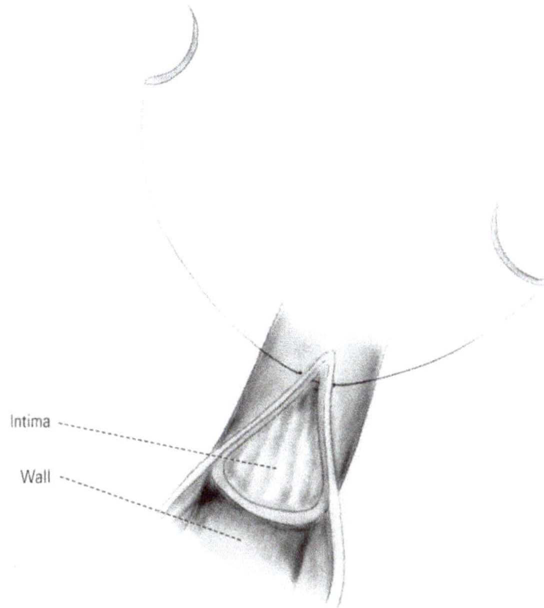

Figure 41-9. Arteriotomy closure. The initial sutures in the internal carotid artery may be placed with a microneedle holder, with care taken to suture both intimal and wall layers on both sides. (*Adapted from* Ojemann *et al.* [1].)

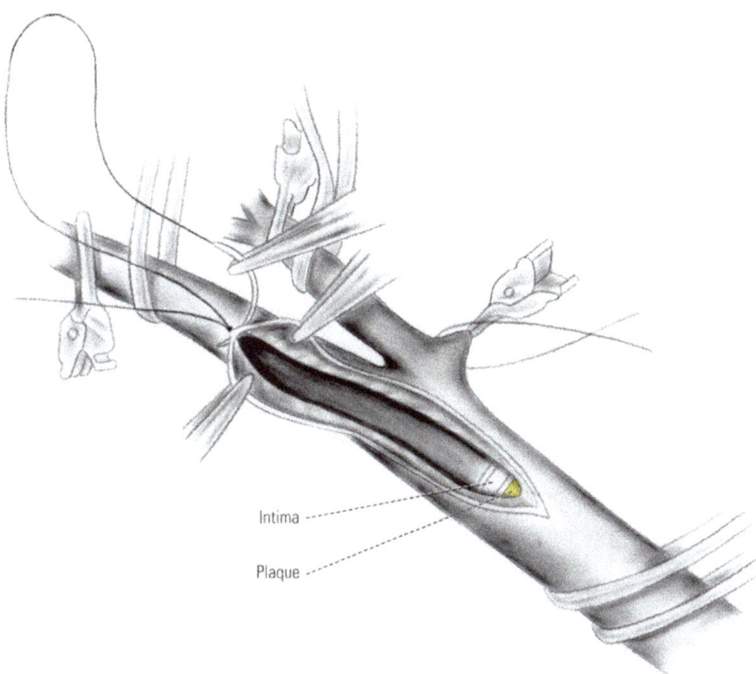

Figure 41-10. Tacking sutures with double-armed 6-0 prolene are placed at 120° angles. (*Adapted from* Ojemann *et al.* [1].)

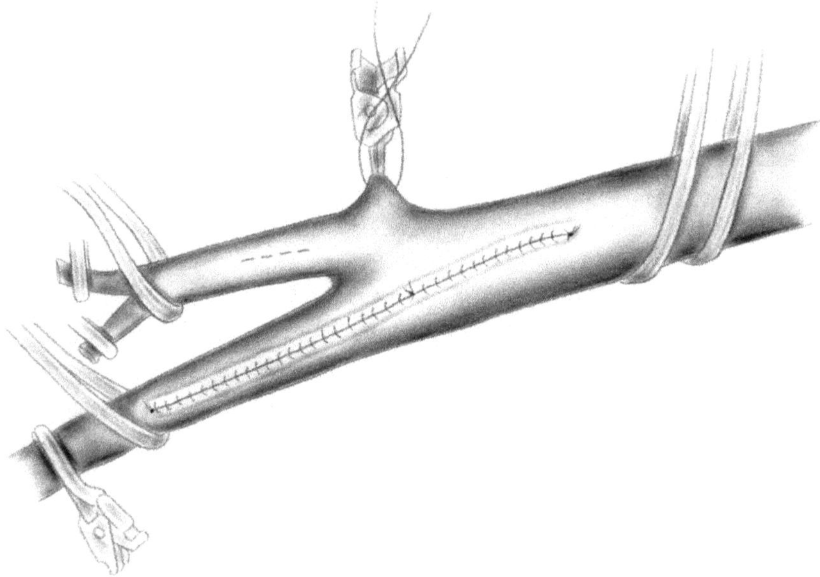

Figure 41-11. Arteriotomy closure continued. The sutures are gradually placed farther apart. The thick wall of the common carotid artery requires a standard needle holder. (*Adapted from* Ojemann *et al.* [1].)

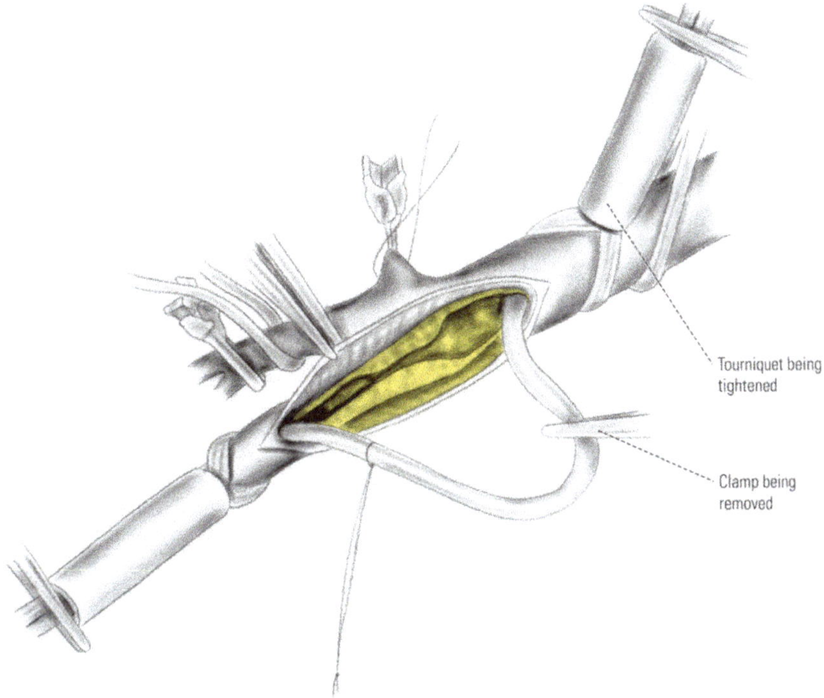

Figure 41-12. Placement of shunt. The proximal portion of the shunt has been placed in the common carotid artery. (*Adapted from* Ojemann *et al.* [1].)

Reference

1. Ojemann RG, Heros RC, Crowell RM: *Surgical Management of Cerebrovascular Disease*, edn 2. Baltimore: Williams & Wilkins; 1998:35–75.

CHAPTER

42

Surgery of Peripheral Nerves

Principles of Peripheral Nerve Surgery

Because trauma is responsible for most peripheral nerve injuries, it is understandable that times of war have produced much of the knowledge upon which the principles of peripheral nerve surgery are based. Since peripheral nerve injuries are not life threatening, other system injuries are usually of primary concern. Once the cardiorespiratory condition of the patient is stabilized, attention may then be directed to compound extremity injuries. Prior to any operative debridement, a careful examination should be done to ascertain the extent of neurologic dysfunction. At the time of initial surgery, the nerve injury is inspected and described as to its nature, location, and severity. Surgical repair of the nerve is deferred at the time of initial surgery if the wound is contaminated; today's improved surgical technique with aseptic and antiseptic measures has not decreased the risk of an apparently "clean" wound becoming infected with extensive secondary loss of tissue, making reconstructive surgery even more difficult. Separated nerve ends may be tagged with radiopaque sutures to aid localization at the time of a delayed neurorrhaphy.

In any patient awaiting delayed nerve repair, the care of denervated tissue is of paramount importance. The paralyzed muscle must not be overstretched. Thermal and pressure injuries must be prevented. Unnecessary long-term immobilization with attendant stasis, degeneration of muscle fibers, formation of excessive *fibrous tissue* and adhesions are to be avoided. Patients with fractures requiring immobilization benefit from physiotherapeutic measures such as massage and from rotating beds to prevent circulatory stasis. All of these efforts result in a more normal limb at the time of reinnervation. If, at the time of initial debridement, the nerve is found to be severed, eventual surgical repair is obviously indicated. Pathoanatomic studies have shown that the ideal time for secondary suture is about 20 days following injury. The neurorrhaphy can be done at that time only if no evidence of local or systemic sepsis is present and no other injury precludes operative intervention.

Surgical treatment of an injured nerve is also required when the pathology of the lesion is unknown and clinical evidence points to a complete or partial nerve lesion. Clinical assessment of such situations requires accurate anatomic knowledge of the level of the nerve branches to various muscle groups. Electrodiagnostic studies are also important in the evaluation of questionably complete nerve injuries. Electromyography with search for denervation fibrillations, positive sharp waves, and other muscle action potentials as well as the determination of chronaxie and strength-duration curves is often of value. Nerve conduction velocities are sometimes of aid in partial nerve injuries. For more details the reader is referred to one of the standard texts on electrodiagnosis. The often discussed Tinel's sign provides an opportunity to observe the rate of growth of some regenerating sensory fibers. However, a positive Tinel's sign tells us only that some sensory axons are moving peripherally from the proximal side of an area of trauma. A positive sign is no justification for delay of surgical exploration if other evidence of motor or sensory reinnervation fails to appear within the expected time.

The operative approach to the traumatized nerve must provide a wide exposure, and the preoperative skin preparation should allow for extension of the incision either proximally or distally. Skin scars should be excised or avoided, and the skin incision is made in normal skin creases over joints. The incision is planned so that the nerve repair does not lie directly beneath the suture line. Local infiltration with 1:200,000 epinephrine in normal saline is helpful to reduce oozing. The use of a tourniquet is not necessary. Thorough anatomic knowledge, delicate handling of tissues, and dissection parallel to normal tissue planes will reduce blood loss and obviate the need for a tourniquet. The risk of postoperative hematoma formation and ischemic necrosis by using a tourniquet far outweigh the danger of intraoperative hemorrhage.

The surgical exposure at the time of a delayed nerve repair must be done through normal anatomic planes above and below the area of injury. Having identified the nerve proximal and distal to the lesion, dissection is carried into the area of injury. A detailed understanding of the regional anatomy is imperative. Without this knowledge there is great danger of further damage to the nerve trunk or its branches. Electrical stimulation may be of help in locating functional nerve fibers within a large mass of scar tissue, thus guiding further dissection. After the nerve has been completely freed from surrounding scar tissue, an often difficult decision must be made as to whether or not a neuroma in continuity should be resected. Inspection and palpation, although helpful, may be misleading in this regard. The presence of a neuroma is not incompatible with excellent spontaneous recovery. Conversely, a nerve which appears normal may have severe intrafascicular damage precluding regeneration. In these situations, electrical stimulation, with or without in vivo recording of evoked potentials, is a valuable guide. Such stimulation is most reliably done above and below the area of injury before the neurolysis is completed since manipulation can cause a temporary conduction block. Surgeons most experienced in peripheral nerve surgery agree that the results of incision and end-to-end anastomosis of peripheral nerves are not good enough to justify the risk of performing such a procedure on a nerve that might recover spontaneously.

The underlying pathology necessitating surgical intervention may be pressure on or tension of the nerve with impairment of function and a variable potential for recovery. The indicated surgical procedure for such lesions is a neurolysis with rerouting of the nerve and removal of constricting bone or ligament. Neurolysis is defined as the removal of constricting scar which has been preventing regenerating axons from growing through the area of constriction or causing a physiological conduction block at the area of constriction. A neurolysis may be either external or internal.

In performing an external neurolysis, the entire nerve trunk is dissected carefully from its surrounding bed of scar tissue. Again it is emphasized that this procedure is done after first exposing the nerve through normal anatomic planes both above and below the site of injury while sparing all branches by dissecting with the aid of magnifying lenses. Bleeding points on the nerve proper are not electrocoagulated. If the neurolysis obviously interferes with the vascular supply of the nerve, no benefit can be expected from the surgical procedure.

The performance of a proper internal neurolysis is most difficult. The objective is to free the individual fascicles within the nerve. This is done either by microscopic dissection or by injection of warm saline solution. Both techniques are designed to disrupt constricting scar tissue. Avoiding damage to the delicate intrafascicular vascular network is most difficult. Only the epineurium is incised while avoiding disruption of the perineurium and especially avoiding injection of saline into a fascicle.

A majority of traumatized nerves, however, require more than either an internal or an external neurolysis and need to be repaired by an end-to-end anastomosis. To obtain a tension-free anastomosis, extensive mobilization of a nerve may be required. Transposition of the nerve to a new bed may also be necessary. Effective mobilization may necessitate stripping of branches from the parent nerve even though this may cause loss of some blood supply to the nerve (see Figs. 42-7 and 42-8). To prevent damage to adjacent fascicles, this stripping is done only under magnification and only as far as the branch can be easily separated. Ease of dissection alone is not a sufficient guide for this procedure. Magnification is essential because without it small fascicles may be overlooked. In mobilization of a nerve, nutrient vessels are encountered which unavoidably must be sacrificed. In this situation the nutrient vessel must be ligated well away from the nerve trunk to prevent damage to the intrinsic vessels of the nerve. The longitudinally oriented superficial arterial system cannot be adequately visualized and preserved if the limb is made ischemic by the use of a tourniquet. The tourniquet also enhances the risk of postoperative bleeding from these vessels with attendant hematoma and scar formation.

Correct axial orientation of nerve ends prior to neurorrhaphy is essential for optimal apposition of fascicles (Fig. 42-1). Nerve ends must be cut at precise right angles as the distal and proximal ends are resected back to healthy appearing bundles. Ideally a similar cross-sectional arrangement of the bundles can be recognized in the two ends. Reapproximation is performed using a fine suture material, such as 5-0 to 8-0 nylon, which causes the least fibroblastic proliferation.

To facilitate apposition of nerve ends, various joints of the extremity may need to be flexed. Experience gained from two world wars, Korea, and Vietnam has established that flexion of greater than 90° at the elbow and knee must be strictly avoided. Flexion should not exceed 40° at the wrist nor 10° at the ankle.

Whenever possible a direct end-to-end anastomosis of the nerve should be performed. However, nerve autografting has proved to be a preferable method of treatment in bridging irreparable gaps.

The ideal autograft is one with a similar size and fascicular pattern. This is rarely possible, however, so that a nerve with a simple parallel fascicular pattern is most often used. Thin grafts are more successful than thick ones because vascularization is more easily achieved. The shorter the graft the better the chance it will be bridged by sprouting axons. Grafts greater than 15 cm in length universally fail. The superficial radial and the sural nerves are the best donors for free nerve grafts. The medial and lateral antebrachial cutaneous nerves as well as the lateral femoral cutaneous nerve are often used.

Pedicle grafting is also a valuable adjunct in the repair of peripheral nerves. In Figure 42-2, an adjacent uninjured nerve serves as a pedicle graft. The dorsal cutaneous nerve, a branch of the ulnar nerve, may serve as a donor for a median nerve injured in the forearm. This procedure has not been of great value in our experience. On the other hand, the use of a full-thickness pedicle graft from the ulnar nerve to repair a median nerve when both nerves have been injured, has resulted in good sensory recovery. Figure 42-3 demonstrates this technique. The ulnar and median nerves are both cut back to normal appearing fascicles and are then sutured together. The gap in the injured median nerve is measured and the ulnar nerve is then transected this same distance proximal to the ulnar-median anastomosis. The ulnar nerve is not further dissected at this time, but rather the distal anastomosis is delayed for a 3-week period. This delay allows development of new vasculature to the pedicle graft and also gives time for wallerian degeneration to occur in the graft. By this same method the common peroneal nerve may be used to repair the tibial nerve.

A pedicle graft using a cutaneous forearm nerve may also be used to bridge a gap in the median nerve. In Figure 42-4, the lateral antebrachial cutaneous nerve serves as the donor. To accommodate the larger median nerve, a double strand of graft is used.

Another method of repairing injured nerves is illustrated by the nerve crossing procedure used in repairing the facial nerve. Figure 42-6 demonstrates a hypoglossal-facial nerve anastomosis in which the descendens hypoglossi is anastomosed to the distal hypoglossal nerve.

The results of peripheral nerve repair are dependent on many factors that have already been mentioned. Additional variables include the age of the patient and the site of the lesion. The younger the patient, the better the return of function will be. The more distal a nerve is injured, the more effective regeneration will be. The closer a lesion is to the nerve cell body, the more profound will be the effect on this trophic center. Sensory nerve cells are affected more by this retrograde phenomenon than are motor nerve cells.

The surgeon is often confronted with a patient whose injury is many months old. The question then arises as to whether surgical repair is still justified. From our experience it can be said that good results are commonly observed with repair of nerves after delays of 12 to 14 months. This in no way, however, should be construed as evidence that a much earlier repair is not preferable.

Operative Exposures

Brachial Plexus

Because the results of brachial plexus surgery have been disappointing, exploration should be delayed until spontaneous recovery has had a chance to occur. This implies a 3- to 6-month period of observation with electrical testing. The anatomy of the brachial plexus is reviewed in Figures 42-9 and 42-10.

In general, upper plexus lesions have a better prognosis than lower plexus injuries. This is obviously related to the distance from site of injury to the end organs. Current experience with brachial plexus injuries would indicate that perhaps our morbid outlook with regard to these lesions is no longer completely justified.

Ascertaining the clinical level of a brachial plexus lesion preoperatively is imperative since the entire plexus is not readily demonstrated with one operative exposure. For this reason the brachial plexus will be discussed under the following four surgical exposures: 1) supraclavicular (Figs. 42-11 and 42-12), 2) transclavicular (Figs. 42-13 and 42-14), 3) infraclavicular (Figs. 42-15 through 42-17), and 4) axillary (Figs. 42-18 and 42-19).

In all peripheral nerve surgery, the patient should be positioned and draped so that complete mobility of the extremity is available.

The *supraclavicular incision* is made with the patient in the supine position and the operating table flexed so that the patient almost assumes a semi-Fowler's position. This will place the site of the incision uppermost and will prevent stooping of the surgeon. The incision (Fig. 42-11) is about 6-cm long and is made parallel to and 2-cm above the clavicle. The medial extent of the incision extends over the clavicular head of the sternocleidomastoid muscle. This exposure through the base of the lateral triangle of the neck provides easy access to the upper trunks of the brachial plexus (Fig. 42-12). The platysma muscle is incised and branches of the external jugular system are ligated and divided as they pierce the superficial fascia. The areolar tissue overlaying the deep cervical fascia is separated to expose the inferior belly of the omohyoid muscle. This muscle, which runs transversely through the exposure, can be mobilized medially and downward to expose the transverse cervical and suprascapular arteries. It may be important to preserve these vessels especially in the face of an injured axillary artery since they may serve as an important collateral circulation. In Figure 42-12 the medial retractor displaces the sternocleidomastoid muscle and internal jugular vein to expose the anterior scalene muscle. The deep fascia must be incised along the lateral border of the anterior scalene muscle taking care not to injure the phrenic nerve which is embedded in this fascia. The phrenic nerve follows a course downward and medially on the anterior surface of the anterior scalene. The accessory nerve may be identified by bluntly dissecting upward along the lateral border of the sternocleidomastoid muscle until approximately half way up the muscle where an obstruction will be felt due to the nerve which leaves the lateral cervical triangle at that point to enter the muscle. Just beneath the lateral border of the anterior scalene muscle, the trunks of the brachial plexus can be identified. If additional proximal exposure is necessary, the anterior scalene muscle may be transected taking care to preserve the phrenic nerve. It is important to remember the steep angulation at which the lower trunk of the brachial plexus passes inferiorly and anteriorly. The lower trunk is normally kept in a posterior position by the free posterior border of Sibson's fascia. When the anterior scalene muscle is divided without dividing the free border of Sibson's fascia, angulation of the inferior trunk of the brachial plexus may result and produce additional neurological impairment. This relationship may be difficult to visualize in a traumatized brachial plexus but is readily appreciated in approaching this area for a cervical sympathectomy.

The transclavicular incision allows the most complete exposure of the brachial plexus (Fig. 42-13). The position of the patient is identical to that used in the supraclavicular exposure. The incision is made from the lateral border of the sternocleidomastoid across the lateral third of the clavicle and the pectoralis major muscle downward to the axilla just medial to the cephalic vein. The supraclavicular portion of the dissection has already been described. The clavicle is exposed by subperiosteal dissection taking care not to injure the neurovascular structures nearby. The clavicle is obliquely divided using a saw, and the bony ends are gently elevated. Dissection distal to the clavicle proceeds in the deltoid-pectoral groove parallel to the cephalic vein. The fibers of the pectoralis major muscle are separated to expose the cords of the brachial plexus as they pass diagonally into the axilla. The upper portion of the pectoralis minor muscle as well as the lateral half of the pectoralis major muscle may be retracted downward to gain added exposure (Fig. 42-14).

The infraclavicular incision is used to explore the lower third of the brachial plexus. The position of the patient is changed from the previous exposures only in that the arm is abducted approximately 90°. Beginning at the lateral third of the clavicle, the incision is made along the deltopectoral groove in the shape of a lazy reversed *S* to end at the anterior axillary line (Fig. 42-15). The anterior thoracic nerves which cross the operative field in a vertical direction are identified and protected during the exposure of the superficial fascia. The cephalic vein is also identified and retracted superiorly. The fibers of the pectoralis major muscle are separated to expose the deep fascia covering the cords of the brachial plexus. Once again care must be taken to preserve the anterior thoracic nerves. If the deep fascia is opened in a vertical direction, the chance of injuring these nerves is minimized. The pectoralis minor is either retracted medially or transected at its insertion into the coracoid process (Figs. 42-16 and 42-17). Immediately beneath the pectoralis minor muscle, covered only by a very thin fascia, are the lateral, medial, and posterior cords of the brachial plexus. The axillary artery at this level is between the medial and lateral cords and in front of the posterior cord.

The *transverse axillary incision* (Fig. 42-18) is used to expose the cords of the brachial plexus and the nerves arising from them. The patient is placed on the operating table in the supine position and the upper extremity is abducted 135°. The incision is made through an axillary skin flexion crease. Figure 42-19 demonstrates the anatomical relationships after the fascia has been opened and the pectoralis major and latissimus dorsi muscles have been retracted. The posterior cord and radial nerves are located immediately behind the axillary artery. In dissection of these nerves, it must be remembered that the motor branches to the long and lateral heads of the triceps muscle leave the radial nerve high in the axilla. Preservation of these branches can be most difficult if the radial nerve is encased in scar tissue. Figure 42-19 also illustrates the thoracodorsal nerve and other branches of the posterior cord of the brachial plexus. The thoracodorsal nerve is surrounded by lymphatics and is easily damaged inadvertently resulting in paralysis of the latissimus dorsi muscle. Also located behind the brachial plexus in these same lymphatics is the long thoracic nerve as it passes medially and inferiorly on the surface of the serratus anterior muscle. Unexpected winging of the scapula is seen all too frequently following axillary surgical procedures if this nerve is not identified and protected as it always should be.

Axillary Nerve

The axillary nerve arises from the posterior cord of the brachial plexus in the axilla (Fig. 42-16) and passes through the quadrangular space accompanied by the posterior circumflex humeral artery (Fig. 42-19). The nerve lies deep to the deltoid muscle and passes between the teres major and minor muscles. The most frequent isolated injury of this nerve is seen with inferior dislocations of the shoulder or fractures of the surgical head of the humerus, which result in stretch injury of the nerve. The conservative treatment of such a nerve injury is splinting of the upper extremity in abduction. If surgical exploration becomes necessary, the patient is placed on the operating table in the supine position with the arm placed against the chest wall (Fig. 42-20). A skin incision is made along the posterior margin of the deltoid muscle. The nerve is located on the inferior surface of the deltoid muscle where it lies between the teres major and minor muscles. If a neurorrhaphy is performed, the shoulder joint is immobilized with the arm abducted. Surgical results have been gratifying, but return of function may require 6 to 7 months.

Musculocutaneous Nerve

The transaxillary incision (Fig. 42-18) may also be used to expose the musculocutaneous nerve. This nerve is the continuation of the lateral cord of the brachial plexus after its contribution to the median nerve is given off. In exposing the musculocutaneous nerve surgically (Fig. 42-19), it can most easily be located by following the median nerve proximally. Close to its origin this nerve gives off one or two branches to the coracobrachialis muscle, and these branches may be easily injured if dissection is not begun high enough in the axilla. The nerve pierces the coracobrachialis muscle only a few centimeters later and then descends in the arm between the biceps and brachialis muscles.

Radial Nerve

The surgical exposure of the radial nerve as it emerges from the posterior cord of the brachial plexus has been described in the section on brachial plexus surgery (Figs. 42-18 and 42-19).

The radial nerve is exceptionally prone to injury at the point where it passes around the lateral aspect of the humerus and through the lateral intermuscular septum. The radial nerve in the arm is exposed by an incision along the posterolateral aspect of the arm (Fig. 42-20). The patient is supine on the operating table with the arm adducted at the shoulder and flexed at the elbow. The incision is made from the level of the neck of the humerus along the posterior border of the deltoid muscle to just above the lateral epicondyle at the elbow. The brachial fascia is opened over the entire length of the wound. The plane between the long and lateral heads of the triceps muscle can be easily palpated and dissection is carried out in this direction. These muscles are separated by blunt dissection to expose the radial nerve and the radial collateral artery (Fig. 42-21), which actually lies deep to the long head of the triceps muscle in a groove in the humerus between the lateral and medial heads of this muscle. As the nerve reaches the distal third of the humerus, it pierces the lateral intermuscular septum and runs between the brachialis and brachioradialis muscles (Fig. 42-22) across the front of the lateral epicondyle. In this area the nerve should be approached from the medial side to preserve the motor branches to the supracondylar muscles. In retracting the long head of the triceps muscle, as depicted in Figure 42-21, it must be remembered that the ulnar nerve is located just beneath this muscle. External rotation of the arm greatly facilitates mobilization of the radial nerve in the supracondylar region.

To expose the radial nerve from the supracondylar region distally the arm must be extended and externally rotated. A skin incision is made beginning 6 cm above the elbow along the anterior margin of the brachioradialis muscle and continuing into the forearm along the extensor carpi radialis muscle (Fig. 42-23). Proximally the nerve is located between the brachioradialis muscle laterally and the biceps and brachialis muscles medially as illustrated in Figure 42-25. In this interval at the level of the elbow, the radial nerve divides into its terminal branches, the superficial and deep radial nerves. Distal to the elbow these branches of the radial nerve are located by blunt dissection between the brachioradialis and extensor carpi radialis muscles. The superficial radial nerve is purely a cutaneous nerve. It descends in the forearm immediately under the brachioradialis and must, therefore, be protected when retracting this muscle. The deep radial nerve (dorsal interosseous nerve) is the larger terminal division of the radial nerve.

The deep radial nerve passes through the supinator muscle as it winds its way around the lateral side of the radius. In fractures of the radius this is a common site for injury to this nerve. The skin incision for exposure of this nerve is made along the extensor carpi radialis muscle (see Fig. 42-26). Dissection is carried out between the extensor carpi radialis brevis and the extensor digitorum muscles (Figs. 42-24, 42-25, and 42-27). Separating these muscles exposes the underlying supinator and abductor pollicis longus muscles. The nerve is identified as it emerges from the supinator muscle. If the nerve has to be followed proximally, the fibers of the supinator muscle must be incised. This incision must always be parallel to the course of the nerve. Distally as the nerve reaches the dorsum of the forearm it divides into many small branches, making surgical repair extremely difficult.

Median Nerve

The median nerve is the most important nerve of the upper extremity; this has been emphasized by using it as an example in discussing nerve grafting (Figs. 42-2 to 42-4) and mobilization of peripheral nerves (Figs. 42-7 and 42-8). In dealing with median nerve lesions, remember that without it the hand is useless.

In exposure of the median nerve in the upper arm, the patient is placed on the operating table in the supine position with the arm abducted to 90° and externally rotated so that the upper extremity lies straight (Fig. 42-28 and 42-29). An incision is made from the axilla to just above the medial epicondyle in the median bicipital groove directly over the neurovascular bundle. In the antecubital fossa the incision is made transversely along a skin flexion crease to the margin of the brachioradialis muscle. To expose the median nerve in the forearm, the incision is carried diagonally across the ventral surface from the medial border of the brachioradialis muscle at the elbow to the ulnar side of the wrist. The skin incision at the wrist follows a transverse skin flexion crease and then extends into the palm along the flexor crease at the base of the thenar eminence. These incisions may be used individually or in combination for exposure of the median nerve.

To expose the median nerve in the arm, an incision is made in the skin over the medial bicipital groove. Having retracted the skin margins, the neurovascular bundle is easily palpable. The deep fascia is incised longitudinally over the coracobrachialis muscle. Retracting this muscle laterally will allow exposure of the nerves and brachial artery (Fig. 42-28); however, in retracting the coracobrachialis muscle, one must always be cognizant of the course of the musculocutaneous nerve (Figs. 42-17 and 42-19). The median nerve from its origin in the axilla to the antecubital fossa has an intimate relationship with the axillary and brachial arteries. In the axilla, the nerve lies at the anterolateral aspect of the artery. The median nerve then diagonally crosses the artery in its course through the arm to assume a position medial to the artery at the elbow (Fig. 42-30). The ulnar nerve lies just medial to the artery and median nerve in the upper arm as far as the insertion of the coracobrachialis, where it pierces the posterior layer of the intermuscular septum and passes posteriomedially toward the medial epicondyle. Also in close proximity to the median nerve in the upper arm are the medial brachial cutaneous and medial antebrachial cutaneous nerves. These nerves lie medial to the median nerve as far as the level of the insertion of the coracobrachialis muscle where they pierce the deep fascia to become subcutaneous. Having reviewed the close relationship of all these structures within the neurovascular bundle, it is easy to understand why missile wounds so often result in injury to more than one structure.

In exposing the median nerve at the elbow, a Z-shaped incision is made beginning 5 to 7 cm above the medial epicondyle and then following a flexion crease transversely across the antecubital fossa to the margin of the brachioradialis muscle, where it is continued distally along the medial margin of this muscle (Figs. 42-29 and 42-31). Taking care to preserve the medial and lateral antebrachial cutaneous nerves, the skin margins are undermined and widely retracted (Fig. 42-32). The fascia is incised longitudinally and the lacertus fibrosus (bicipital aponeurosis) is transected as shown in Figs. 42-33 and 42-34. Thus, the median nerve and brachial artery are exposed on the brachialis muscle as they pass into the antecubital fossa medial to the bicipital tendon. Branches of the nerve to the pronator teres muscle must be carefully identified and protected. Having crossed the antecubital fossa, the nerve disappears between the two heads of the pronator teres muscle, which is a possible site for entrapment of this nerve ("honeymoon paralysis"). Just above the upper margin of this muscle, the brachial artery divides into the radial and ulnar arteries.

Exposure of the median nerve in the forearm requires a longitudinal incision along the volar aspect of the forearm (Fig. 42-29). The nerve after passing between the two heads of the pronator teres muscle proceeds under the tendinous arch of the flexor digitorum superficialis muscle and descends through the middle of the forearm adherent to the fascia on the underside of this muscle. Dissection is carried out between the pronator teres and the flexor carpi radialis muscles (Fig. 42-35) and the fibers of the flexor digitorum superficialis muscle are separated to expose the nerve immediately beneath it. Small short muscular branches to this muscle must be kept in mind when mobilizing the median nerve in the forearm (Figs. 42-7, 42-8, and 42-35). A great deal of additional mobility of the nerve can be attained by division of the pronator teres muscle (Fig. 42-7), allowing superficial transposition of the nerve.

The median nerve at the wrist is most often exposed in the treatment of carpal tunnel syndrome. A transverse skin incision over a flexion crease of the nerve is made under local anesthesia (Fig. 42-36). The thin superficial fascia is divided to expose the transverse carpal ligaments (flexor retinaculum). The ligament is incised parallel to the median nerve and perpendicular to the fibers of the ligament (Fig. 42-37). It is of utmost importance that the ligament is transected in its entire width (Fig. 42-36). The median nerve is superficial to the flexor tendons in the carpal tunnel. An external neurolysis is not indicated in the treatment of the carpal tunnel syndrome because the entrapment is relieved by section of the transverse carpal ligament. Therefore, it is not necessary to dissect out the nerve as long as the incision of the ligament is done on the ulnar half of the wrist.

Surgical exposure of the median nerve in the palm is performed through an *S*-shaped incision illustrated in Figures 42-29 and 42-38. The superficial fascia and the transverse carpal ligament are opened, permitting wide retraction of the skin flaps (Fig. 42-39). At the distal border of the transverse carpal ligament, a large branch leaves the radial side of the median nerve and curves sharply into the muscles of the thenar eminence. This is the motor branch of the median nerve (recurrent thenar branch), and it represents the only hazard to exposure of the median nerve in the hand. Having given off its motor branch, the median nerve then divides into three common palmar digital nerves (Fig. 42-40). The ulnar nerve may be exposed by this same incision. In dissection at the ulnar side of the wrist it is crucial to remember that although the ulnar nerve is deep to the volar carpal ligament and the palmaris brevis muscle, it is superficial to the transverse carpal ligament.

The median and ulnar nerves at the wrist and hand are exposed using a slightly different skin incision in Figures 42-41 and 42-42.

Ulnar Nerve

Exposure of the ulnar nerve as it arises from the medial cord of the brachial plexus is gained by the previously described transaxillary approach (Figs. 42-18 and 42-19). The operative approach to the ulnar nerve in the arm has also been discussed in the section on the median nerve (Figs. 42-29 and 42-30) since these nerves share a common fascial compartment in the upper arm. It must be remembered, however, that the ulnar nerve leaves the neurovascular bundle, at the level of the insertion of the coracobrachialis muscle passing posteriorly to lie on the medial head of the triceps muscle on its way toward the medial epicondyle. Having left the neurovascular bundle the nerve is covered only by the deep fascia. The ulnar nerve has no branches in the arm until just above the medial epicondyle where several fine articular branches leave the nerve. The nerve then passes the back of the elbow between the olecranon and the medial epicondyle of the humerus. The ulnar nerve in the arm is accompanied by the superior ulnar collateral branch of the brachial artery, the ulnar collateral branch of the radial nerve, and the ulnar collateral veins.

Preserving this vascular accompaniment is usually the only difficulty in the dissection of the ulnar nerve in the arm.

Anterior transposition of the ulnar nerve at the elbow is a very common neurosurgical exercise. This operation is done either for a tardy ulnar palsy or to gain additional length in performing a neurorrhaphy. The arm is positioned in extension and is externally rotated

(Fig. 42-43). An incision is made from the medial bicipital groove 10 cm above the medial epicondyle to the lateral surface of the flexor carpi ulnaris muscle of the forearm in a lazy S-shaped curve. An incision behind the medial epicondyle should be avoided because this is a common pressure point. The deep fascia is initially opened proximally and the nerve identified. The deep fascia is then incised following the course of the nerve over the entire length of the skin incision (Fig. 42-44). The secret to a successful transposition of the ulnar nerve lies in the management of the dissection at the two extremes of the wound. Dissection proximally must be carried as high as the insertion of the coracobrachialis muscle where the ulnar nerve leaves the neurovascular bundle to be certain that the nerve is transposed anteriorly and not angulated over the firm intermuscular septum. Distally the nerve must be mobilized between the two heads of the flexor carpi ulnaris muscle (Fig. 42-45). The fibrous arch between these two parts of the muscle must be completely divided so that when the nerve is anteriorly transposed, no angulation will occur. Having completed these two crucial steps, the remaining mobilization of the nerve is simply done. Muscular branches to the flexor carpi ulnaris muscle should be preserved, and stripping of these branches from the parent nerve easily provides enough mobility so that the nerve can be transposed without any tension. A few sutures in the antecubital fascia over the nerve will secure its new position anterior to the medial epicondyle.

The forearm incision for exposure of the ulnar nerve is made along the flexor carpi ulnaris muscle (Fig. 42-43). The course of the ulnar nerve in the forearm can be traced by drawing a straight line between the medial epicondyle of the humerus and the lateral edge of the pisiform bone at the wrist. The deep fascia is incised along the lateral border of the flexor carpi ulnaris muscle, and this muscle is bluntly dissected from the flexor digitorum superficialis muscle laterally and the flexor digitorum profundus muscle below. The nerve is exposed lying on the anterior surface of the flexor digitorum muscle (Figs. 42-46 and 42-47). At the mid forearm level, the nerve is joined by the ulnar artery, which assumes a position on the lateral side of the nerve. Figure 42-46 also illustrates muscular branches of the nerve which supply the flexor carpi ulnaris and the ulnar portion of the flexor digitorum profundus muscles and the dorsal cutaneous branch, which leaves the nerve in the distal third of the forearm, to supply sensation to the ulnar side of the back of the hand. In the distal third of the forearm the ulnar nerve emerges at the radial side of the flexor carpi ulnaris tendon and is covered only by the antebrachial fascia. This superficial position of the nerve at the wrist makes it vulnerable to injury, particularly by laceration.

To expose the ulnar nerve at the wrist a curvalinear incision is made beginning at the base of the hypothenar compartment, curving medially at the wrist to avoid cutting across flexion creases and then continuing into the forearm along the radial side of the flexor carpi ulnaris tendon (Fig. 42-48). The ulnar nerve is identified proximally just beneath the antebrachial fascia and dissection then proceeds distally. The volar carpal ligament (palmar carpal ligament) and the palmaris brevis muscle are incised as the ulnar nerve is followed in its course past the radial side of the pisiform bone (Fig. 42-49). Once again it must be emphasized that the ulnar nerve is superficial to the transverse carpal ligament (flexor retinaculum) as it crosses the wrist to enter the palm. Along the radial aspect of the pisiform bone the ulnar nerve divides into its terminal branches to the hand, the superficial and deep branches.

Obturator Nerve

The obturator nerve is rarely injured by missile wounds, but it may be damaged by a fracture of the superior ramus of the pubis. It may be compressed against the bony pelvis by a tumor or, during pregnancy, by the fetal head. Certainly the commonest reason for exposing this nerve is in the treatment of adductor spasm or intractable hip pain. Having mentioned obturator neurectomy for intractable hip pain, a word of caution is in order. Because the obturator nerve supplies sensory branches to the hip joint, this procedure does give relief of pain in such conditions as chronic arthritis; however, one must be certain of the diagnosis since an irritative lesion of the nerve in the pelvis can give pain in the identical distribution.

Only the exposure at the obturator foramen is described here. A transabdominal extraperitoneal approach is used. A 6-cm incision is made 4 cm above and parallel to the inguinal ligament (see Fig. 42-52). A muscle-splitting incision is made through the abdominal muscles to expose the preperitoneal fat. Obviously, this approach must be made with the urinary bladder empty. An index finger is inserted through the abdominal wall and then directed inferiorly in the preperitoneal space (Figs. 42-53 and 42-54). The pulsations of the external iliac artery are easily identified signifying that the probing finger is beneath the inguinal ligament. The bony rim of the superior pelvic ramus cannot be missed, and immediately below it the internal aperture of the obturator canal is palpable with its characteristic groove and medial half-moon shaped rim (Fig. 42-54). A sponge stick is inserted over the finger and used to retract the peritoneum posteriorly. The nerve can then be visualized. It is elevated with a blunt nerve hook and sectioned. The surgical principle of cutting only what is clearly visualized is of utmost importance in this procedure because, as Figure 42-54 illustrates, many nearby structures could easily be injured.

Lateral Femoral Cutaneous Nerve

Meralgia paresthetica is a syndrome consisting of paresthesias, pain, and sensory loss over the anterolateral surface of the thigh. This affliction of the lateral femoral cutaneous nerve is often caused by entrapment of the nerve at the level of the inguinal ligament. The lateral femoral cutaneous nerve arises from the posterior branches of the second and third lumbar nerves along the lateral border of the psoas muscle. It crosses the iliacus muscle and passes into the thigh immediately beneath the lateral extent of the inguinal ligament at the anterior superior spine of the ilium. Once again it must be emphasized that more proximal lesions of the nerve must be distinguished before treatment is undertaken. Lesions of the ilium, cecum or sigmoid colon may compress the nerve at the level of the psoas muscle. A herniated intervertebral disk at Ll-2, or L2-3, will occasionally cause symptoms indistinguishable from meralgia paresthetica. Therefore, prior to surgical treatment of this syndrome, a nerve block using local anesthetics is indicated. The needle is inserted one finger breadth medial to and below the anterior superior iliac spine. Ten cubic centimeters of a 1% solution are sufficient. Most unsuccessful attempts are the result of inserting the anesthetic too deeply.

The operative exposure of the lateral femoral cutaneous nerve is made under local anesthesia. A three cm incision immediately beneath the lateral extent of the inguinal ligament (Fig. 42-55) is carried down to the fascia lata which is incised in the same direction (Fig. 42-57). By retracting the fascia lata the nerve can be identified by blunt dissection as it passes just medial to the anterior superior iliac spine (Fig. 42-58). Actually the nerve passes through a triangle in most instances which has as its borders the inguinal ligament anterosuperiorly, the bone laterally and the attachment of the iliacus fascia to the inguinal ligament inferiorly. Having exposed the nerve it can be pulled downward and transected (Fig. 42-58) or transposed medially by incising the shelving border of the inguinal ligament (Fig. 42-59). This latter procedure gives the nerve a more direct course, as can be appreciated from Figure 42-56, and removes the nerve from its bony boundary by the ilium.

Femoral Nerve

The femoral nerve, formed by the posterior divisions of the second, third and fourth lumbar nerves, is the largest branch of the lumbar plexus. Passing inferiorly in a groove formed by the adjacent psoas and iliacus muscles, it is joined by the external iliac artery (Fig. 42-54). Together they pass beneath the inguinal ligament into the femoral triangle. At this level the external iliac artery becomes the femoral artery, and it is separated from the laterally situated femoral nerve by psoas muscle fibers and the iliacus fascia (Fig. 42-62).

In the pelvis the femoral nerve is exposed by the transabdominal retroperitoneal approach described for the obturator nerve (Figs. 42-53 and 42-54).

The femoral nerve in the thigh is approached through a vertical incision which is made beginning at the mid portion of the inguinal ligament and continued inferiorly along the medial border of the sartorius muscle (Fig. 42-60). Camper's fascia is incised and retracted widely. A *T*-shaped incision is made into the fascia lata and the falciform margin of the fossa ovalis, as shown in Figure 42-61. The fascia lata incision is parallel to the medial margin of the sartorius muscle. On retracting the incised fascia, the femoral artery and vein and deep inguinal lymph nodes become visible. Figure 42-62 illustrates these structures without showing the femoral sheath. The artery is then gently retracted medially and a vertical incision is made into the iliacus fascia (deep layer of the fascia lata) to expose the femoral nerve in its groove between the iliacus and psoas muscles (Fig. 42-62). Three to 5 cm below the inguinal ligament the nerve divides into terminal muscular, articular and sensory branches.

Sciatic Nerve

The sciatic nerve is actually two nerves contained within a common connective tissue sheath—the common peroneal and the tibial nerves. This large mass of nerve fibers arises from spinal cord segments L4 to S3. The tibial division is formed from the anterior division of the entire series of nerve roots, and the common peroneal is formed from the posterior branches of nerves L4 through S2. Occasionally the separate identity of the two nerves is clear throughout the thigh. The tibial division is the medial part of the sciatic nerve; the common peroneal is lateral in the nerve. The sciatic nerve leaves the pelvis through the lower part of the greater sciatic foramen and extends straight down the thigh until its two parts bifurcate at the level of the distal one-third of the femur.

The sciatic nerve roots are exposed to possible traumatic injury as they pass over the ala of the sacrum in direct contact with it. Since the common peroneal nerve arises from the posterior divisions of the rootlets, it is not surprising that trauma in this area results in a selective injury to this nerve. The sciatic nerve roots are separated from the hollow of the sacrum only by the piriformis muscle. For this reason it must be emphasized that a complete rectal examination should be performed on any patient who has symptoms suggesting sciatic nerve pathology.

Operative treatment of sciatic nerve lesions in the gluteal region usually yields disappointing results. This, as has been shown by Sunderland, is due to the large number of small fascicles which are separated by large amounts of epineural connective tissue and due to the relatively long distance from target organs of many of the fascicles. Even though the prognosis is not good, lesions at this level should have the benefit of surgical exploration. Because of the long delay in spontaneous recovery of function following axonotemesis or neuronotemesis, early exploration of these injuries is indicated.

The exposure of the sciatic notch is performed with the patient prone by making a curvalinear incision from above the greater trochanter to the insertion of the gluteus maximus muscle at the mid thigh (Fig. 42-63). After opening the fascia, the gluteus maximus muscle is transected close to its insertion into the iliotibial band of the fascia lata (Fig. 42-64). The gluteus maximus is then hinged medially to expose the sciatic nerve beneath the piriformis muscle as it leaves the pelvis (Fig. 42-65). The surgeon should be aware that anatomical variations in the relationship of the nerve to the piriformis muscle are not uncommon. The piriformis muscle occasionally passes between the two divisions of the nerve. Rarely the entire sciatic nerve will pass over the piriformis muscle. These anatomic variants may constrict the nerve and result in irritative symptoms. The surgeon must be aware that important vascular contributions are made to the sciatic nerve at the level of the notch from the inferior gluteal artery and lower in the thigh from many perforating branches of the deep femoral artery.

In the thigh, the sciatic nerve is exposed through a vertical midline incision which is curved laterally at the gluteal fold and medially at the popliteal fossa (Fig. 42-66). The fascia must be carefully opened and gently retracted to avoid injury to the posterior femoral cutaneous nerve which is located immediately beneath the fascia. The cleft between the semitendinosis and biceps femoris muscles is opened to expose the sciatic nerve deep within this groove (Fig. 42-67). In this dissection, care must be taken to avoid injuring small muscular branches to the hamstring muscles. To overcome a gap in the sciatic nerve, additional length may be obtained by extending the thigh at the hip and flexing the leg at the knee. As previously mentioned, the leg must not be flexed greater than 90° at the knee, and after the cast is removed the leg must be very gradually straightened. The common peroneal nerve is especially sensitive to stretch injury because, as Sunderland points out, it has more small fascicles and less adipose tissue in the epineurium than the tibial nerve. An additional difference in these two nerve components is that the common peroneal nerve has an angular course and is fixed not only at the fibular head but also at the sciatic notch. Many excellent surgical repairs of this nerve have resulted in no functional recovery because of postoperative stretch injuries.

The sciatic nerve usually bifurcates at the lower one-third of the thigh as it enters the popliteal space; however, occasionally the separate identity of the tibial and common peroneal nerves is maintained throughout the thigh. At the popliteal space these nerves separate, and the common peroneal nerve follows the tendon of the biceps femoris muscle to wind around the head of the fibula, whereas the tibial nerve continues the straight course of the sciatic nerve vertically through the popliteal space.

To expose the bifurcation of the sciatic nerve as well as the common peroneal and tibial nerves within the popliteal fossa, a Z-shaped incision is made (Fig. 42-68). The horizontal limb of the incision crosses the popliteal space transversely along a flexion crease. The proximal extension is made upward parallel to the hamstring tendons. The distal limb curves downward along the fibula. Figure 42-69 illustrates the fascial exposure after retracting the skin margins. The popliteal fascia is incised vertically taking care once again to preserve the posterior femoral cutaneous nerve. The biceps femoris muscle is separated from the semitendinosus and semimembranosus tendons at the superior extent of the incision. The common peroneal nerve is identified as it follows along the medial margin of the biceps femoris muscle (Fig. 42-70) and followed distally to the neck of the fibula. This dissection is carried out on the lateral surface of the nerve to avoid injury to the lateral sural nerve which leaves its medial aspect within the popliteal space and to muscular and articular branches which leave at the level of the head of the fibula. The tibial nerve is identified in the midline lateral as well as posterior to the popliteal artery and vein. In dissection of the tibial nerve in the popliteal space, articular, muscular and the medial sural branches must be preserved. Within the popliteal space both the common peroneal and tibial nerves receive nutrient arteries from the popliteal artery, the tibial nerve, which is closely approximated to the artery, by small perforating vessels and the common peroneal nerve from more laterally placed genicular and muscular branches.

Common Peroneal Nerve

Having followed the biceps femoris tendon through the popliteal space to the back of the head of the fibula, the common peroneal nerve enters the leg by turning forward around the neck of the fibula beneath the uppermost fibers of the peroneus longus muscle, where it divides into its superficial and deep branches. The anatomical relationship of this nerve in this area cannot be overemphasized because this site requires the most frequent surgical exposure of a peripheral nerve in the lower extremity. The vulnerability of the common peroneal nerve to stretch injury has already been emphasized. Its superficial position while held against a bony structure makes it a frequent victim of direct trauma. Not only is the nerve easily compressed in this area but its nutrient vessels may also be compromised leading to ischemic damage to the nerve.

Exposure of the common peroneal nerve at the fibular head requires a complete knowledge of the anatomy of the popliteal space, since the nerve often has to be exposed as far proximally as the sciatic bifurcation. The surgical incision demonstrated in Figure 42-71 represents an inferior extension of the popliteal fossa incision shown in Figure 42-68, and these two incisions often must be used together. After incising the fascia the nerve is identified at the level of the fibular head. The nerve is followed distally as it penetrates the peroneus longus muscle, then passes between the superficial and deep heads of this muscle and, at this point, divides into its superficial and deep branches (Fig. 42-72). The superficial head of the muscle may have to be partially reflected to expose the bifurcation of the nerve. The common peroneal nerve is securely fixed during its course below the head of the fibula even before entering the peroneus longus muscle by the deep fascia which attaches to the fibula. This means that additional length cannot be gained in this nerve by mobilization distally. Gaps in the common peroneal nerve must be made up by proximal mobilization of the nerve and flexion of the knee joint.

Deep Peroneal Nerve

The deep peroneal nerve continues the forward and downward course of the common peroneal nerve, passing through the upper part of the origin of the extensor digitorum longus muscle to the lateral border of the tibialis muscle. At this point in the anterior compartment of the leg, it takes up a position along the lateral aspect of the anterior tibial artery and descends with it to the ankle.

In addition to direct injuries, this nerve is not infrequently involved in an ischemic nerve lesion—the "anterior tibial syndrome"—particularly in the military. This syndrome is characterized by severe pain, swelling and discoloration over the anterior compartment of the leg after strenuous activity. Neurologically there is a foot drop and loss of sensation over the first interdigital space. The treatment of this condition is to enlarge the osseo-fascial compartment and relieve obstructed circulation by surgical incision.

The skin incision for the operative exposure of the deep peroneal nerve is shown in Figure 42-73. The incision is made parallel to the palpable tibialis anterior muscle. Having incised the crural fascia, dissection is carried between the tibialis anterior and the extensor hallucis longus tendons to expose the deep peroneal nerve lateral to the anterior tibial artery and vein (Fig. 42-74).

Tibial Nerve

The anatomy and surgical exposure of the tibial nerve within the popliteal fossa have been described with the sciatic nerve. Leaving the popliteal area, the nerve passes under the tendinous arch of the soleus muscle and descends immediately beneath the transverse intermuscular septum, where it overlies the tibialis posterior muscle as it proceeds toward the medial malleolus.

The tibial nerve in the leg is exposed by an incision along the medial border of the gastrocnemius and soleus muscles (Fig. 42-75). A posterior midline muscle-splitting incision is contraindicated. The fan-like arrangement of the muscles prevents separation of the fibers without extensive destruction of muscle tissue. The crural fascia is incised parallel to the skin incision. The medial border of the gastrocnemius muscle is retracted to reveal the popliteus and soleus muscles. It is necessary to go through some fibers of the soleus muscle medially to expose the transverse intermuscular septum. This fascial layer is then opened vertically to expose the tibial nerve and the tibial artery on its medial border (Fig. 42-76). To obtain additional proximal exposure, the soleus muscle may be mobilized from the popliteus muscle. However, it must be remembered that the popliteus muscle while crossing over the soleus muscle passes under the tibial nerve.

Exposure of the distal tibial nerve at the ankle may be indicated for laceration, painful neuroma, or external compression of the nerve. Entrapment of this nerve causes a painful condition analogous to the carpal tunnel syndrome. It is relieved by incision of the retinaculum over the tibial nerve. The skin incision follows the course of the flexor digitorum longus tendon posterior to the medial malleolus and curves anteriorly over the medial surface of the navicular bone (Fig. 42-77). This incision must stay well above the sole of the foot. The fascia and flexor retinaculum are incised parallel to the skin incision (Fig. 42-78) to expose the tibial nerve and posterior tibial vessels. The nerve and vessels enter the foot by passing deep to the origin of the abductor hallucis muscle and, under that muscle, divide into medial plantar and lateral plantar nerves and vessels. By retracting the flexor digitorum longus tendon dorsally and the abductor hallucis and flexor digitorum brevis muscles plantarward, these structures are easily seen and can be dissected well into the sole of the foot (Fig. 42-79). Following repair of the tibial nerve at the ankle, sensory return has been quite rewarding, but reinnervation of intrinsic foot muscles is a rare event.

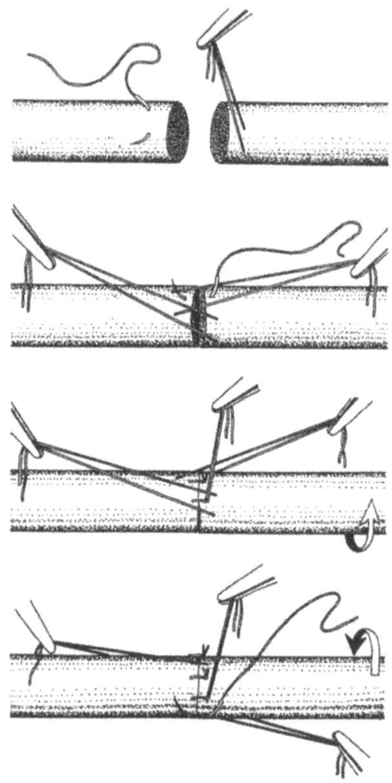

Figure 42-1. Technique of nerve suture. A, Tension sutures are placed into the epineurium to approximate the nerve ends during the anastomosis and to aid in proper alignment. B, Traction and tension sutures apposes the nerve ends. The anastomosis is done with 5-0 to 8-0 nylon or silk depending on the size of the injured nerve. C and D, Rotation of the tension sutures permit completion of the suture line.

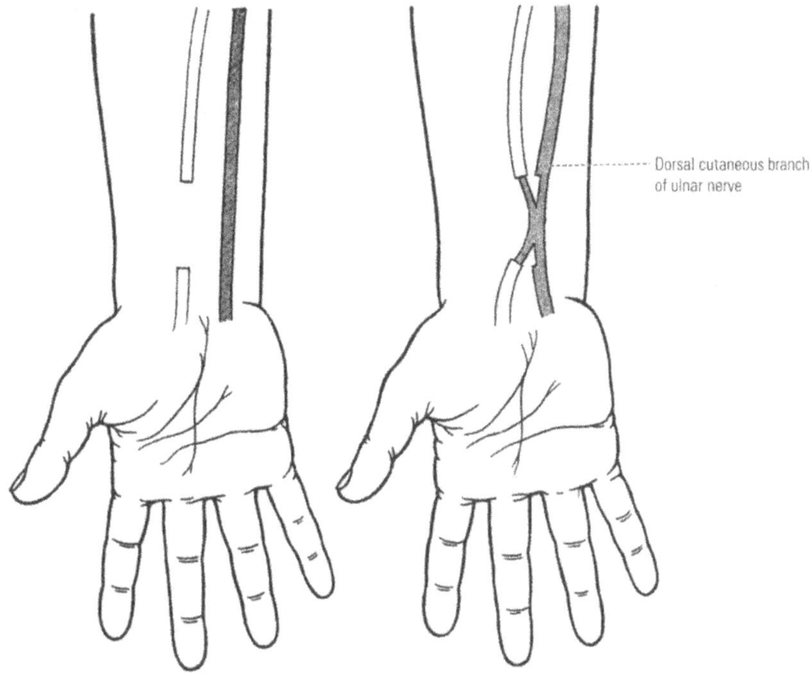

Figure 42-2. Methods of bridging gaps: lateral pedicle grafting from adjacent normal nerve. *Observe*: Cutaneous nerves provide the most readily available donors. In this instance, the dorsal cutaneous branch of the ulnar nerve is used to repair a defect in the median nerve.

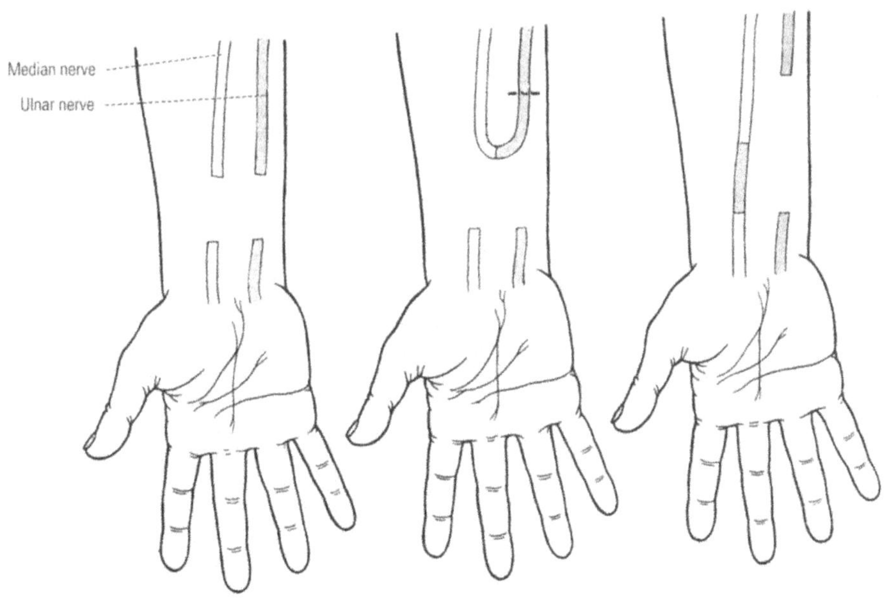

Figure 42-3. Full-thickness pedicle grafting from an adjacent injured nerve. *Observe*: 1. In this example both the ulnar and median nerves have been damaged to the extent that neither are reparable by the end-to-end anastomosis. 2. The ulnar nerve is sacrificed in favor of the median nerve because of their respective sensory and motor distributions. 3. The proximal stump of the ulnar nerve is used as a full-thinkness pedicle graft.

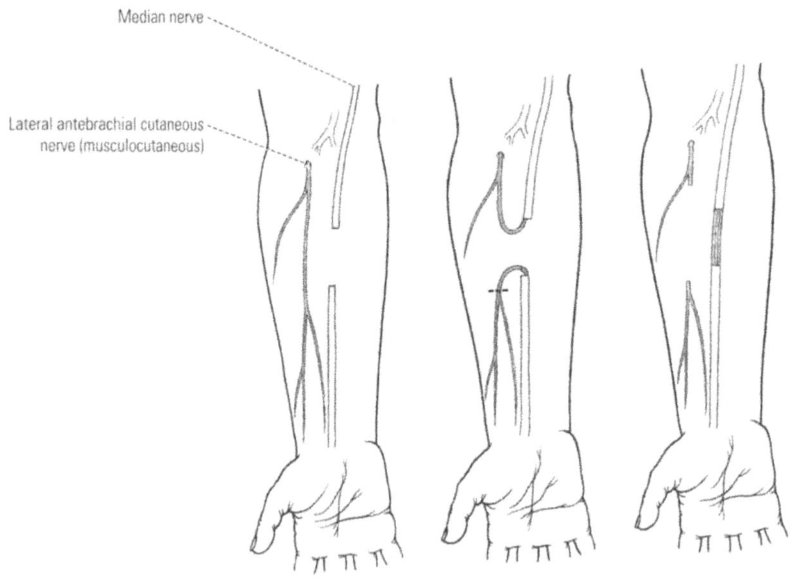

Figure 42-4. Full-thickness pedicle grafting from an adjacent normal nerve. Observe: A less important uninjured nerve, *ie,* the lateral antebrachial cutaneous nerve, is sacrificed. The donor nerve is divided at the level of the gap. These ends are then sutured into the proximal and distal stumps of the injured nerve, i.e. the median nerve. A length of graft is taken both distally and proximally from the donor nerve and fashioned into a cable graft.

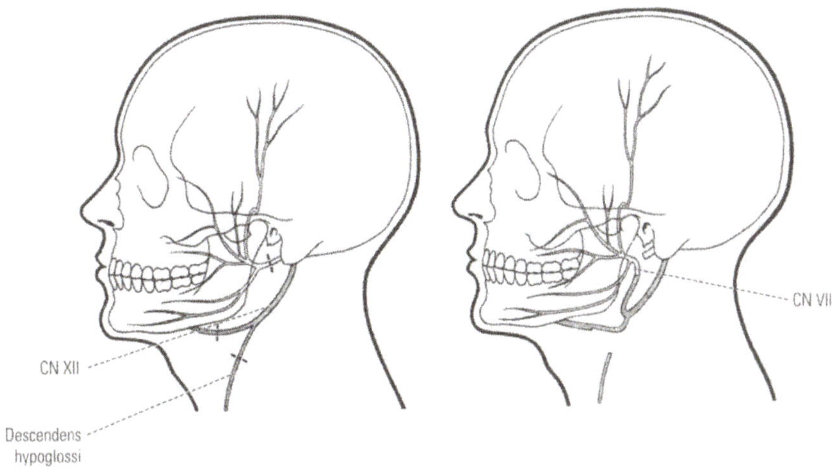

Figure 42-5. Full-thickness nerve crossing graft as in facial-hypoglossal anastomosis. *Observe*: Not only is the hypoglossal nerve anastomosed to the distal facial stump, but the descendens hypoglossi is sutured to the distal hypoglossal nerve.

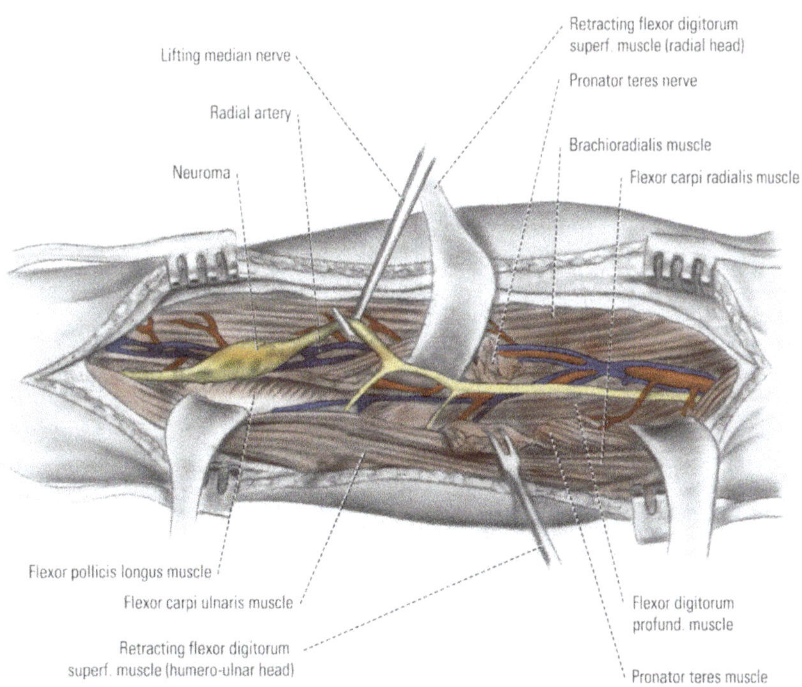

Figure 42-6. Mobilization. The median nerve in the forearm serves as an example to illustrate this method. *Observe*: 1. The median nerve is freed throughout its course in the forearm. 2. The pronator teres muscle is divided without injury to its innervation. 3. The flexor digitorum superficialis muscle is divided at the fibrous arch between the humeral and radial heads. 4. The lacertus fibrosus is incised parallel to the pronator teres muscle and retracted with the skin.

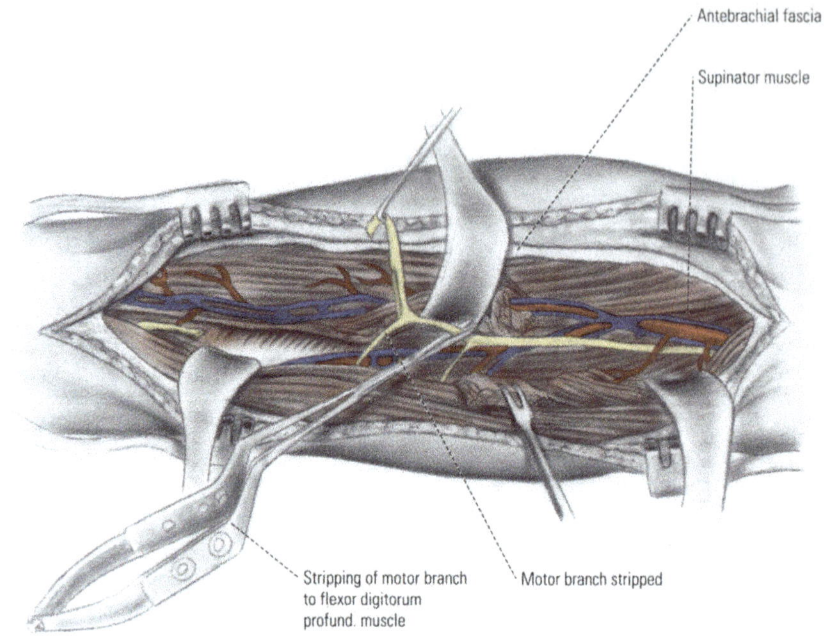

Figure 42-7. **Stripping of the branches mobilizes the nerve from its muscular bed. Stripping is always done under magnification to prevent fascicular damage and to preserve the longitudinal blood supply.**

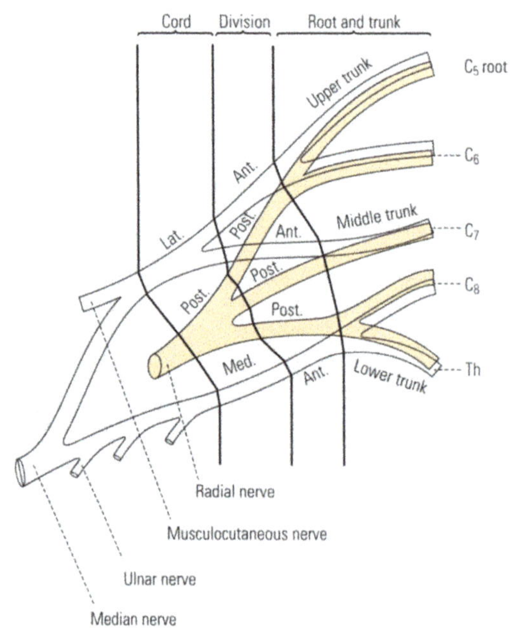

Figure 42-8. **The brachial plexus. This illustration delineates the areas of the roots, trunks, divisions, and cords.**

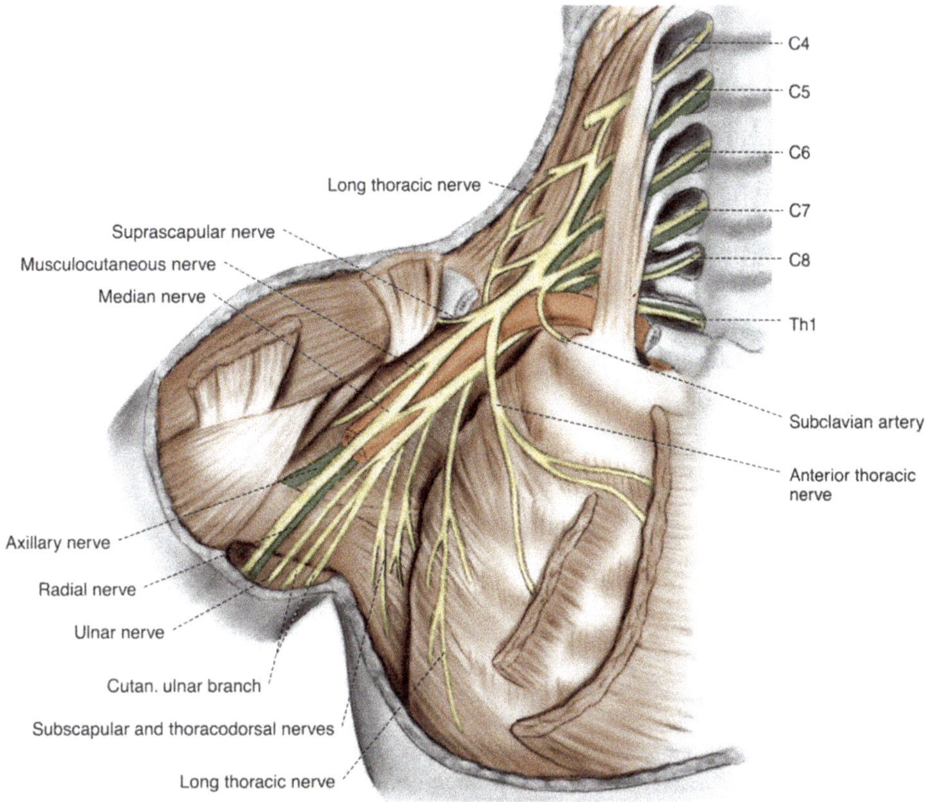

Figure 42-9. Anatomy of the brachial plexus.

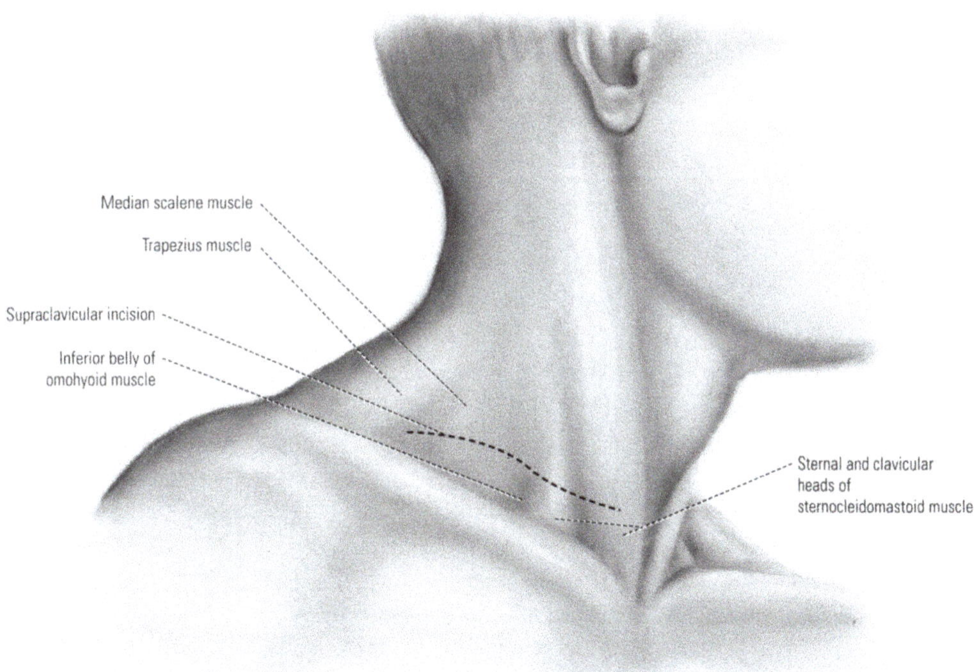

Figure 42-10. Exploration of the brachial plexus: supraclavicular incision. ***Observe***: 1. The position of the patient for supraclavicular exposure of the proximal brachial plexus. 2. A 6-cm incision is made 2 cm above and parallel to the clavicle.

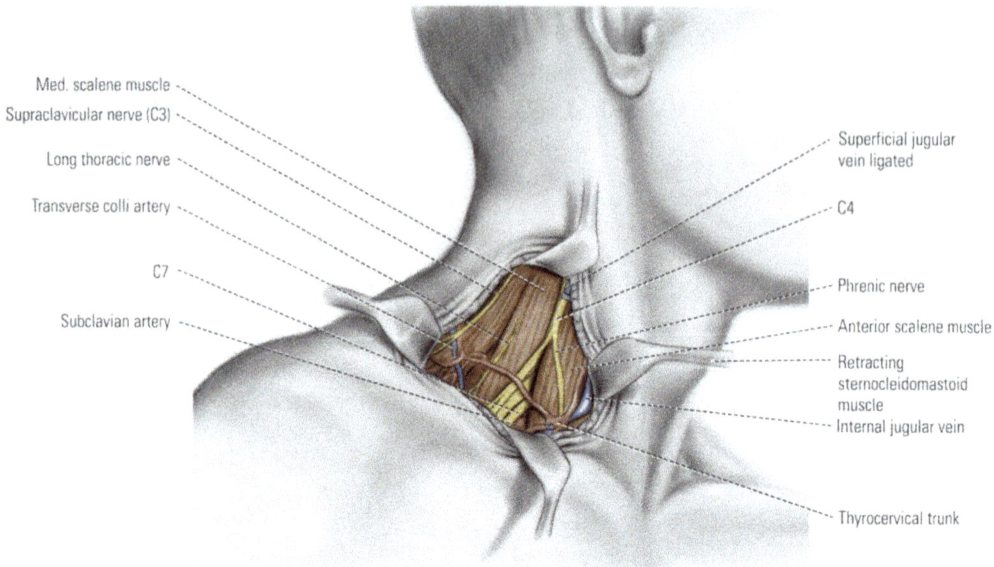

Figure 42-11. Exposure of the posterior cervical triangle. *Observe*: 1. The relationship of the phrenic nerve to the anterior scalene muscle. 2. The long thoracic nerve, after being formed by branches from C5, C6, and C7, emerges between the fibers of the medial scalene muscle. 3. The fifth and sixth cervical nerve roots converge and join to form the *upper trunk*. 4. The seventh cervical nerve root appears from behind the lateral rim of the anterior scalene muscle to become the *middle trunk* as it crosses the medial scalene muscle. 5. The *lower trunk* is formed by the union of the eighth cervical and first thoracic nerve roots and is not seen in this supraclavicular exposure. The structures being held posteriorly by Sibson's fascia are behind and occasionally beneath the subclavian artery.

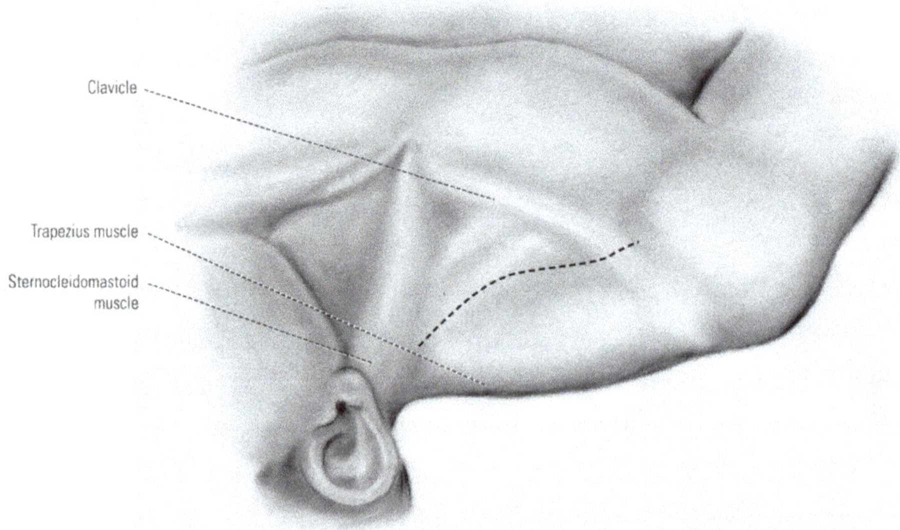

Figure 42-12. Transclavicular approach: skin incision. *Observe*: The incision crosses the clavicle in its outer third.

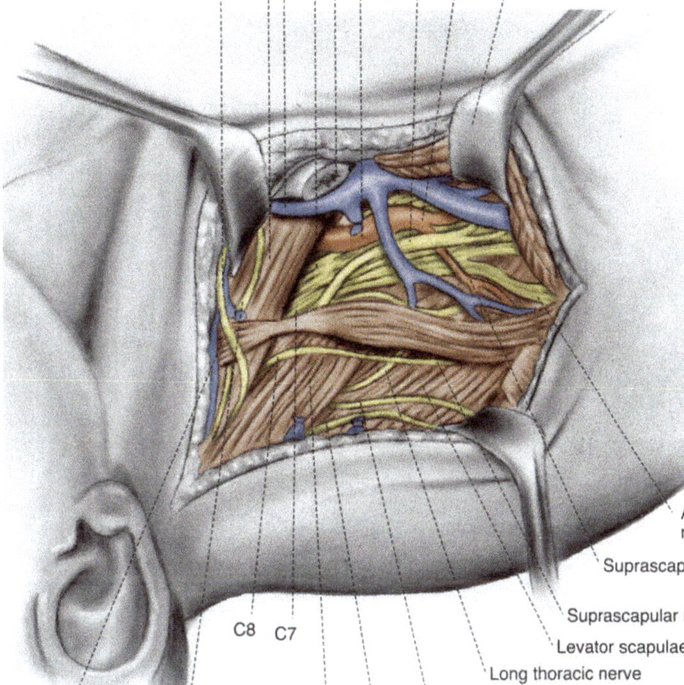

Figure 42-13. In the transclavicular approach, all trunks of the brachial plexus are exposed. The lower trunk is deep to the subclavian artery. Lateral to the first rib, which is palpable, the trunks lie above and behind the first part of the axillary artery where they separate into anterior and posterior divisions. The posterior divisions join to become the posterior cord, which gives origin to the axillary and radial nerves. The lateral cord is formed by the anterior divisions of the upper and middle trunks along the lateral side of the axillary artery. It gives rise to the musculocutaneous nerve (not seen here) and the lateral portion of the median nerve. The medial cord is a continuation of the anterior division of the lower trunk and lies along the medial border of the axillary artery. The ulnar nerve and the medial portion of the median nerve arise from this cord.

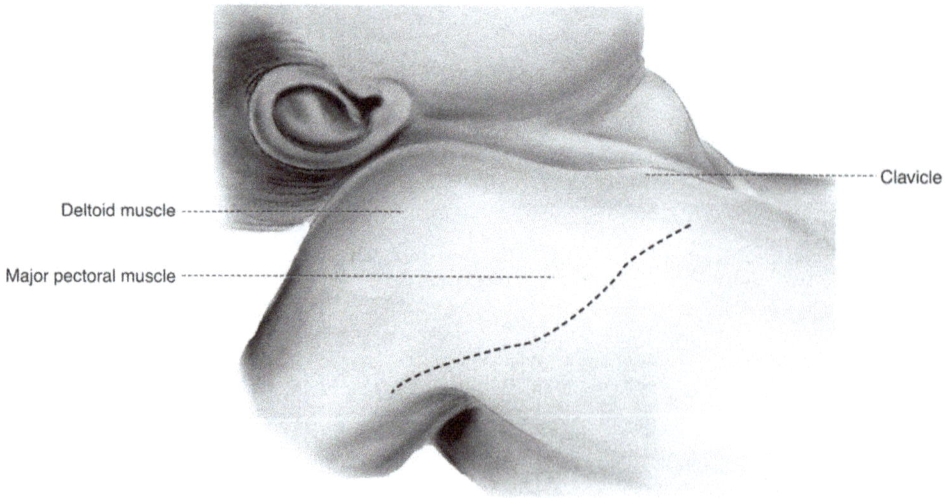

Figure 42-14. Infraclavicular incision. The skin incision begins below midportion of the clavicle and extends laterally toward the insertion of the pectoralis major muscle. The arm is abducted to 90°.

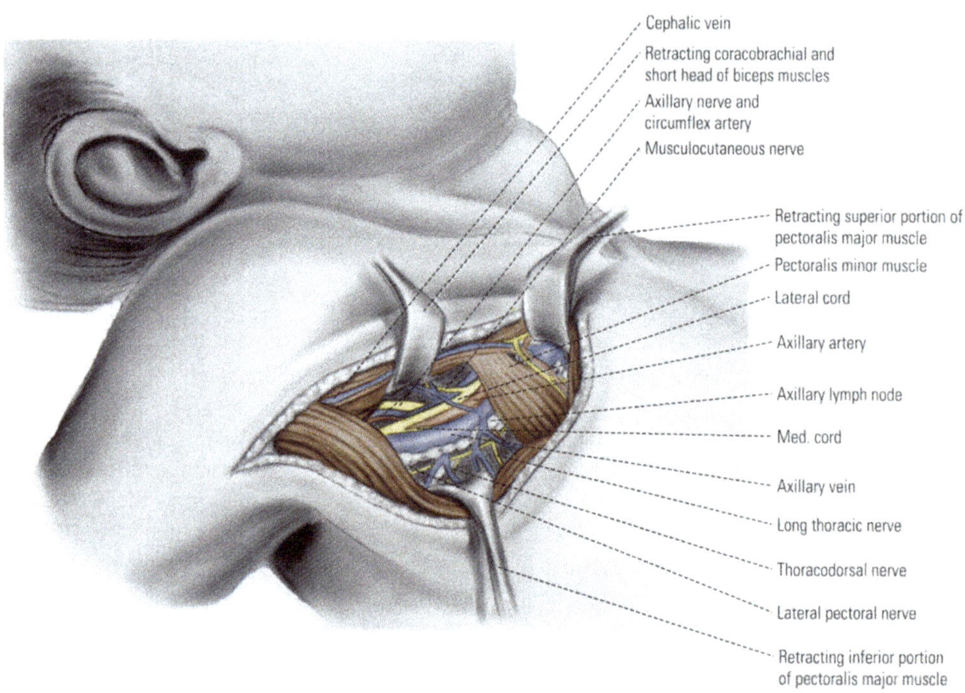

Figure 42-15. Infraclavicular approach. *Observe*: 1. The pectoralis major muscle is separated in the direction of the fibers. 2. The brachial plexus runs perpendicular to the pectoralis muscles. 3. The thin fascia covering the neurovascular bundle is opened. 4. The axillary artery lies above and behind the axillary vein.

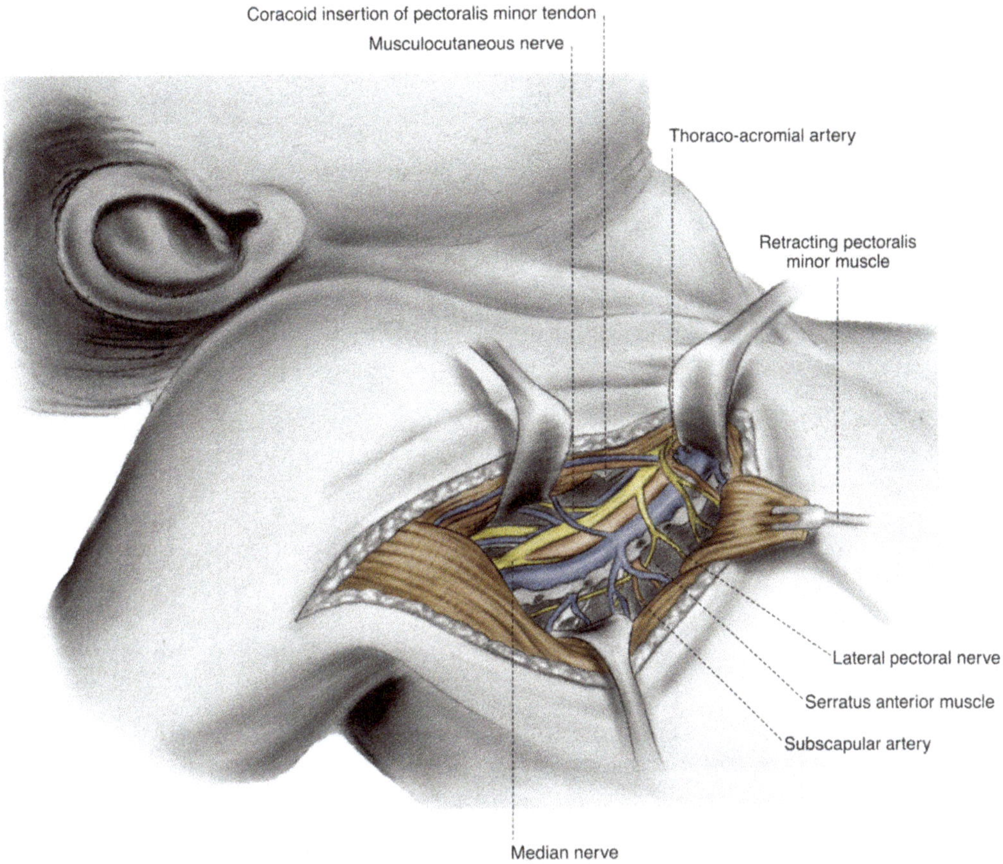

Figure 42-16. The pectoralis minor muscle has been transected at its tendinous insertion to aid in exposure. The thoracoacromial artery lies beneath the pectoralis minor muscle and may be ligated if it cannot be retracted medially. The musculocutaneous nerve arises from the medial cord and passes into the coracobrachialis muscle. The medial and lateral cords are seen uniting to form the median nerve.

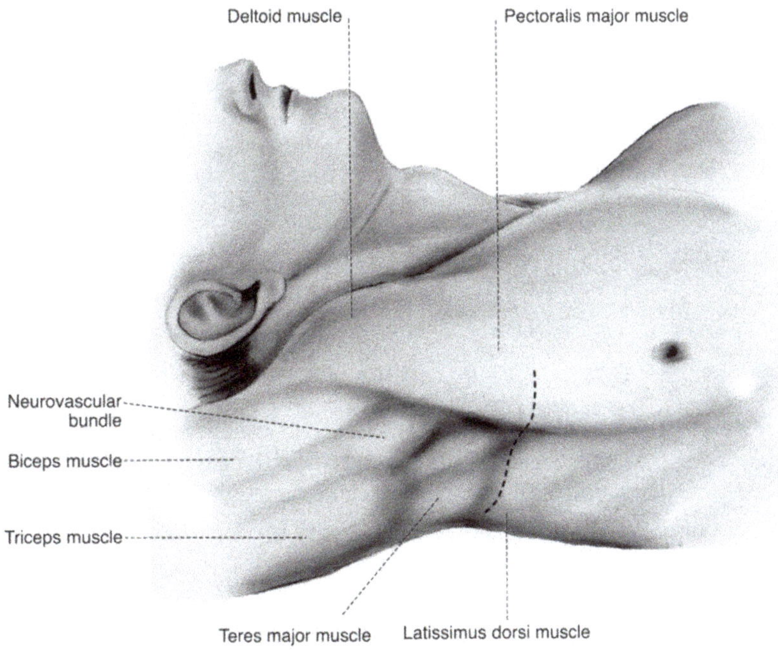

Figure 42-17. Axillary incision for lower brachial plexus. Note that the transverse incision follows axillary skin crease. The arm is abducted 135°.

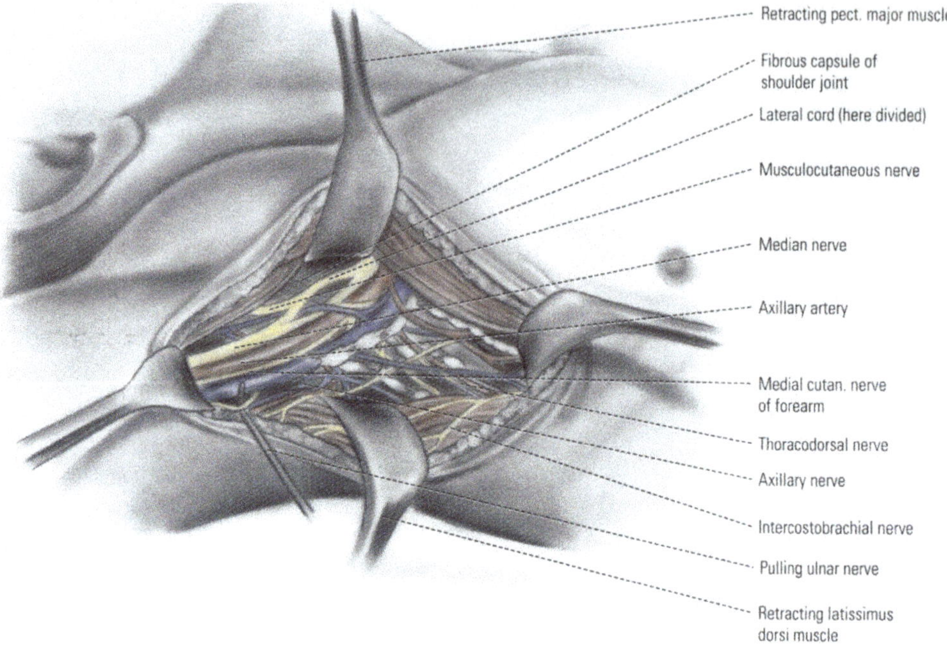

Figure 42-18. Axillary exposure of the lower brachial plexus. This approach is preferred in exposure of the proximal radial and axillary nerves which are hidden behind the brachial artery. When dissecting the radial nerve in the axilla, the motor branches to the long and lateral heads of the triceps must be identified to prevent inadvertent injury. The median nerve closely follows the brachial artery.

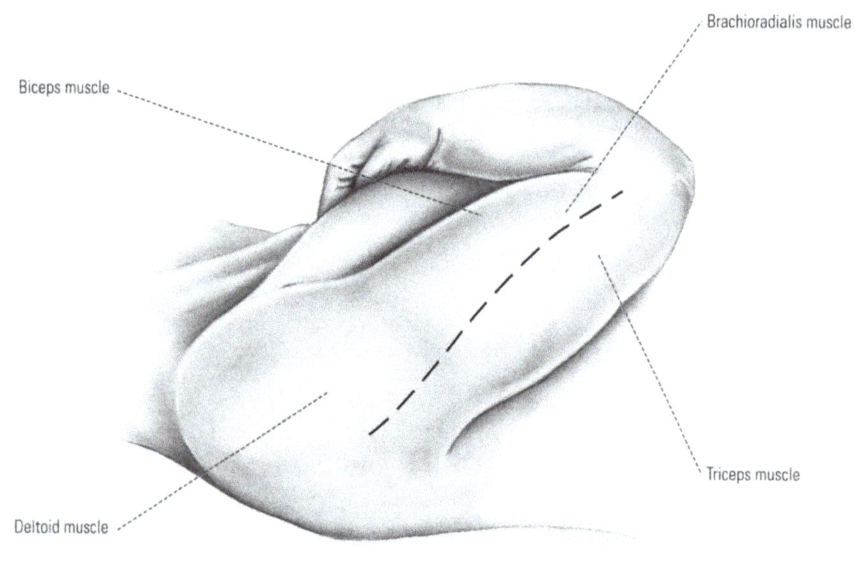

Figure 42-19. Exposure of the radial and axillary nerves in the arm. *Observe*: 1. The position of the arm on the thorax. 2. The incision is made from the posterior margin of the deltoid muscle to just above the lateral epicondyle at the elbow. 3. Compare with transaxillary exposure (Fig. 42-18).

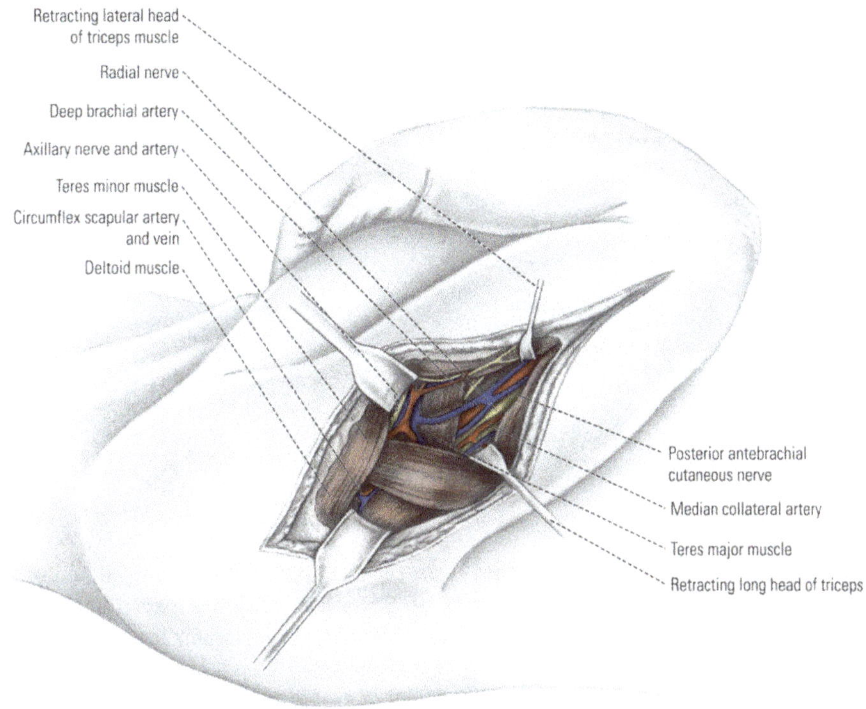

Figure 42-20. Exposure of the radial and axillary nerves in the arm. *Observe*: 1. The radial nerve is exposed between the long and lateral heads of the triceps muscle. It passes behind the lateral head of the triceps muscle where it is intimately related to the humerus. 2. The axillary nerve follows the upper surface of the teres major muscle toward its insertion in the humerus.

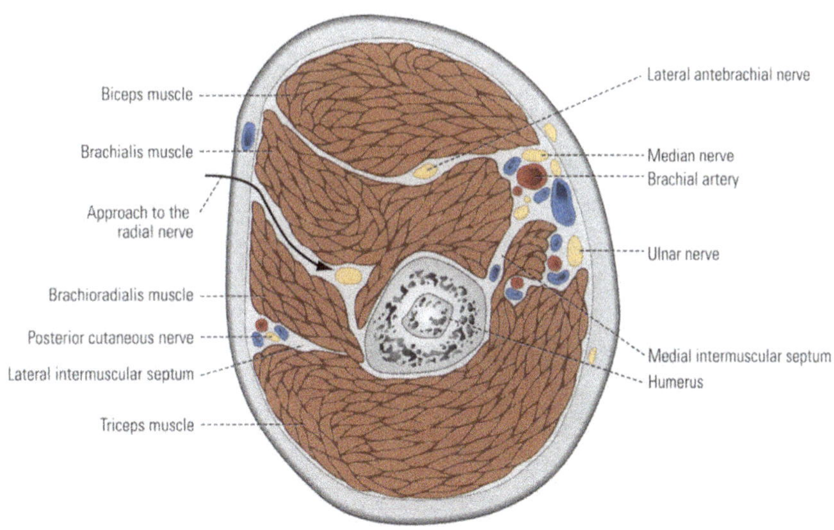

Figure 42-21. Exposure of the radial nerve in the arm. Transverse section of the distal third of the arm. The operative approach to the radial nerve at this level is between the brachialis and the brachioradialis muscles (corresponding to the operative exposure seen in Fig. 42-22).

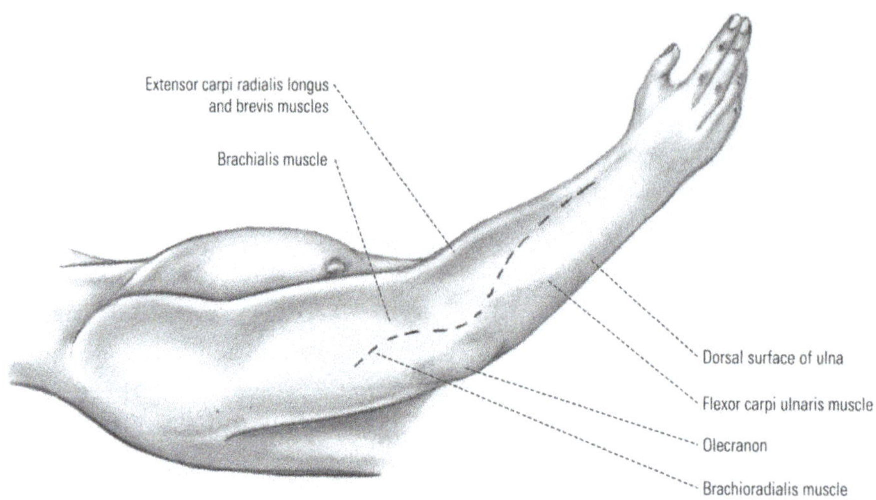

Figure 42-22. **Incision. *Observe*: 1. The arm is extended and externally rotated as compared with Figure 42-18. 2. The skin incision is made from over the groove between the brachialis and brachioradialis muscle to over the extensor carpi radialis muscle.**

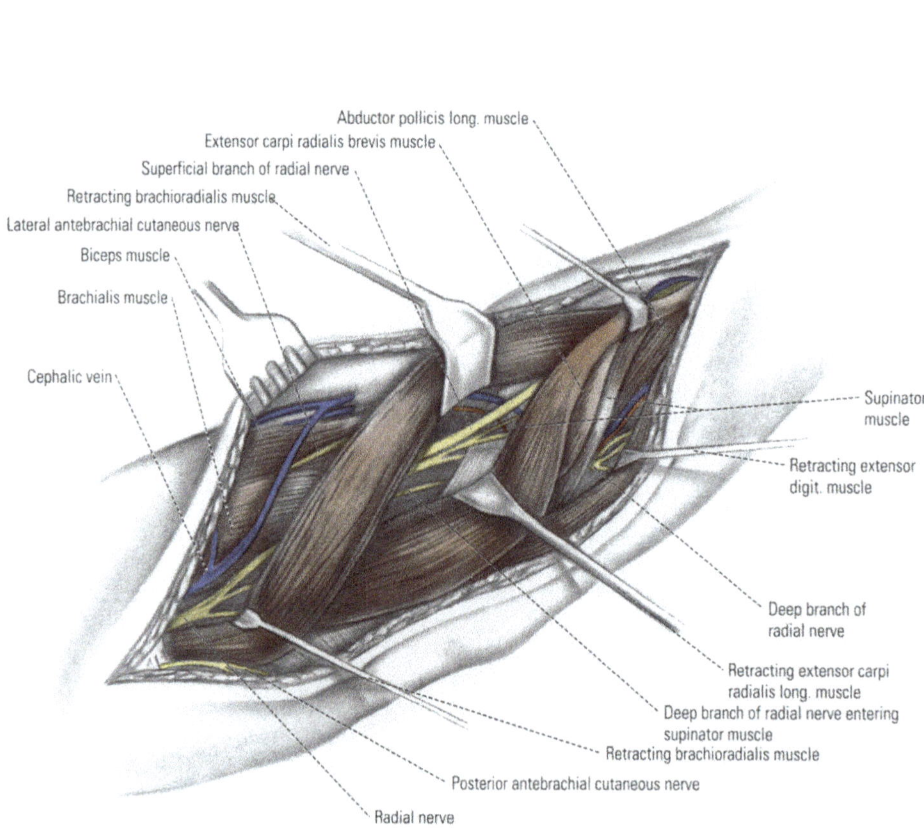

Figure 42-23. **Exposure of the radial nerve in the lower arm and forearm. *Observe*: 1. Prior to entering the groove between the brachialis and brachioradialis muscles, the radial nerve is relatively superficial. 2. The radial nerve divides into the deep and superficial branches as it crosses the capsule of the elbow joint. 3. The deep branch enters the supinator muscle and winds around the lateral aspect of the radius. 4. The superficial branch passes along the extensor carpi radialis muscle to become superficial in the distal third of the forearm.**

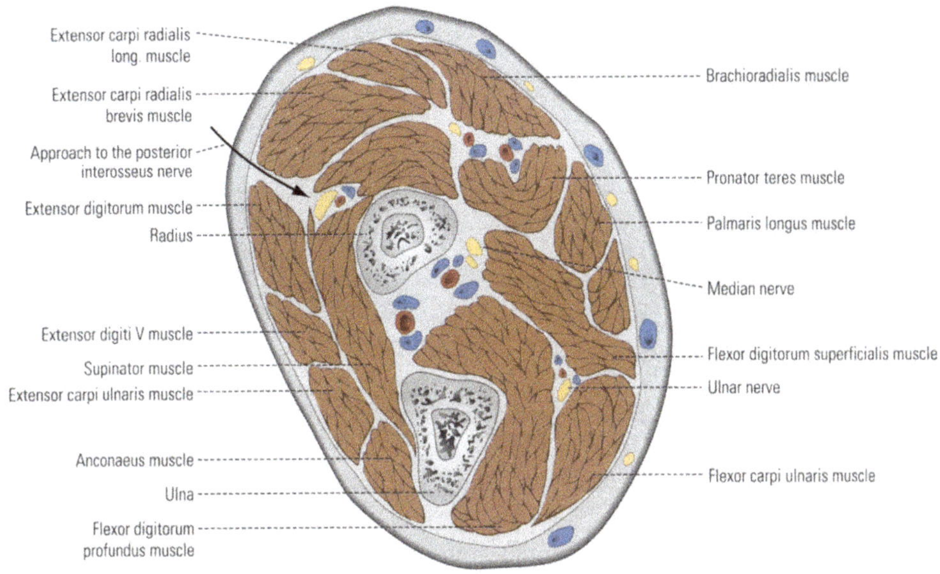

Figure 42-24. **Exposure of the deep branch of the radial nerve in the forearm: transverse section of the proximal third of the forearm. *Observe*: The operative approach to the deep branch (posterior interosseous nerve) at the level is between the extensor carpi radialis brevis and extensor digitorum muscles.**

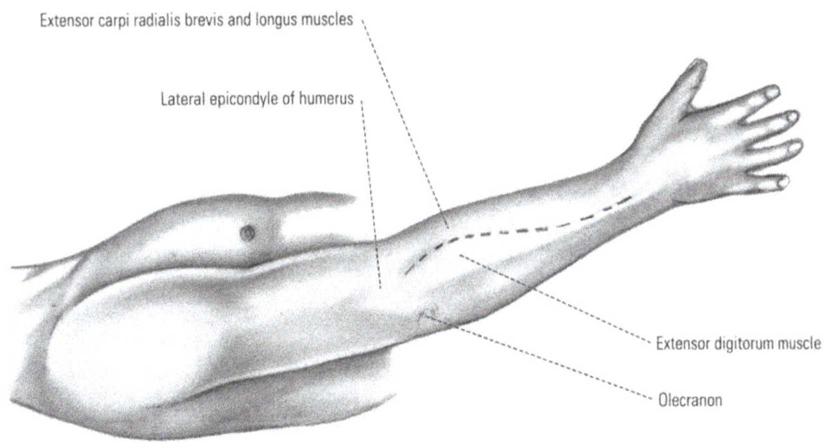

Figure 42-25. **The skin incision is made from just in front of the lateral epicondyle of the humerus and extends distally in the groove between the extensor carpi and extensor digitorum muscles.**

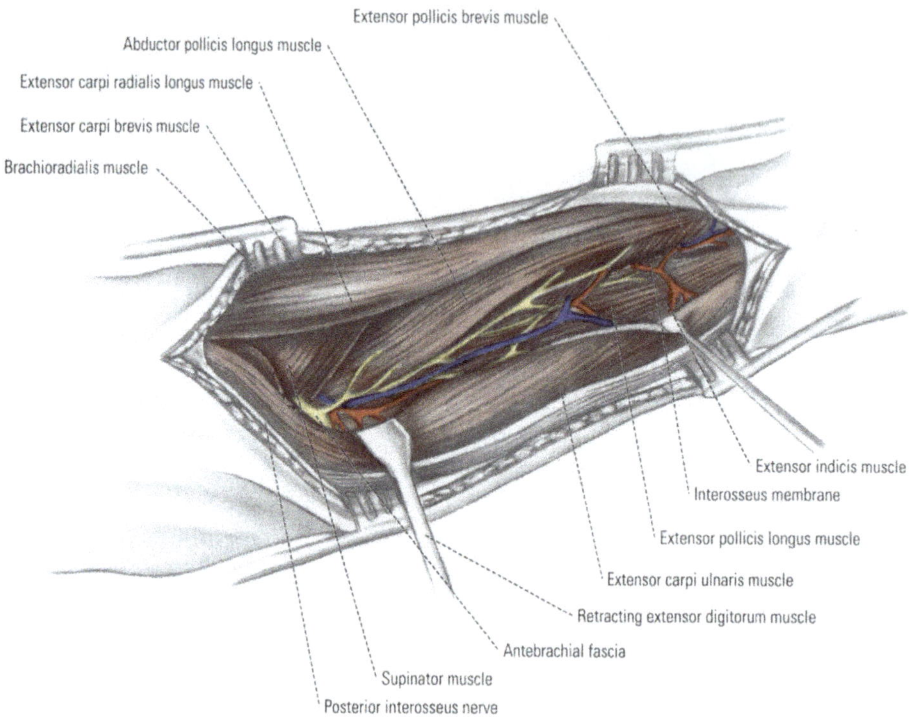

Figure 42-26. Exposure of the deep branch of the radial nerve in the forearm. *Observe*: 1. The deep branch (posterior interosseous nerve) is exposed as it emerges from the supinator muscle by dissecting between the extensor carpi radialis brevis and the extensor digitorum muscles. 2. To visualize the deep branch as it enters the supinator muscle, dissection is carried down between the brachioradialis and extensor carpi radialis longus muscles. This may be necessary if the distal posterior interosseous nerve cannot be identified because of transection or scar tissue.

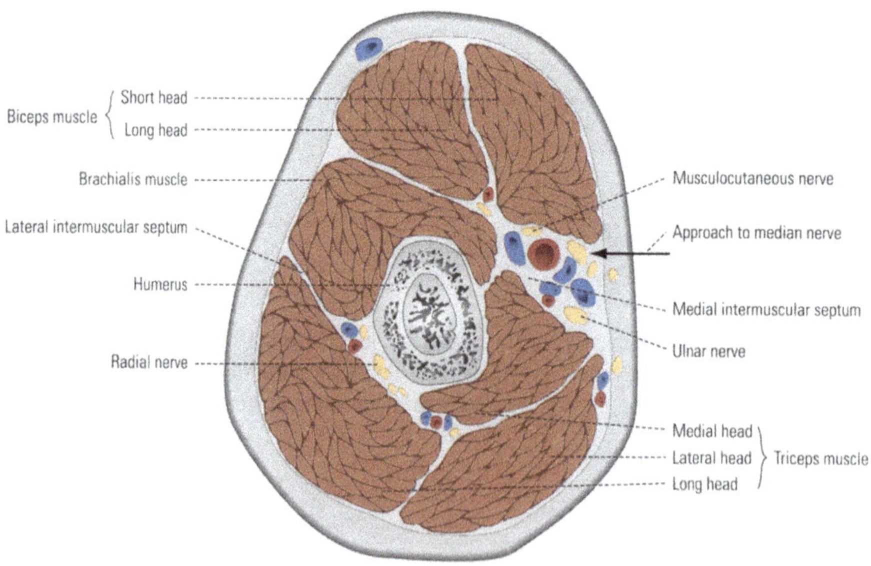

Figure 42-27. Exposure of the median and ulnar nerves in the arm: transverse section of the upper third of the arm. The operative exposure is between the biceps and triceps muscles.

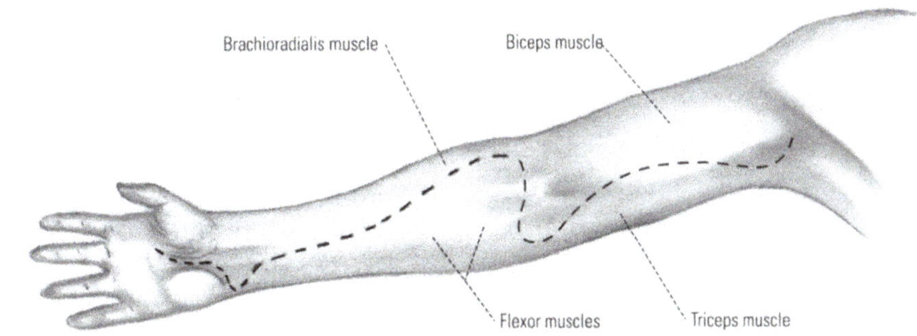

Figure 42-28. Incision. *Observe*: 1. In the arm the median nerve is exposed by an incision over the neurovascular bundle between the biceps and triceps muscles. This same incision is used to expose the ulnar nerve in the arm. 2. In the antecubital fossa a transverse incision is made following a normal skin crease to the medial border of the brachioradialis muscle. 3. In the forearm the incision is made along the medial border of the brachioradialis muscle. The incision is gradually slanted toward the medial side of the forearm so that at the wrist it approaches the pisiform bone. This incision is also applicable for exposure of the ulnar nerve in the distal forearm. 4. At the wrist the incision is made transversely following a flexion crease. 5. The incision in the hand is made through the flexion crease at the base of the thenar eminence.

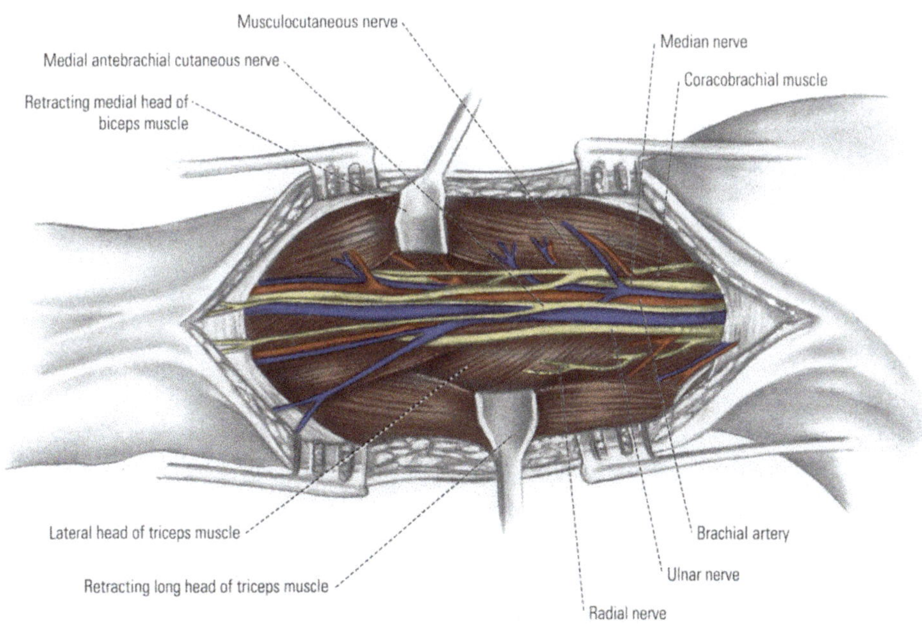

Figure 42-29. Exposure of the median and ulnar nerves in the arm. *Observe*: 1. The median nerve has an intimate relationship to the brachial artery. Proximally it lies lateral to the artery but it crosses the artery anteriorly to assume a medial position at the elbow. 2. The long and lateral heads of the triceps muscle are separated to reveal the radial nerve just before it disappears around the humerus. 3. The musculocutaneous nerve having penetrated the coracobrachialis muscle appears here between that muscle and the biceps muscle.

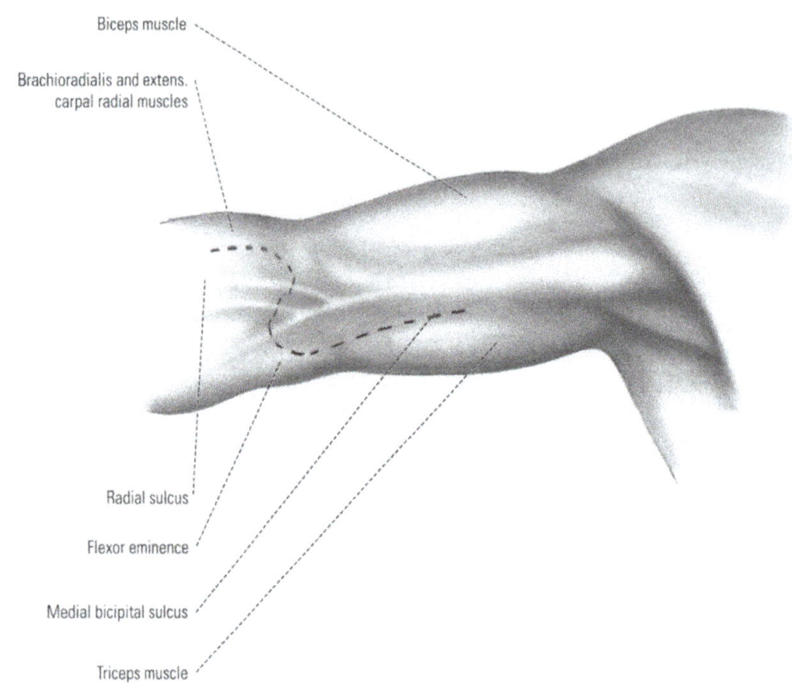

Figure 42-30. Incision. *Observe*: 1. The arm is abducted to 90° and the elbow joint is fully extended. 2. A *Z*-shaped incision is made to avoid crossing a flexion crease.

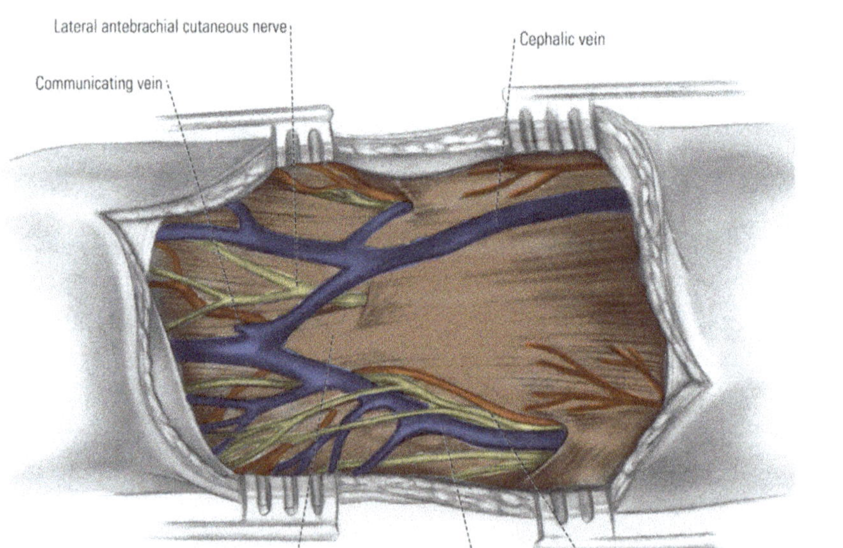

Figure 42-31. Exposure of the median nerve at the elbow. *Observe*: 1. Subcutaneous dissection provides a wide exposure of the antecubital fascia. 2. The medial and lateral antebrachial cutaneous nerves are identified and protected.

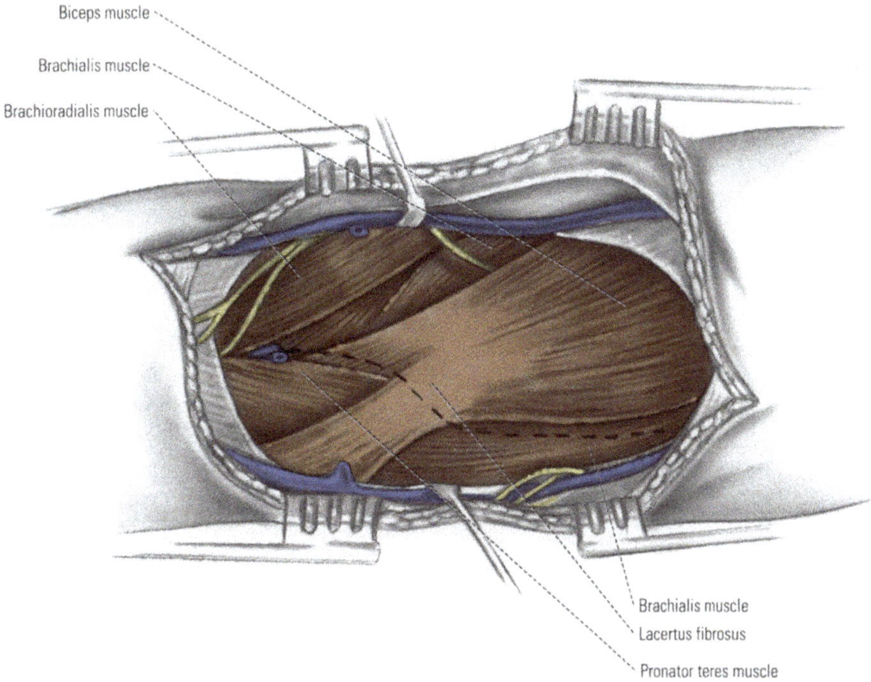

Figure 42-32. Exposure of the median nerve at the elbow. *Observe*: 1. The antecubital fascia has been incised and retracted. 2. *Dotted line* marks the course of the median nerve and brachial artery.

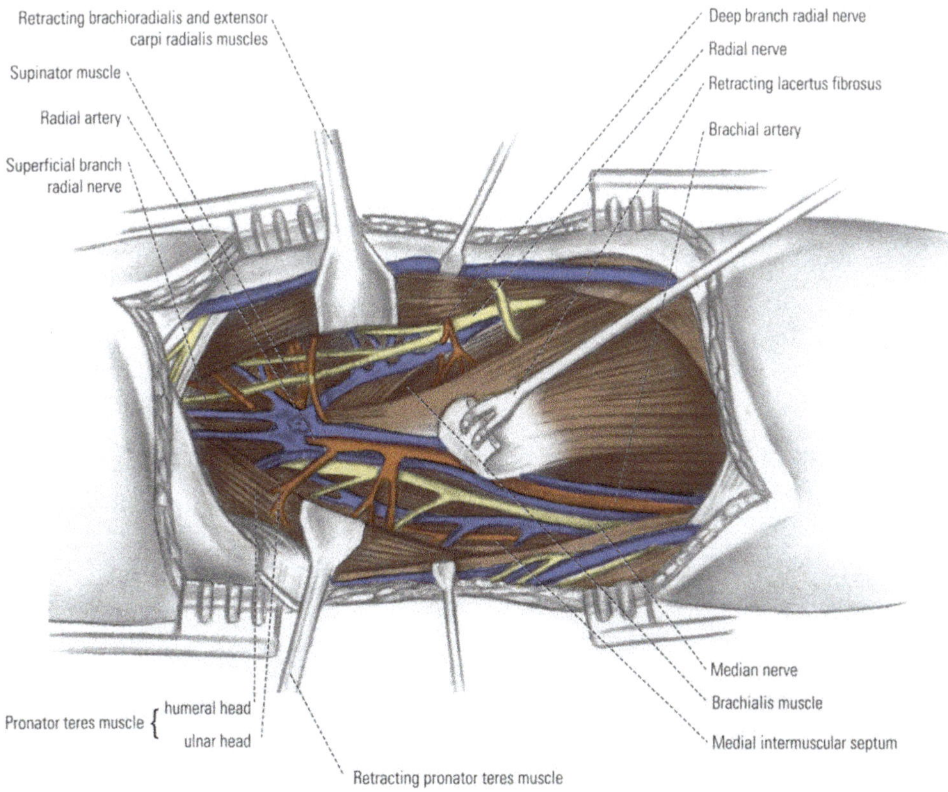

Figure 42-33. The lacertus fibrosus has been transected. The median nerve is separated from the humerus only by the brachialis muscle. The median nerve passes between the two heads of the pronator teres muscle as it proceeds into the forearm. The radial nerve is also seen in this exposure. It perforates the supinator muscle and divides into the deep and superficial branches.

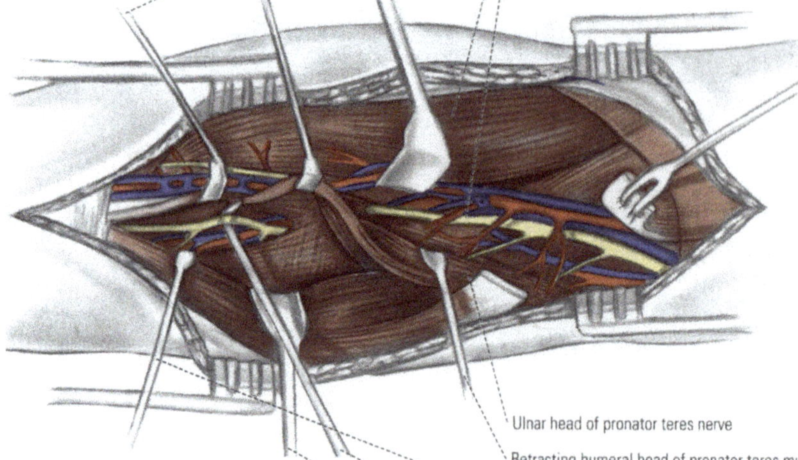

Figure 42-34. Exposure of the median nerve in the forearm. *Observe*: 1. After passing between the two heads of the pronator teres muscle the median nerve assumes an intimate relationship with the deep surface of the flexor digitorum superficialis muscle. 2. Branches to the pronator teres muscle must be identified and protected. 3. Separation of the pronator teres muscle from the flexor carpi radialis muscle inferiorly gives additional exposure of the median nerve.

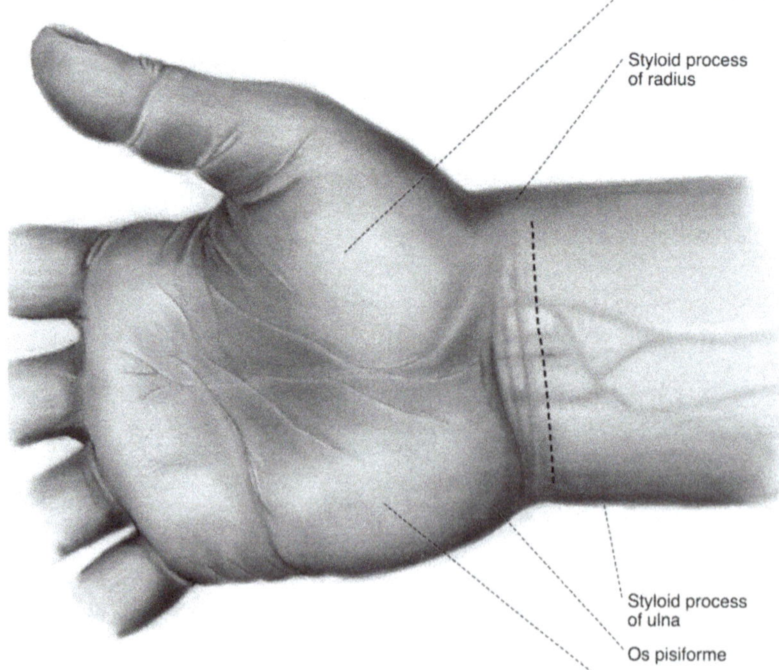

Figure 42-35. Exposure of the median and ulnar nerves at the wrist: incision. Note that a transverse incision is made in a flexion skin crease.

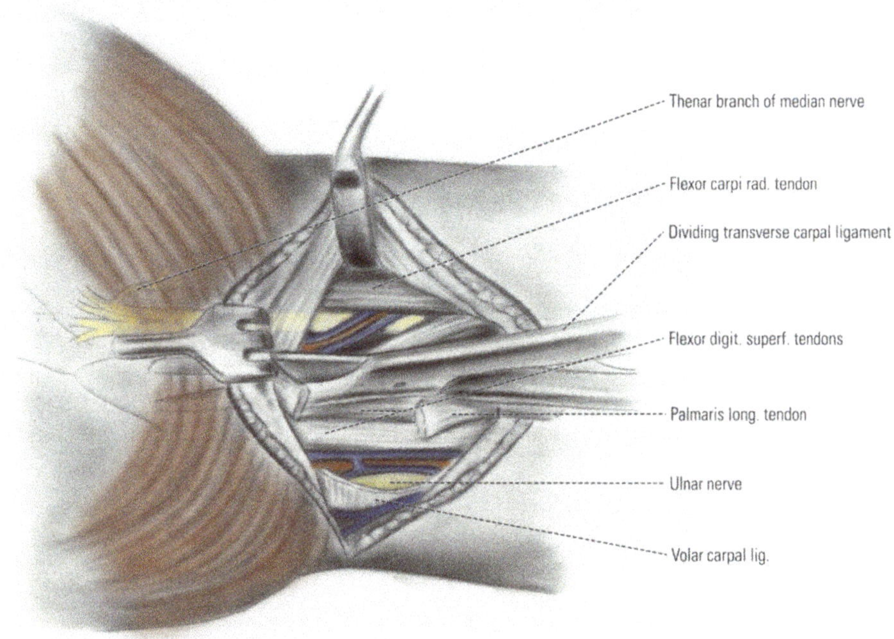

Figure 42-36. Exposure of the median and ulnar nerves at the wrist. Observe: 1. The transverse carpal ligament is divided medial to the median nerve to protect the recurrent branch as well as the two sensory branches to the thumb. 2. If mobilization of the median nerve is required, the incision shown in Figure 42-38 is used.

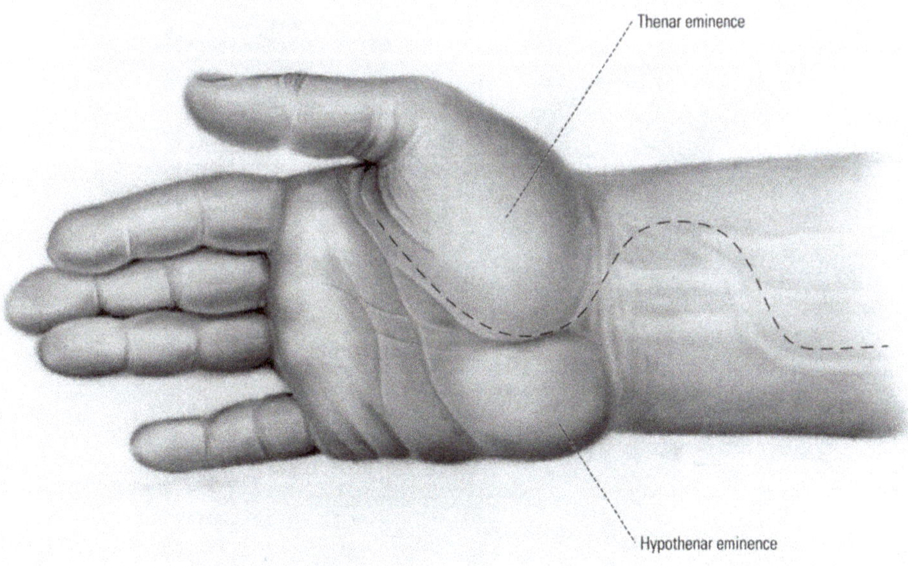

Figure 42-37. Exposure of the median nerve from forearm to palm: incision. Note that a curvilinear incision is used to prevent crossing flexor creases. The palmar extension follows the skin crease at the base of the thenar eminence.

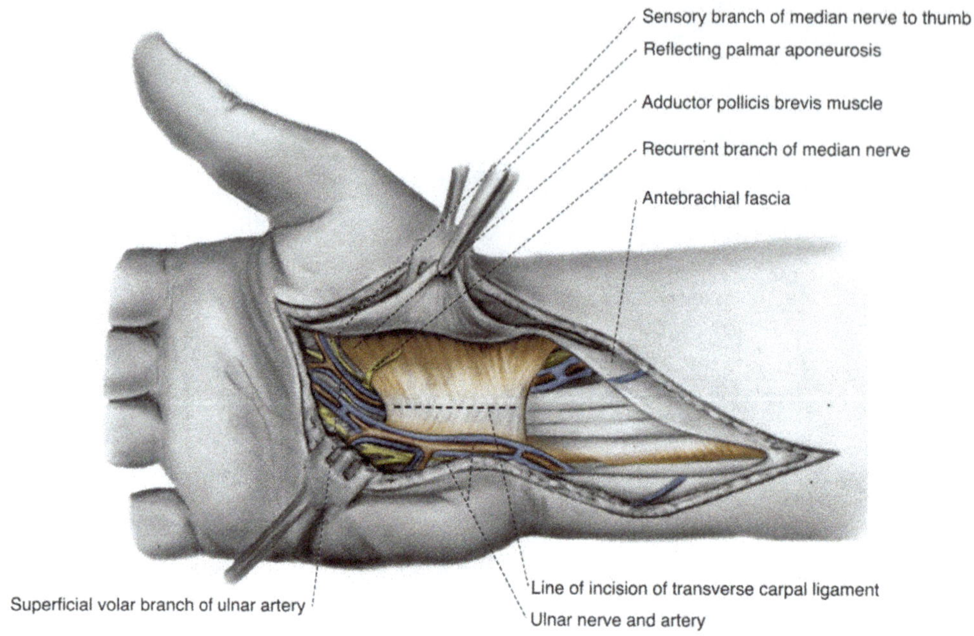

Figure 42-38. Note the superficial position of the recurrent branch at the inner margin of the adductor pollicis brevis muscle and the width of the transverse carpal ligament.

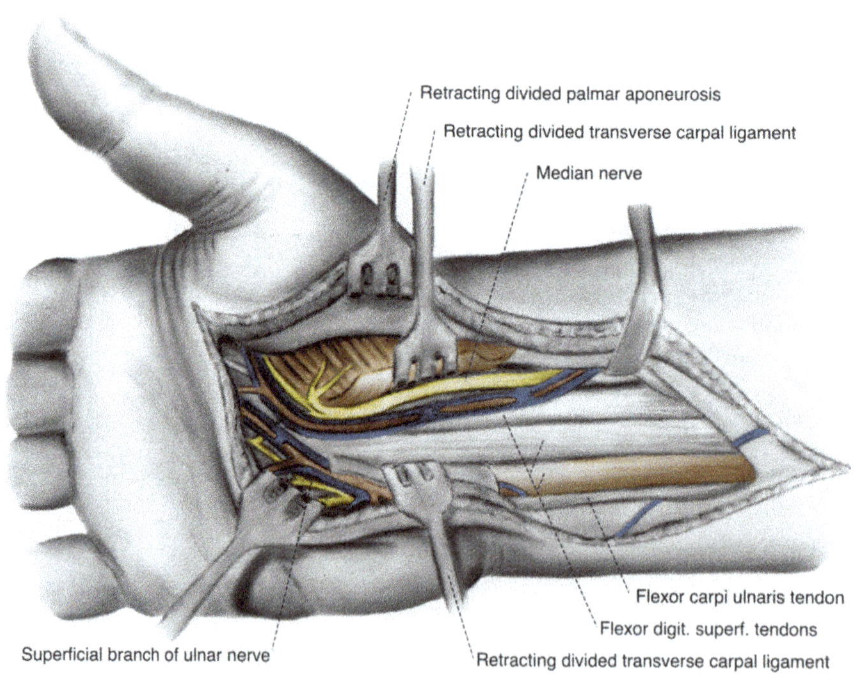

Figure 42-39. Exposure of the median nerve from forearm to palm. Note that the antebrachial fascia and transverse ligament have been incised in the midline. The median nerve and the accompanying artery lie lateral to the flexor digitorum superficialis tendons. The ulnar nerve which has divided into the superficial and deep branches is seen medially.

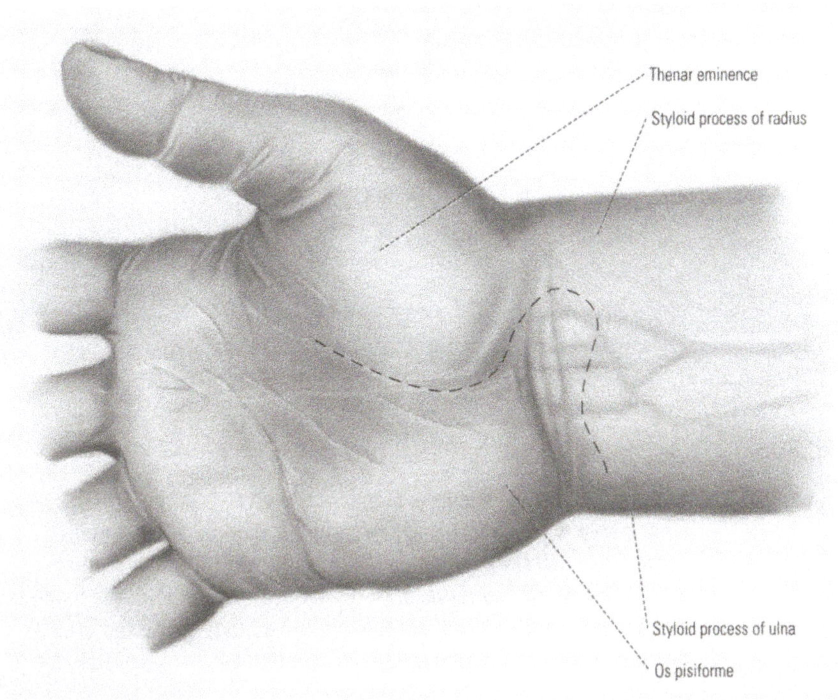

Figure 42-40. Exposure of the median and ulnar nerves in the wrist and palm: incision. Note that no flexion creases are crossed by the incision.

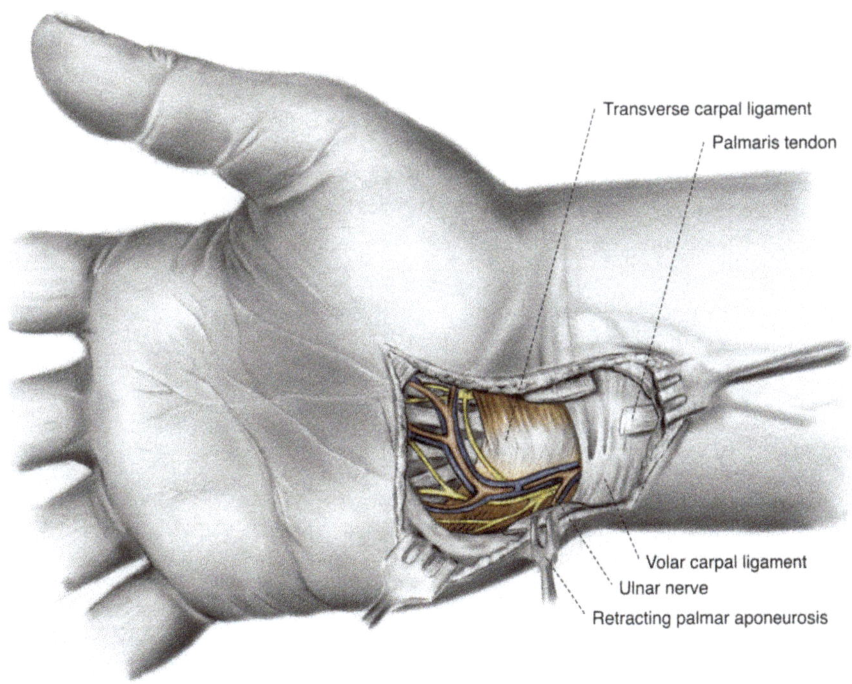

Figure 42-41. Exposure of the median and ulnar nerves in the wrist and palm. Note the ulnar nerve and its accompanying artery are beneath the volar carpal ligament but superficial to the transverse carpal ligament.

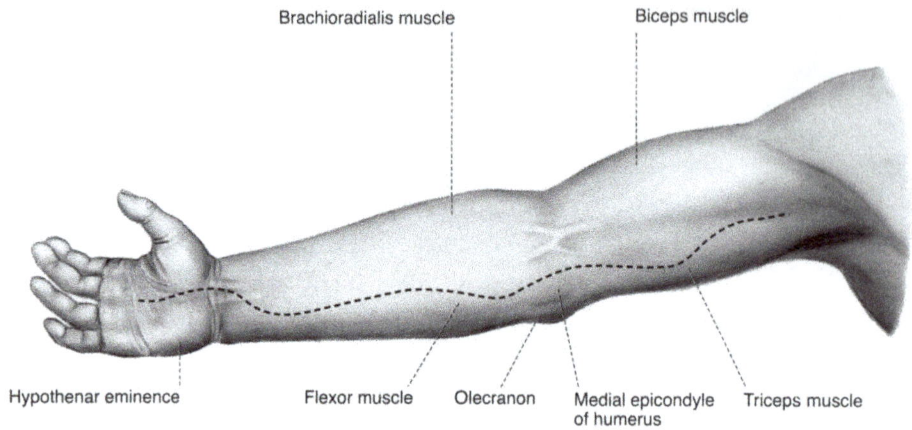

Figure 42-42. Exposure of the ulnar nerve: incision. *Observe*: 1. In the arm the ulnar nerve is exposed using the same incision as for the median nerve. 2. At the elbow the incision is made ventral to the medial epicondyle of the humerus. 3. At the wrist a medial detour is made to avoid crossing the flexion creases before swinging into the crease between the thenar and hypothenar eminences.

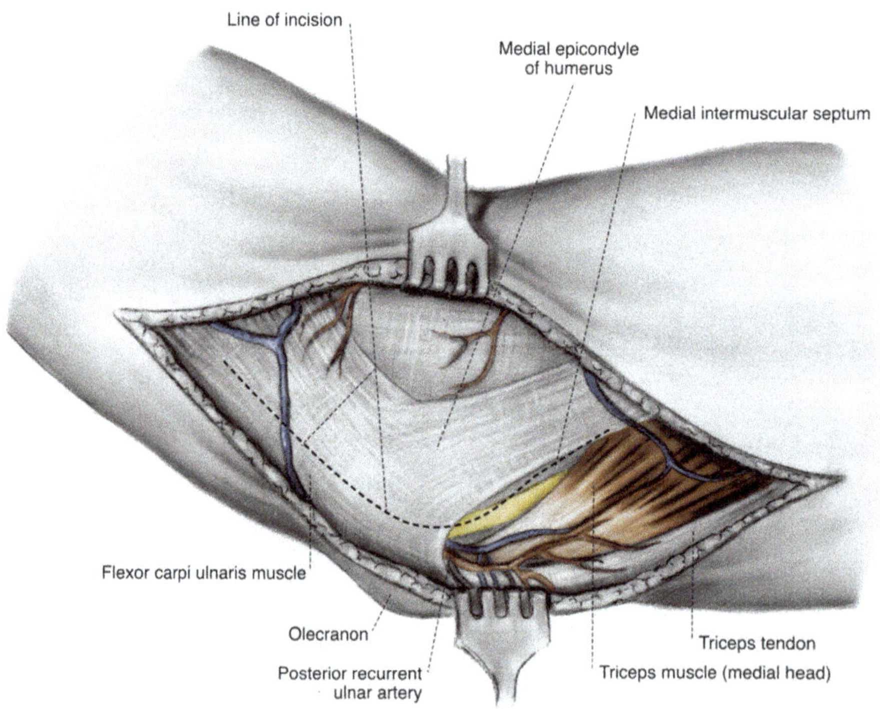

Figure 42-43. Exposure of the ulnar nerve at the elbow: transposition of the ulnar nerve. The fascia is incised directly over the course of the ulnar nerve.

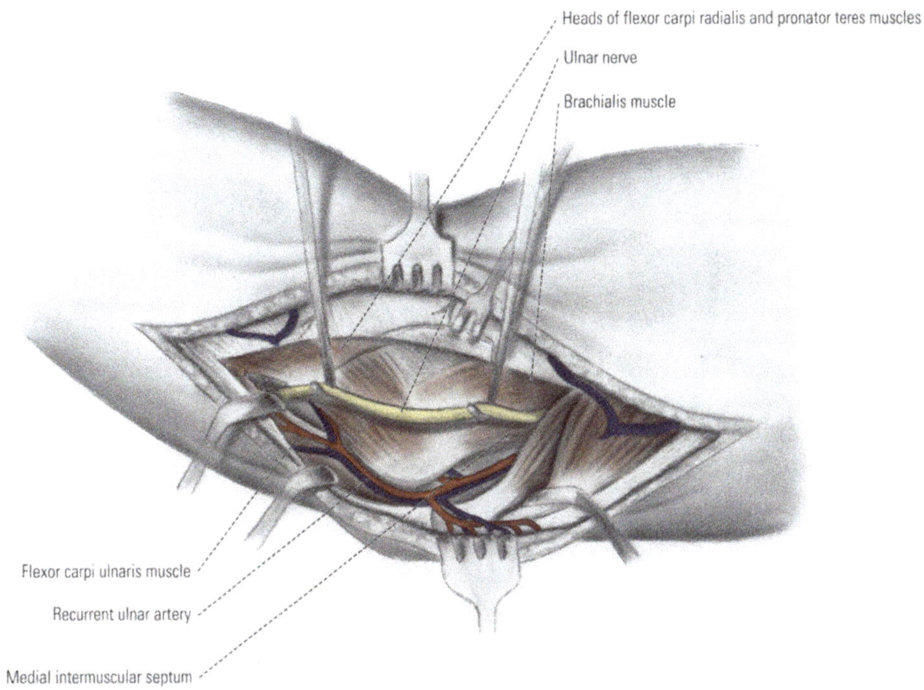

Figure 42-44. Proximal dissection must be to the level of the insertion of the coracobrachialis muscle. Incision of the intermuscular septum is a key step in preventing angulation of the nerve. 2. Distal mobilization must include division of the fibrous arch between the two heads of the flexor carpi ulnaris muscle.

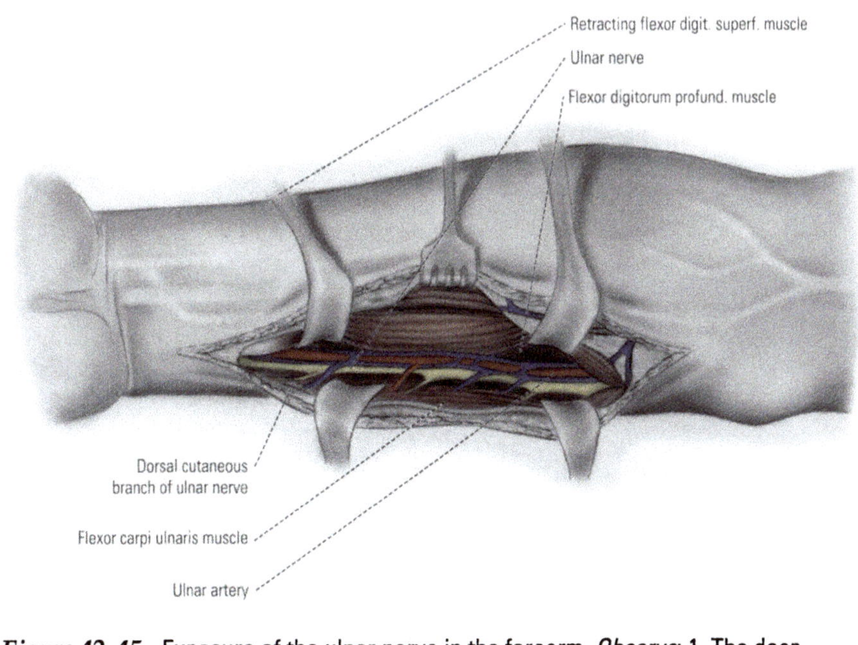

Figure 42-45. Exposure of the ulnar nerve in the forearm. *Observe*: 1. The deep fascia is incised between the flexor carpi ulnaris and the flexor digitorum superficialis muscles. 2. The ulnar artery lies on the radial side of the nerve and supplies many short nutrient branches to the nerve. 3. The dorsal cutaneous branch of the ulnar nerve originates in the distal third of the forearm.

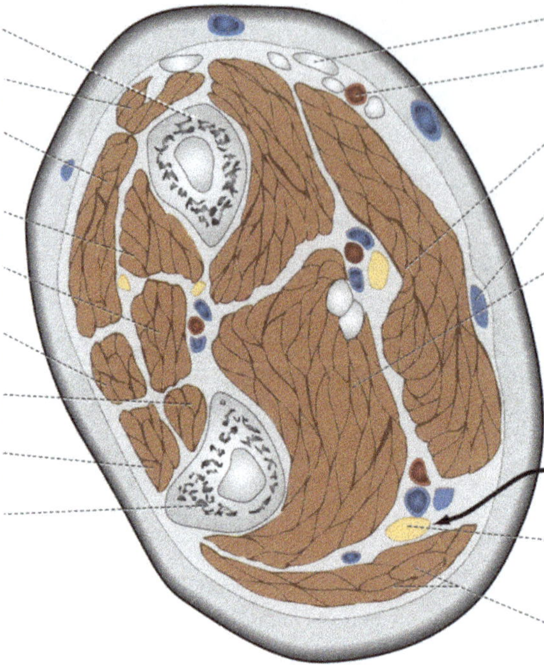

Figure 42-46. Exposure of the ulnar nerve in the forearm: transverse section through the middle third of the forearm. The operative exposure is between the flexor carpi ulnaris and flexor digitorum superficialis muscles.

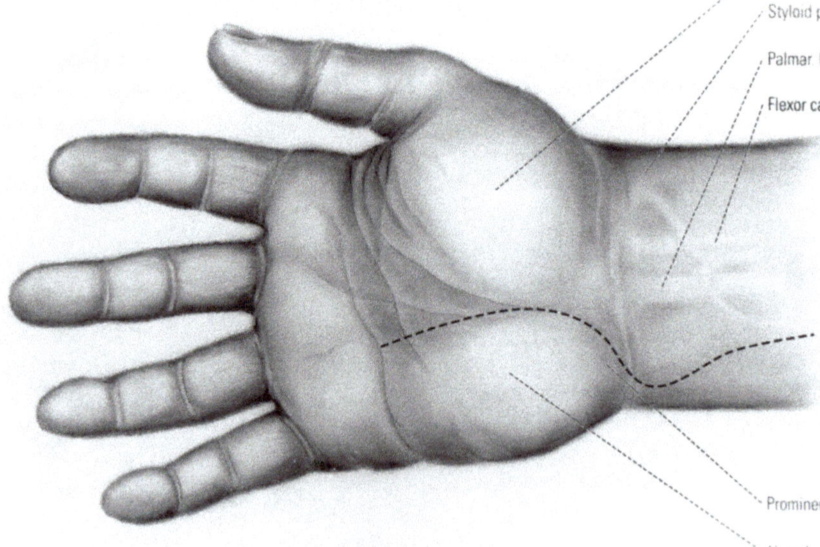

Figure 42-47. Exposure of the ulnar nerve at the wrist and palm: Incision. Note that the lazy S-shaped incision avoids crossing flexion creases.

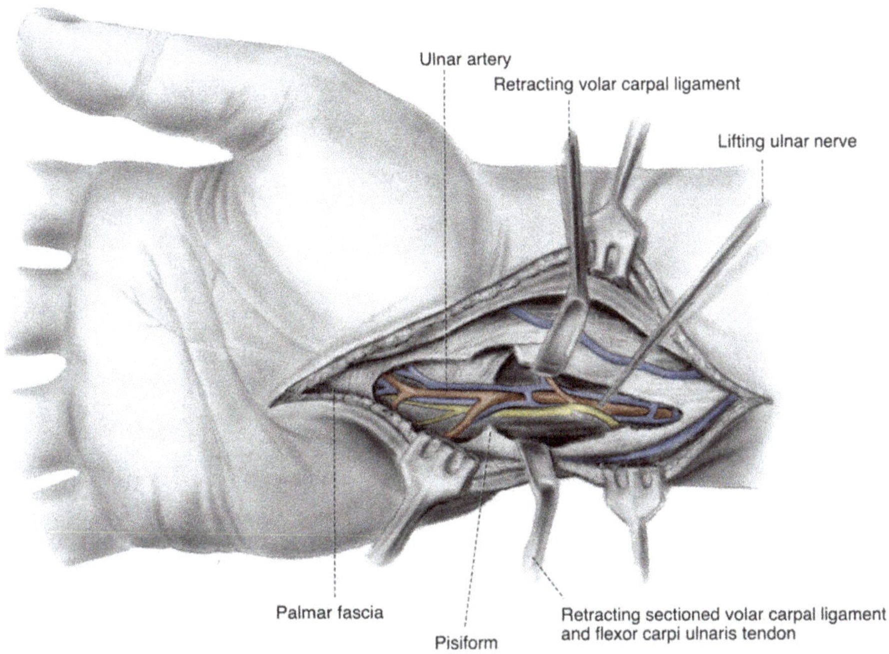

Figure 42-48. Exposure of the ulnar nerve at the wrist and palm. Note that the volar carpal ligament is incised close to the radial side of the pisiform bone and the antebrachial fascia is incised along the radial margin of the flexor carpi ulnaris tendon.

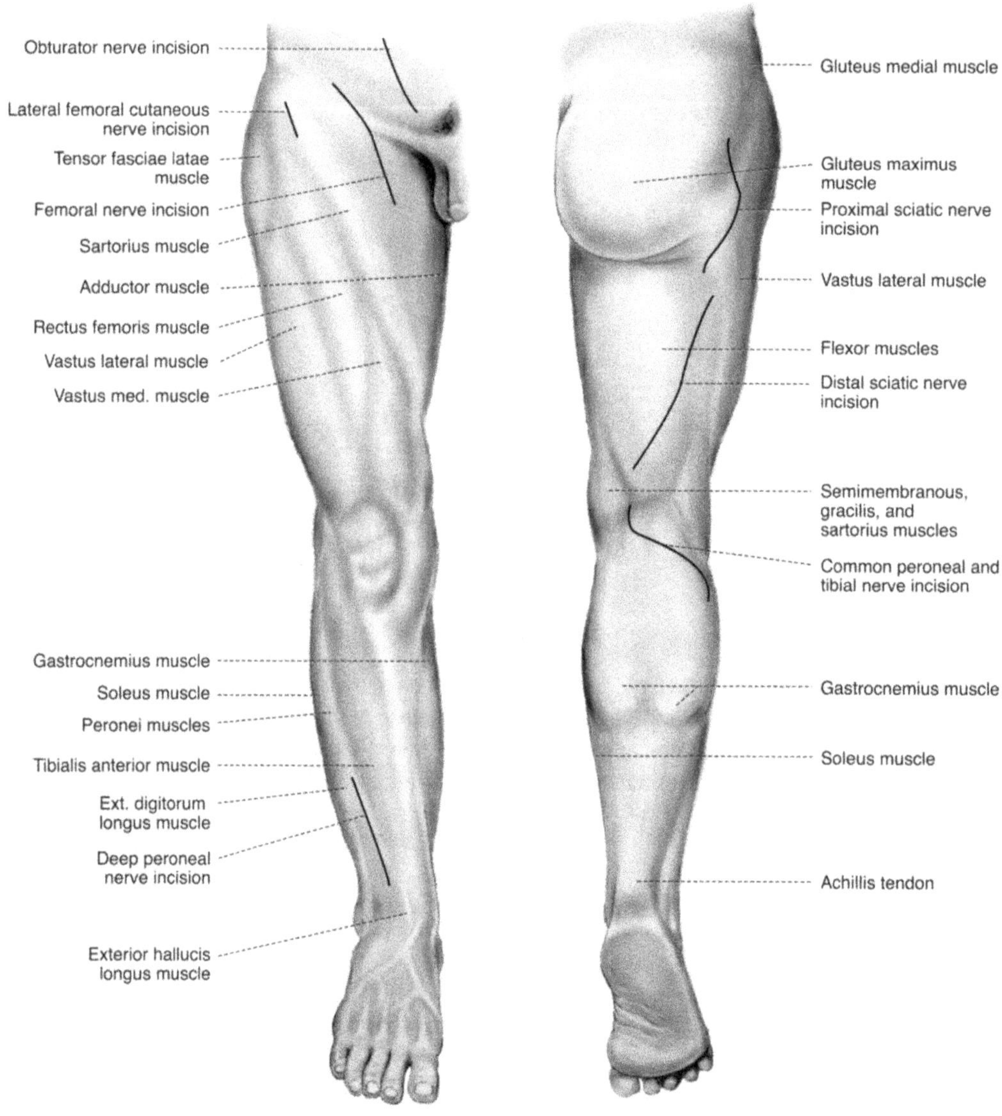

Figure 42-49. Exposure of peripheral nerves in the lower extremity: incisions. Each incision will be discussed in more detail later, but notice that all incisions are made in such a way that maximum exposure will be obtained with the most favorable cosmetic result.

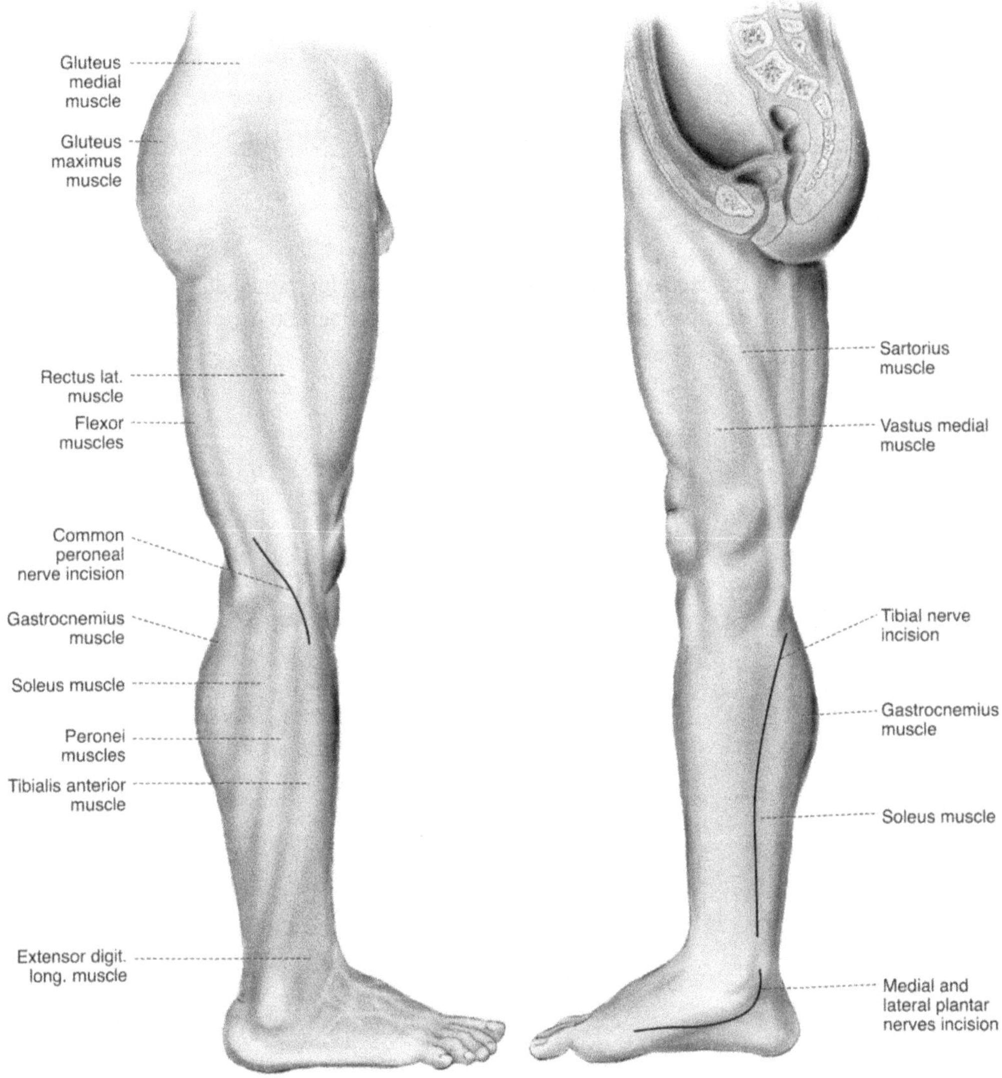

Figure 42-50. Exposure of peripheral nerves in the lower extremity: incisions.

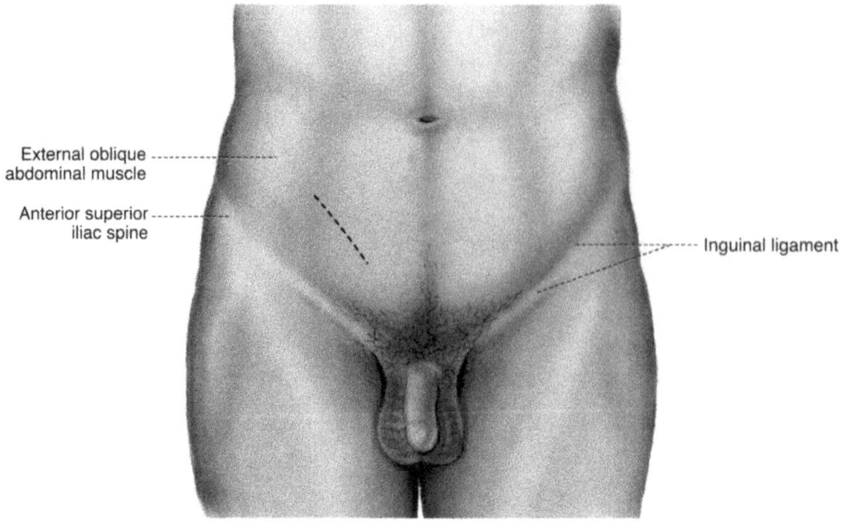

Figure 42-51. Exposure of the obturator nerve: incision for transabdominal extraperitoneal approach. Note that the incision is made 4 cm above and parallel to the inguinal ligament.

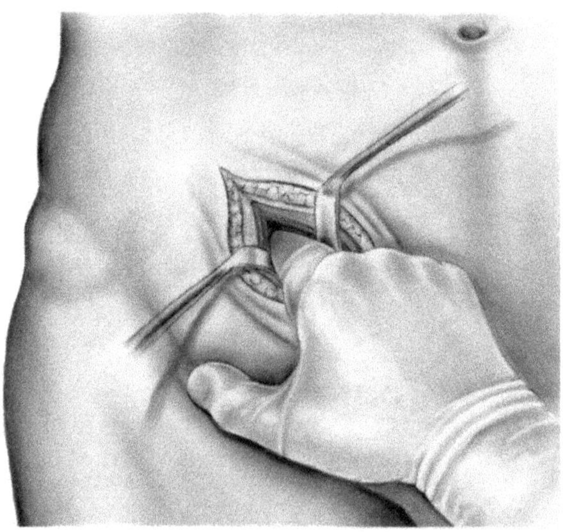

Figure 42-52. Transabdominal extraperitoneal approach. *Observe*: 1. A muscle-splitting incision is used. 2. Having visualized the peritoneum, the index finger dissects it from the abdominal wall.

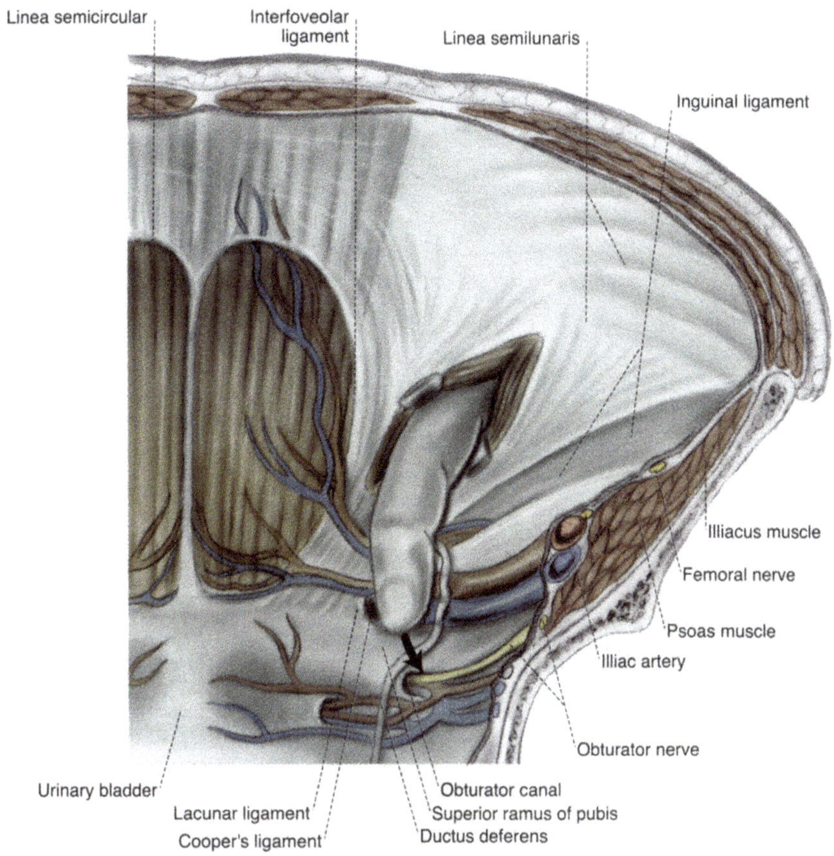

Figure 42-53. Transabdominal extraperitoneal approach as seen from the inside. *Observe*: 1. The index finger in the preperitoneal space covers the deep inguinal ring and the femoral canal. 2. The superior ramus of the pubis is being palpated. The obturator nerve is intimately related to this structure as it passes out the obturator canal. 3. This same approach is used to expose the femoral nerve in the pelvis.

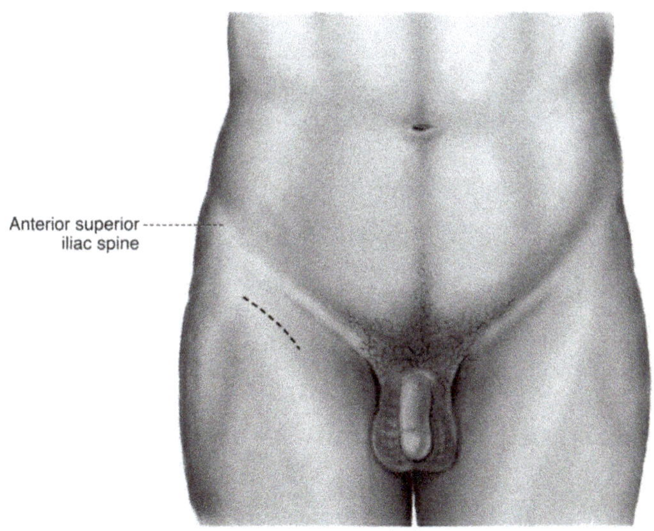

Figure 42-54. Exposure of the lateral femoral cutaneous nerve: incision. The incision is made 3 cm below the anterior superior spine of the ilium and parallel to the inguinal ligament.

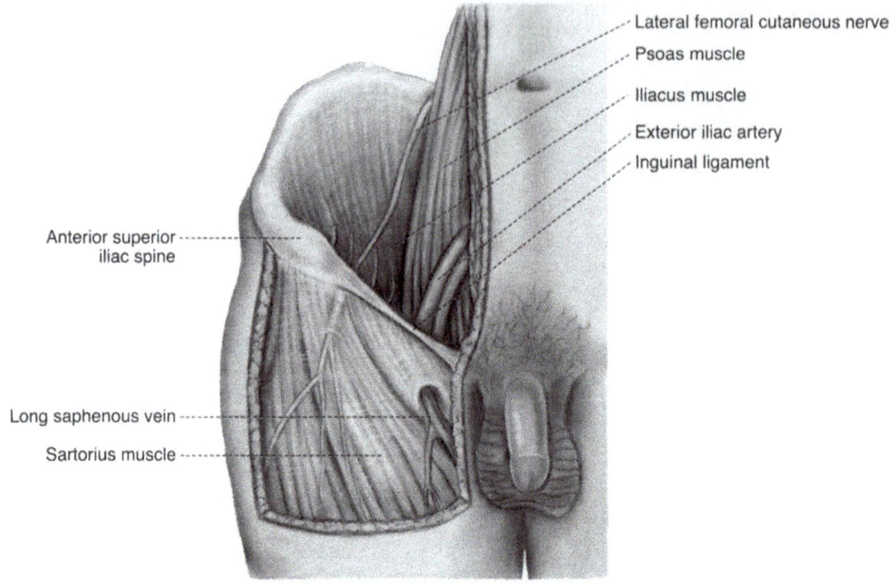

Figure 42-55. Anatomic view to demonstrate the course of the lateral femoral cutaneous nerve. Note that the nerve angulates as it leaves the pelvis at the origin of the inguinal ligament.

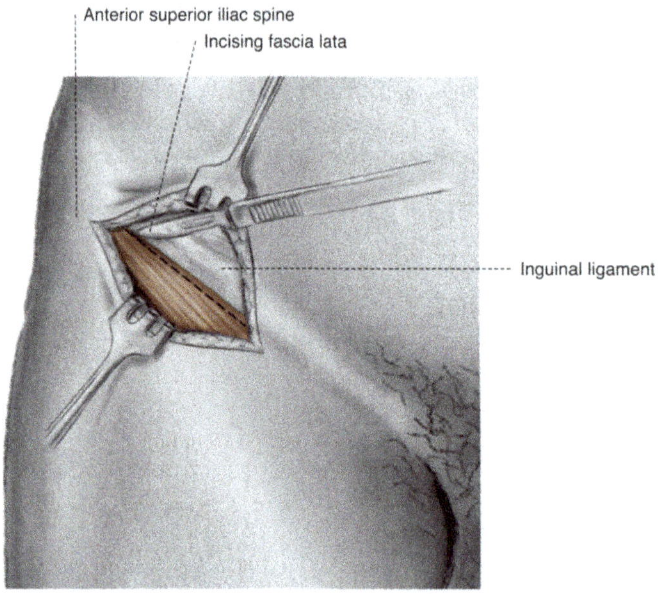

Figure 42-56. The fascia lata is incised parallel to the inguinal ligament.

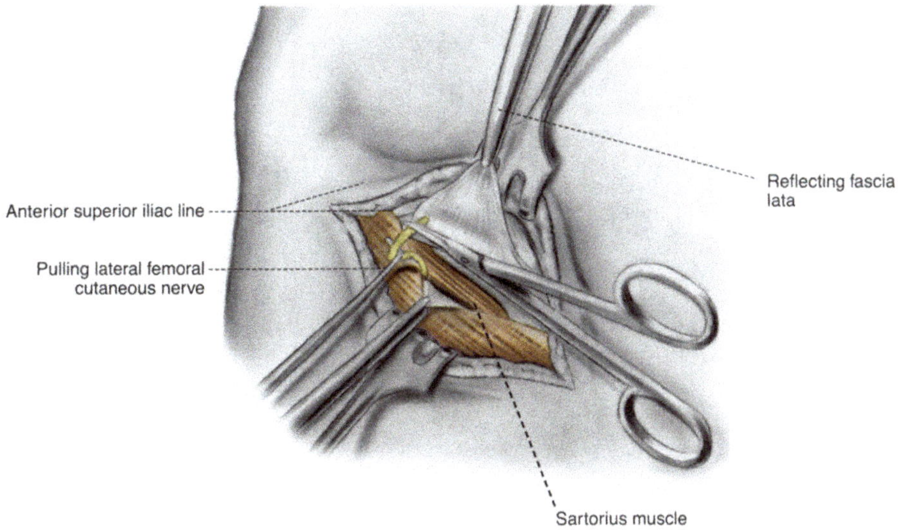

Figure 42-57. Transection of the nerve. *Observe*: 1. The nerve is identified as it passes through a triangle formed by the anterior superior iliac spine and the two origins of the inguinal ligament. 2. Traction is applied to the nerve prior to transection.

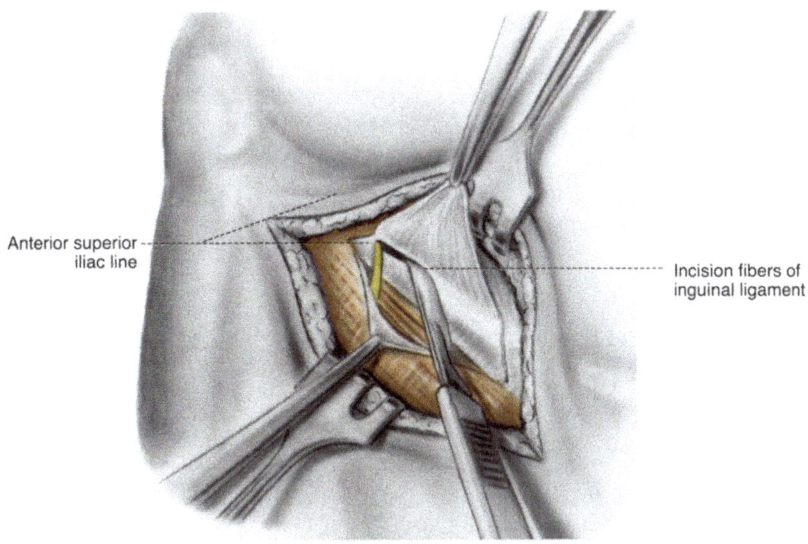

Figure 42-58. Transposition. By transecting the attachment of the inguinal ligament to the iliacus fascia, the nerve can easily be transposed several centimeters medially on the iliopsoas muscle.

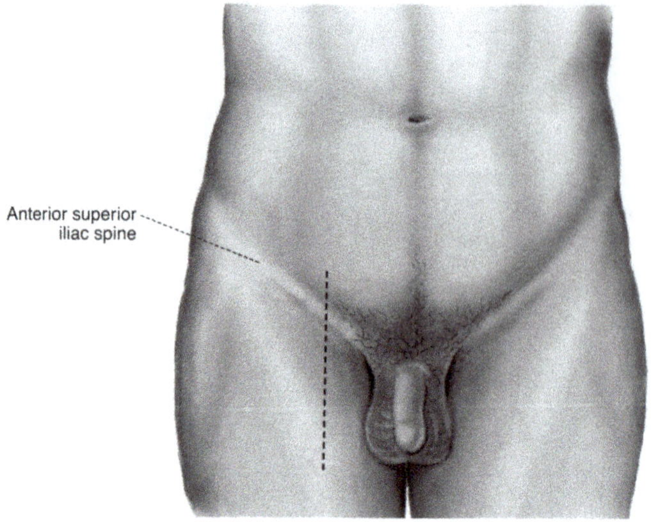

Figure 42-59. Exposure of the femoral nerve. The incision is made from the mid-portion of the inguinal ligament downward following the medial border of the sartorius muscle.

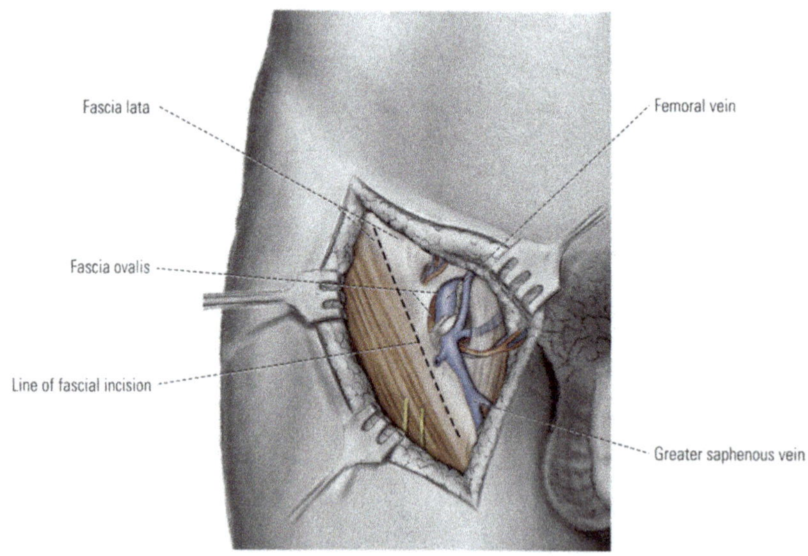

Figure 42-60. Camper's fascia has been incised and retracted. A *T*-shaped fascial incision of the falciform margin of the fossa ovalis and the fascia lata is made parallel to the sartorius muscle.

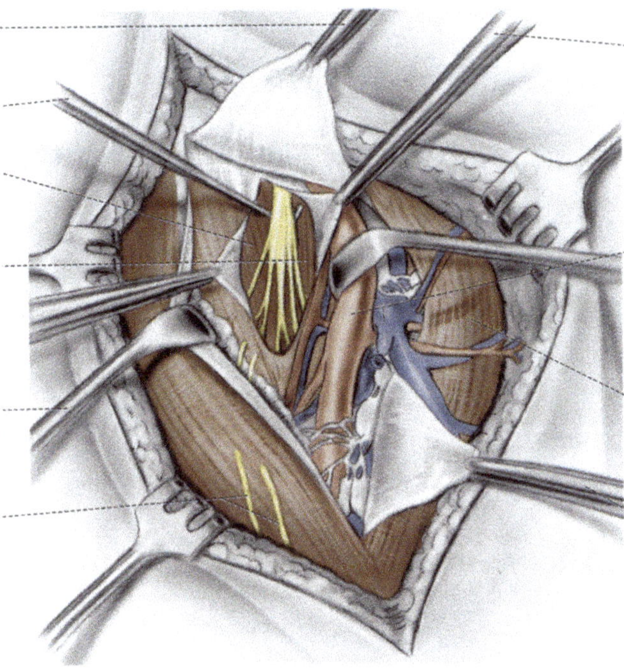

Figure 42-61. The iliacus fascia (deep leaf of the fascia lata) must be incised to expose the femoral nerve in the groove between the psoas and iliacus muscle.

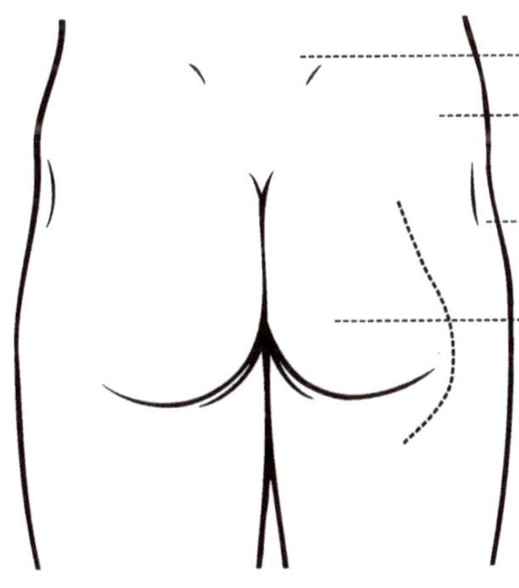

Figure 42-62. Exposure of the sciatic nerve at the sciatic notch. The incision is made from above the level of the greater trochanter medially to below the insertion of the gluteus maximus muscle at the mid-thigh.

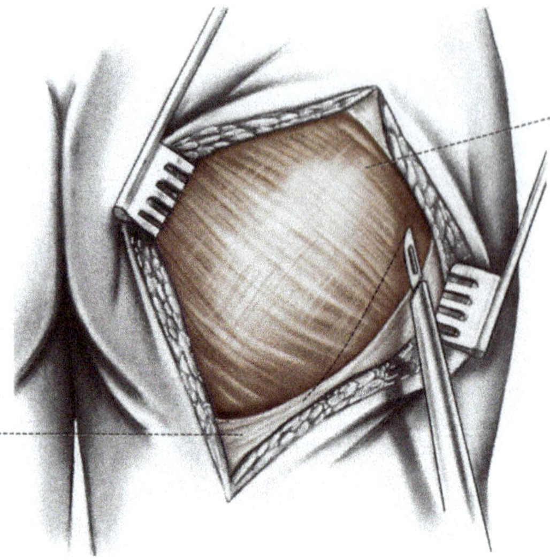

Figure 42-63. **The gluteus maximus muscle is transected close to its insertion into the iliotibial band of the fascia lata.**

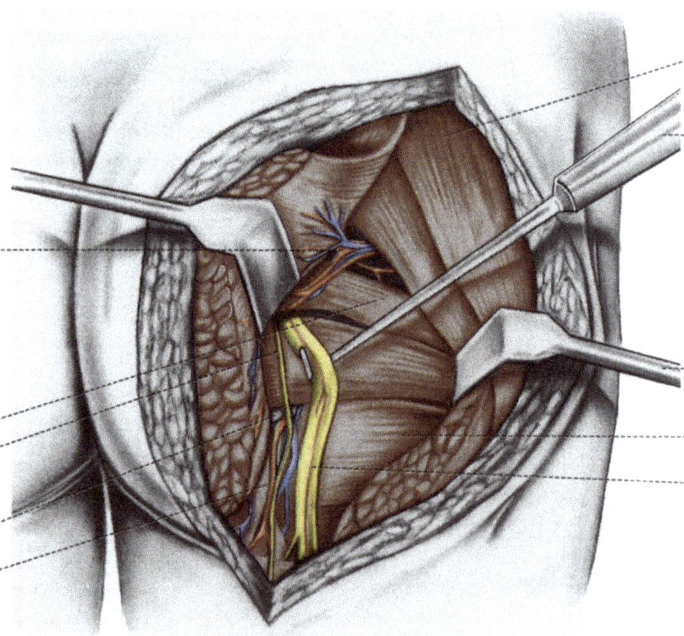

Figure 42-64. **An important arterial supply to the nerve is from the inferior gluteal and medial circumflex femoral arteries. 2. The ischial tuberosity separates the greater and lesser sciatic notches.**

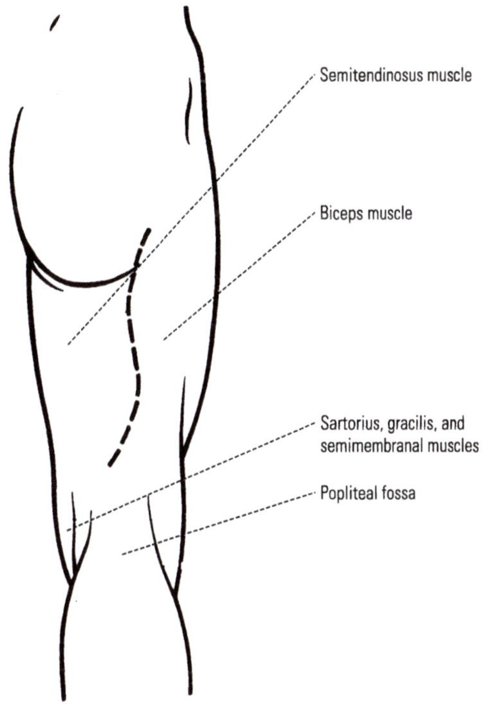

Figure 42-65. Exposure of the sciatic nerve in the thigh: incision. Superiorly the incision curves laterally at the gluteal fold and inferiorly it deviates medially as the popliteal fossa is approached.

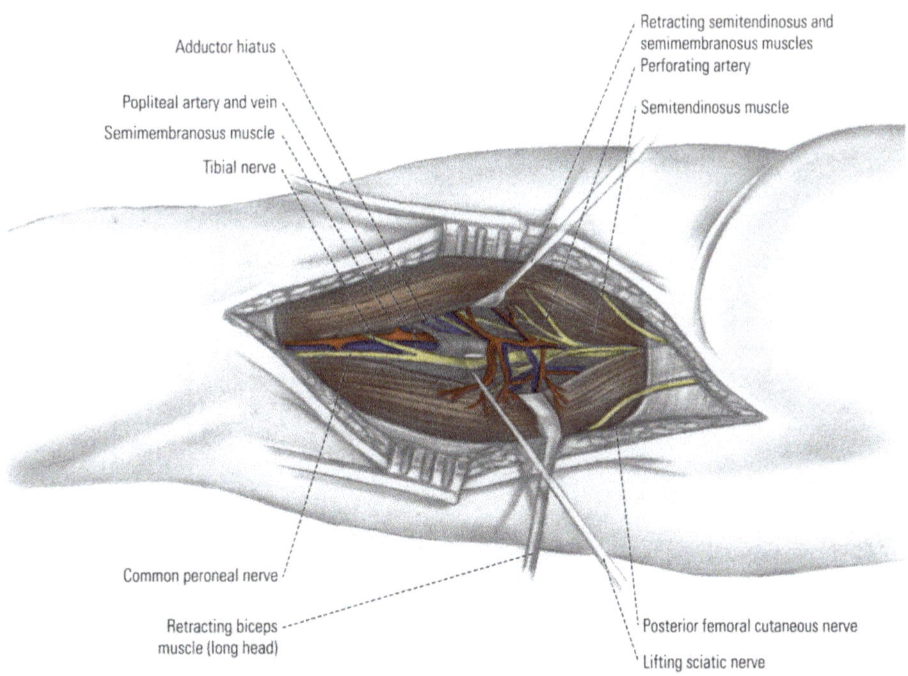

Figure 42-66. In opening the fascia, the posterior femoral cutaneous nerve has been preserved. The dissection is between the biceps femoris and semitendinosus muscles and the muscular branches to these muscles must be preserved. At the level of the adductor hiatus, the nerve is close to the femur.

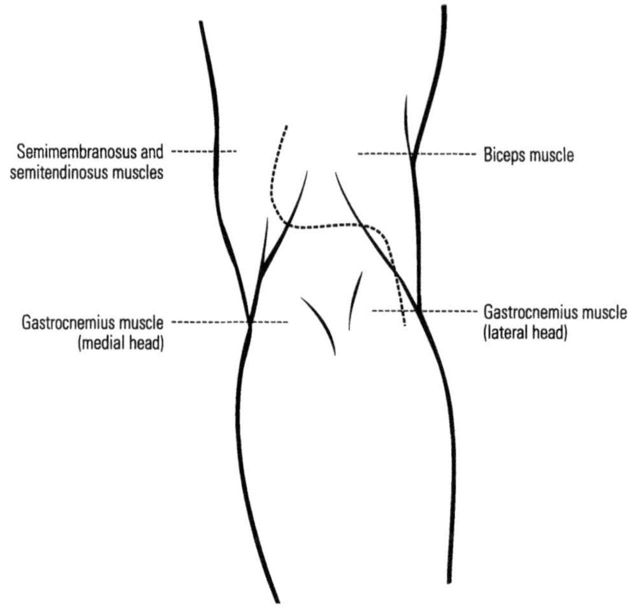

Figure 42-67. Exposure of the tibial and common peroneal nerves at the popliteal fossa: incision. The *Z*-shaped incision allows for healing without contracture.

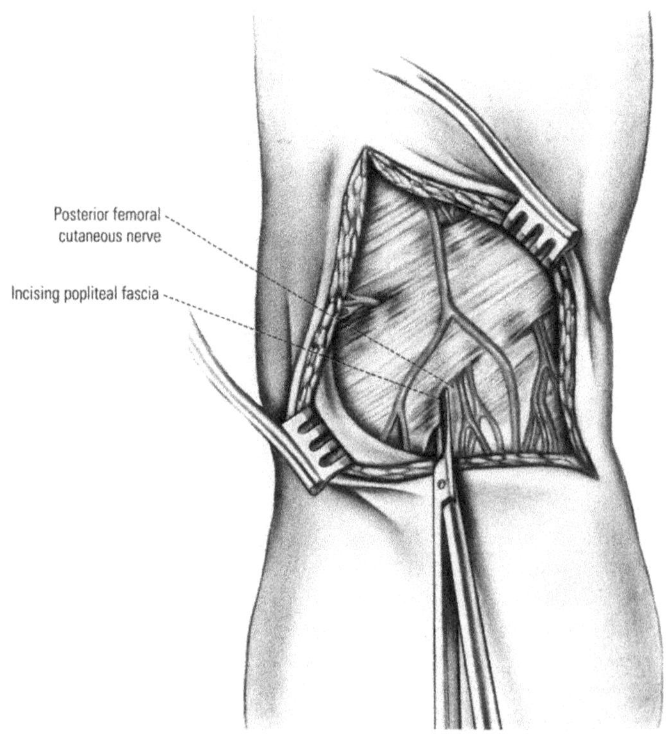

Figure 42-68. The posterior femoral cutaneous nerve is identified and preserved.

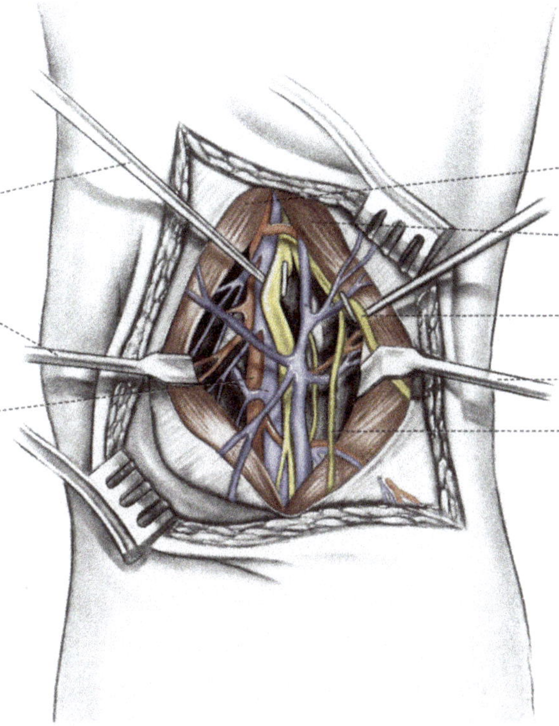

Figure 42-69. The common peroneal nerve follows the tendon of the biceps femoris muscle along the lateral margin of the popliteal space. It gives origin to the lateral sural cutaneous nerve as it crosses the lateral head of the gastrocnemius muscle. The tibial nerve proceeds inferiorly directly in the midline at the lateral side of the popliteal vein.

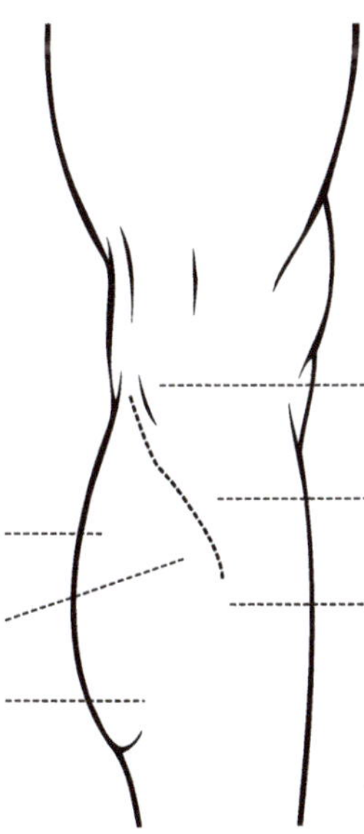

Figure 42-70. Exposure of the common peroneal nerve. This skin incision can be used as an inferior extension of the popliteal fossa incision shown previously.

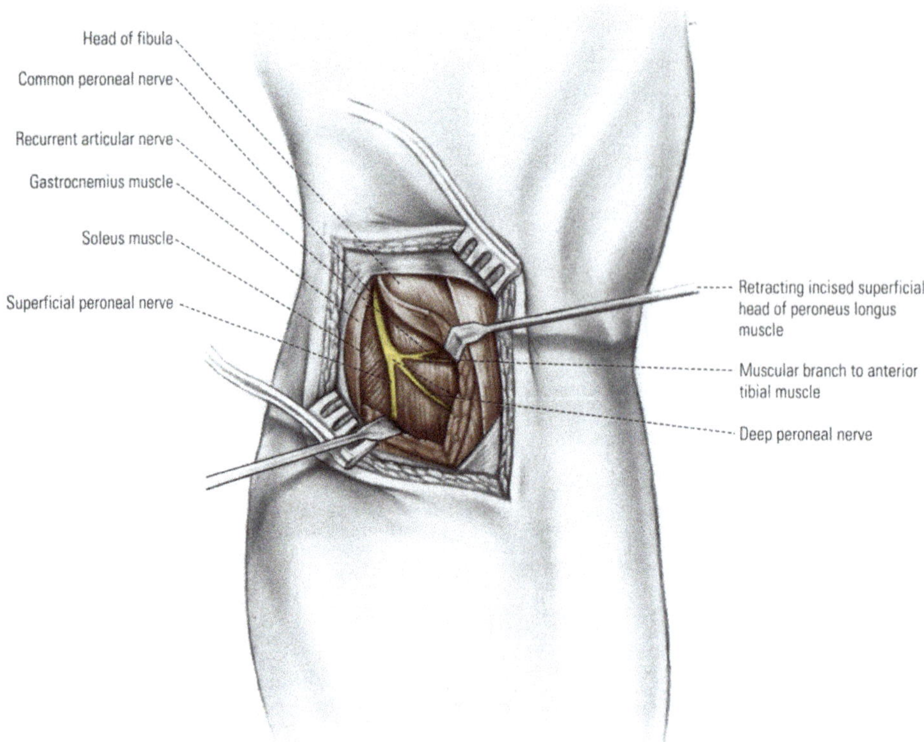

Figure 42-71. The common peroneal nerve crosses the fibers of the gastrocnemius and soleus muscles arising from the head of the fibula. It then passes between the two heads of the peroneus longus muscle where it divides.

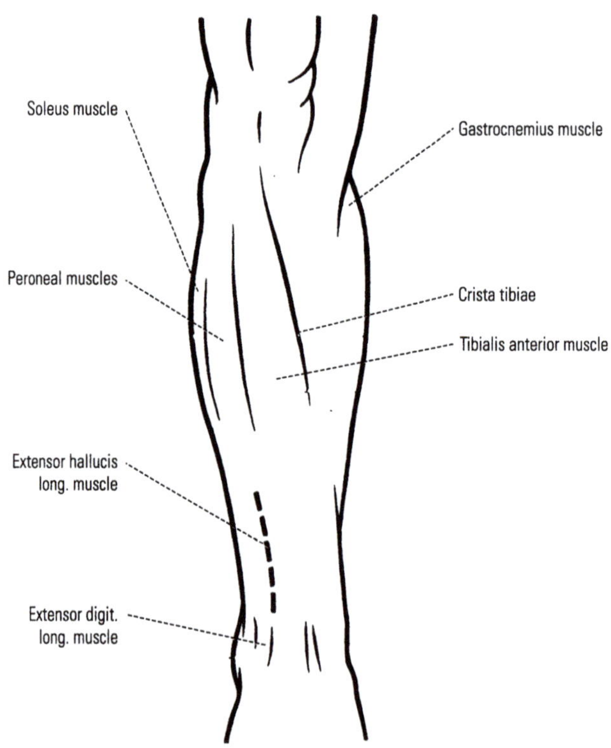

Figure 42-72. Exposure of the deep peroneal nerve in the leg. The skin incision is made between the anterior tibial and extensor hallucis longus muscles. This incision is used for the anterior tibial syndrome.

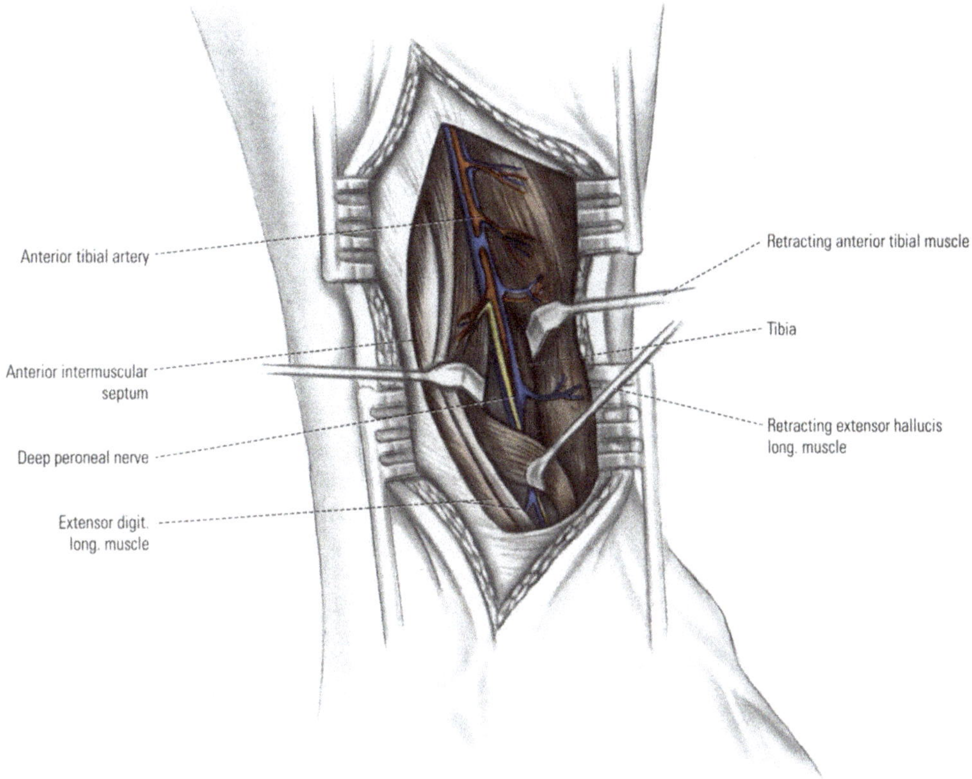

Figure 42-73. Note the relationship of the deep peroneal nerve to the lateral surface of the tibia and the overlying extensor hallucis longus muscle. The intimate relationship between nerve and artery is shown. Nutrient branches must be preserved.

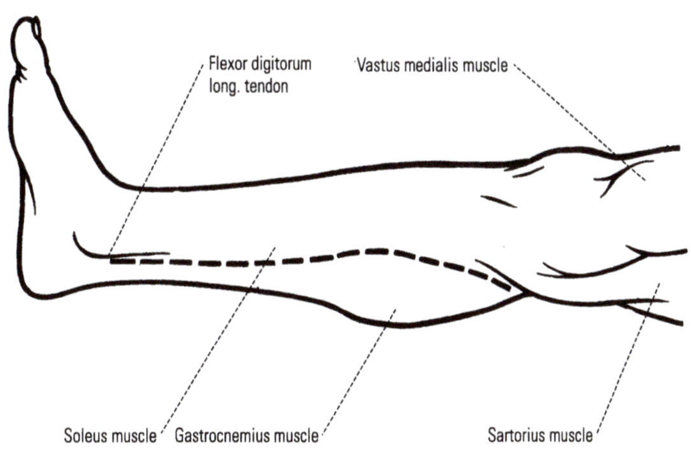

Figure 42-74. Exposure of the tibial nerve in the leg. The skin incision is made along the medial border of the gastrocnemius and soleus muscles. A posterior incision is contraindicated because the fan-like arrangement of the muscles prevents muscle splitting without destruction of the muscle tissue.

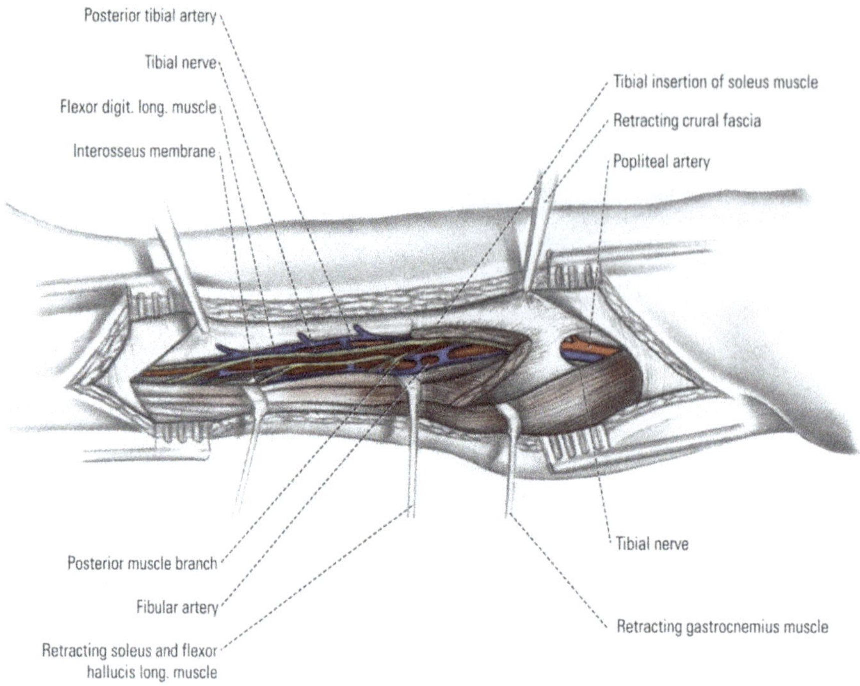

Figure 42-75. Dissection is between the soleus and flexor digitorum longus muscles. The flexor digitorum longus muscle is freed at its origin from the interosseus membrane.

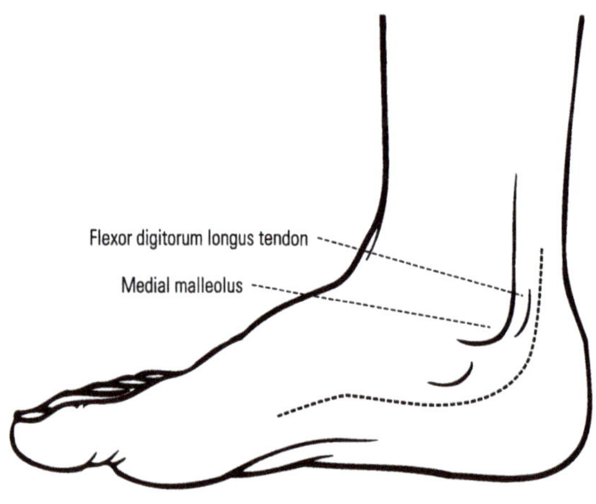

Figure 42-76. Exposure of the medial and lateral plantar nerves. The skin incision is made along the flexor digitorum longus tendon and is curved anteriorly along the medial surface of the navicular bone. The incision stays well above the sole of the foot.

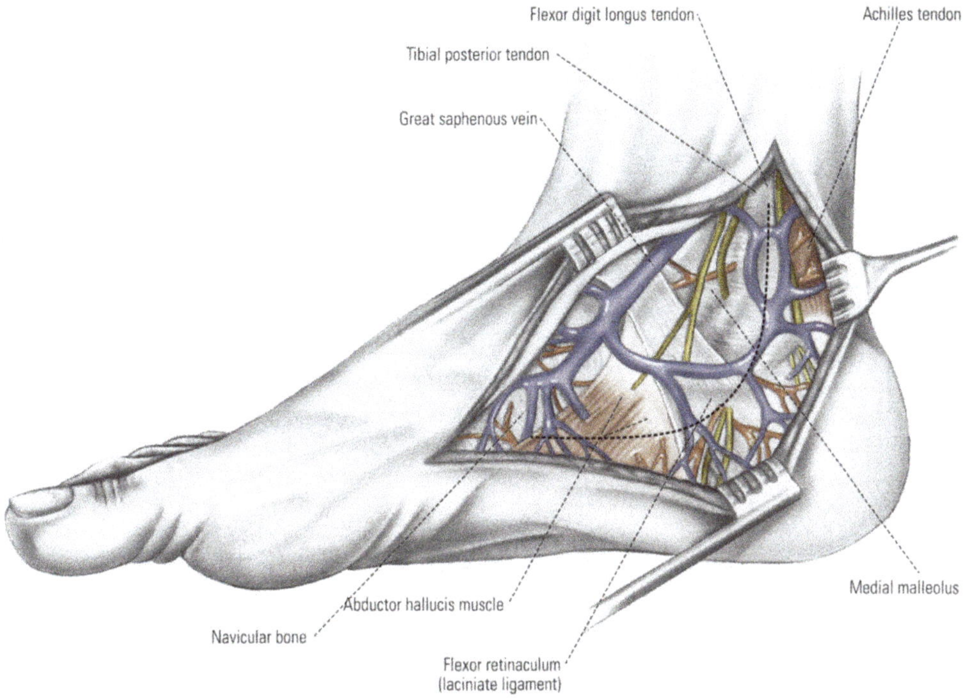

Figure 42-77. The incision of the flexor retinaculum is made in the same direction as the skin incision.

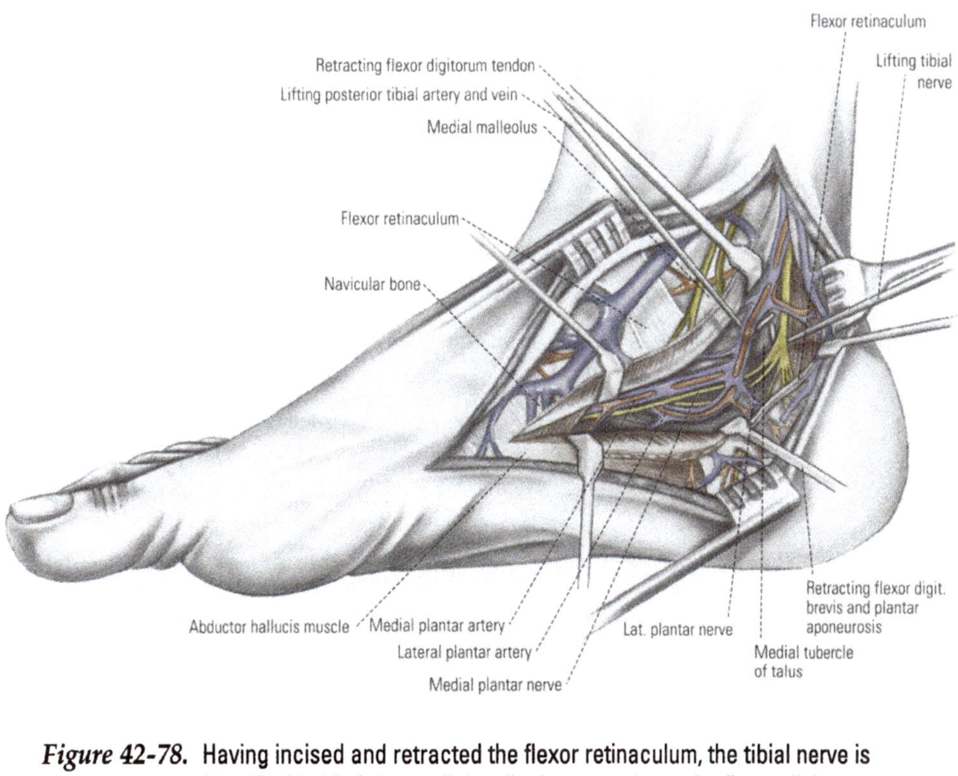

Figure 42-78. Having incised and retracted the flexor retinaculum, the tibial nerve is identified behind the medial malleolus posterior to the flexor digitorum longus tendon. The medial and lateral plantar arteries lie within the fork of the medial and lateral plantar nerves. The flexor digitorum brevis muscle provides a soft cushion for the vessels and nerves.

CHAPTER

43

Hypoglossal-Facial Anastomosis

Paralysis of the facial nerve causes a severe cosmetic deformity. Following intracranial operations in which the facial nerve is found to be irreparably damaged, an early nerve-crossing operation should be done to restore tone to the facial muscles as soon as possible. When the status of the nerve lesion intracranially is unknown, several months of clinical observation with electrical testing should be allowed for spontaneous reinnervation to take place.

The hypoglossal-facial anastomosis is preferred to the accessory-facial combination primarily because of the extensive muscular atrophy of the upper trapezius and sternocleidomastoid muscles, which seems to bother most patients more than hemiatrophy of the tongue. In addition, if the descendens hypoglossi nerve is anastomosed to the distal hypoglossal nerve, the atrophy may be minimal in some patients. It also appears that there are fewer adaptive readjustment difficulties with use of the hypoglossal nerve.

Following hypoglossal-facial anastomosis, the prognosis for return of tone to the facial muscles is excellent in those patients who have had early surgery. This return of tone is crucial for cosmesis and restores a great deal of symmetry to the face at rest. The degree to which voluntary control returns is dependent to a large extent on the motivation of the patient.

This procedure is performed with the patient in the supine position with the head turned slightly away from the operative side. A 6- to 8-cm skin incision is made from 2 cm above the mastoid process obliquely down the neck to 2 cm behind the angle of the jaw (Fig. 43-1). The platysma muscle is divided along the same line and retracted (Fig. 43-2). The tendinous insertion of the sternocleidomastoid muscle is incised over the mastoid process as shown in Figure 43-2, and using a periosteal elevator the tip of the mastoid process is denuded of all tendinous insertions. The deep fascia is incised along the line of the initial incision (Fig. 43-3) while taking care to avoid the capsule of the parotid gland, which often reaches surprisingly far posteriorly. The tail of the parotid gland with its capsule intact is then gently retracted. The tip of the mastoid process is rongeured away, and any exposed mastoid air cells are closed with bone wax. The posterior belly of the digastric is identified as it leaves its origin at the mastoid notch of the temporal bone and is retracted downward and posteriorly. This allows exposure of the facial nerve as it leaves the stylomastoid foramen (Fig. 43-4). On retracting the posterior belly of the digastric, a small branch of the nerve to this muscle may be recognized as it enters the superomedial aspect of the muscle and traced proximally to the parent nerve trunk. In exposing the facial nerve there is a tendency on the part of inexperienced surgeons to search too deeply for the facial nerve, particularly when the tail of the parotid gland has been elevated, since this may also make the facial nerve more superficial. A nerve stimulator may be of aid, especially if the facial nerve has been injured at the stylomastoid foramen and the nerve has to be identified distally. Having identified the nerve, it is divided at the stylomastoid foramen

(Fig. 43-4). Bleeding from the foramen is easily controlled by inserting a short probe and electrocoagulating the small vessels accompanying the nerve.

The simplest method of exposing the hypoglossal nerve is to retract the sternocleidomastoid muscle laterally and expose the carotid sheath at the lower portion of the incision. The hypoglossal nerve is easily identified as it turns forward at this level, loops around the occipital artery, and passes between the internal carotid artery and jugular vein. It is freed upward to the point where it enters the carotid sheath. As the nerve hooks around the occipital artery it gives off the descendens hypoglossi. The hypoglossal nerve is dissected distally until it enters the submandibular triangle beneath the digastric muscle, where it is sharply divided. The descendens hypoglossi is followed down the carotid sheath as far as possible and is also divided sharply (Fig. 43-5).

The proximal hypoglossal nerve is then approximated to the distal facial nerve either above or below the posterior belly of the digastric muscle. Because these nerves are small, this anastomosis should be performed using magnification. The technique of nerve suture does not differ from that described in the chapter on peripheral nerves (see chapter 42).

To put frosting on the cake, the descendens hypoglossi can be anastomosed to the distal hypoglossal nerve (Fig. 43-6). This adds only a few minutes to the operating time and may prevent some of the glossal hemiatrophy.

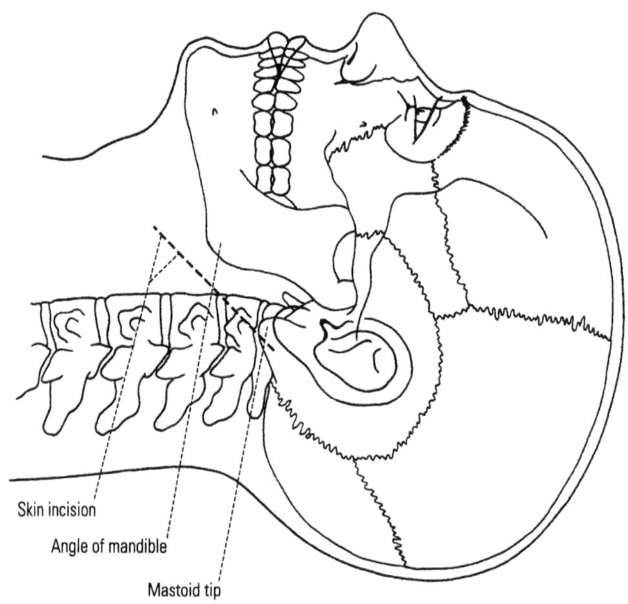

Figure 43-1. Skin incision. A 12-cm oblique incision is made from 2 cm above the mastoid process to 2 cm behind the angle of the mandible.

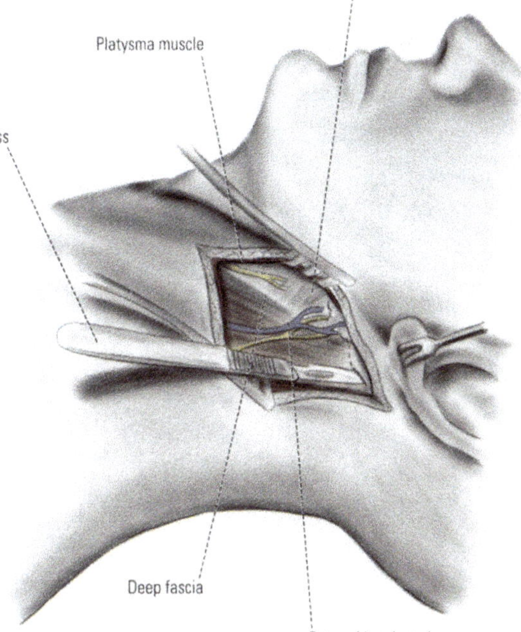

Figure 43-2. Operative exposure after incision and retraction of platysma muscle. Note 1) incision of tendinous insertion of sternocleidomastoid muscle over the mastoid process, and 2) exposure of deep cervical fascia.

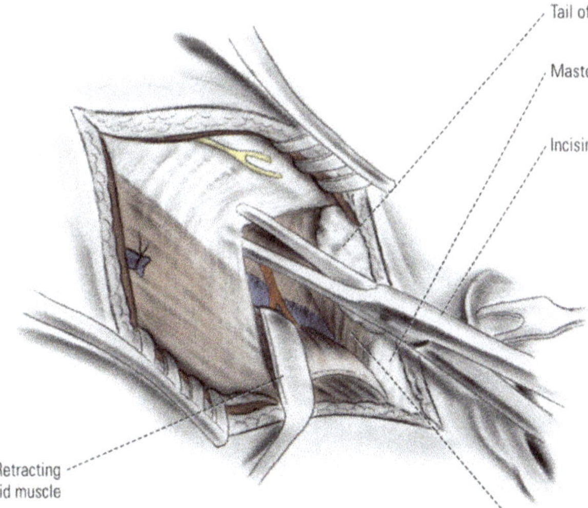

Figure 43-3. Incision of deep fascia parallel to the anterior border of the sternocleidomastoid muscle. The tail of the parotid gland is carefully retracted anteriorly. The posterior belly of the digastric muscle is identified at its origin from the mastoid process.

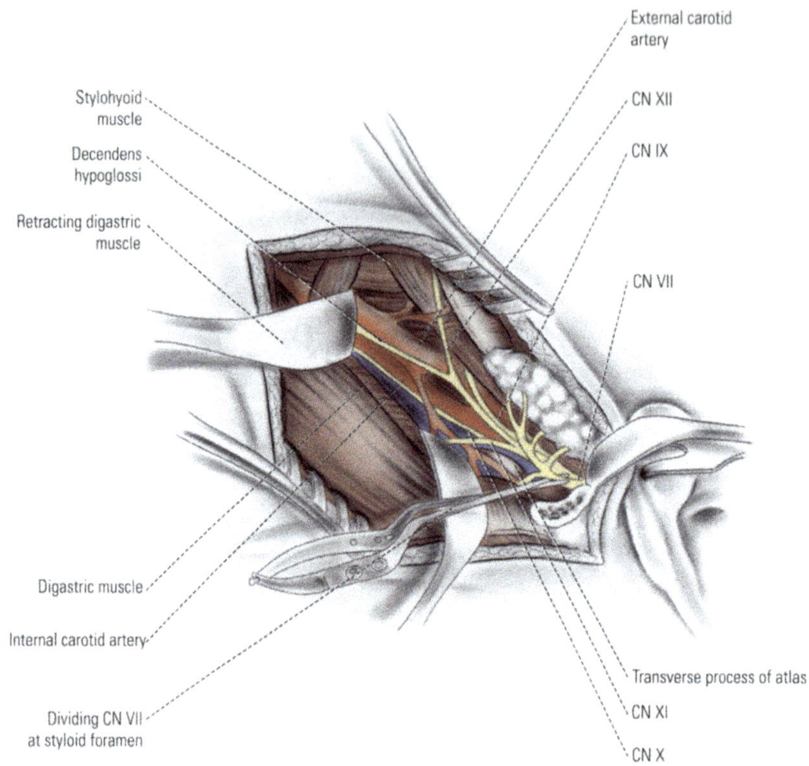

Figure 43-4. **Exposure of the facial nerve. The tip of the mastoid process is removed to help in exposure of cranial nerve VII. All nerves and vascular structures are anterior to the transverse process of the atlas.**

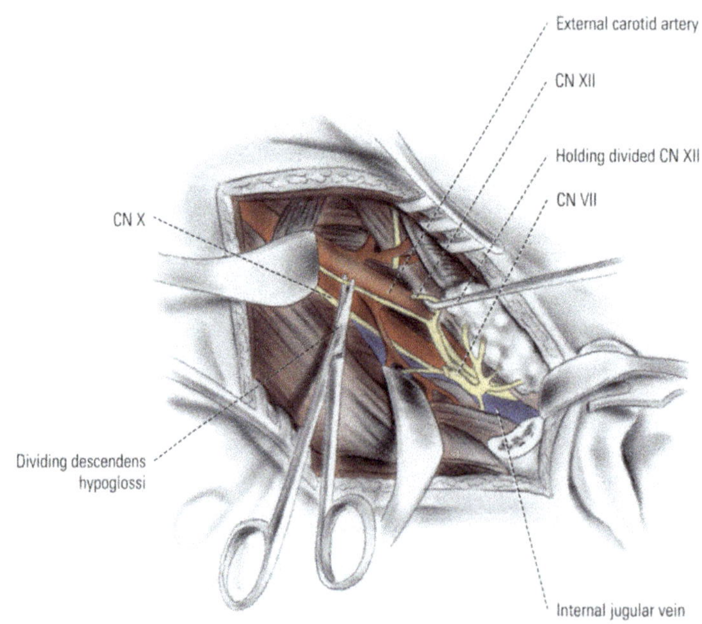

Figure 43-5. **Exposure and division of hypoglossal nerve. The posterior belly of the digastric muscle is pulled downward to expose the distal portion of the hypoglossal nerve traversing the external carotid artery.**

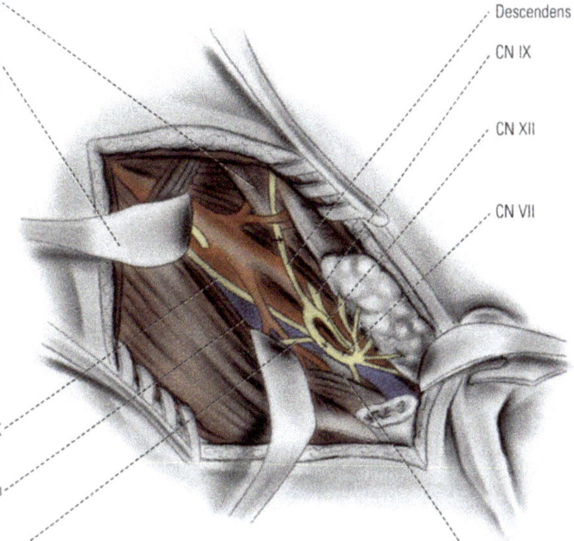

Figure 43-6. Relationship following anastomoses. The hypoglossal nerve is brought medial to the digastric muscle and anastomosed with the facial nerve. The descendens hypoglossi is sutured to the distal end of the hypoglossal nerve.

Index

Note: Page numbers in *italics* indicate illustrations.

D

E

F

G

H

I

J

K

L

M

N

T

U

V

W

Y

GPSR Compliance
The European Union's (EU) General Product Safety Regulation (GPSR) is a set of rules that requires consumer products to be safe and our obligations to ensure this.

If you have any concerns about our products, you can contact us on

ProductSafety@springernature.com

In case Publisher is established outside the EU, the EU authorized representative is:

Springer Nature Customer Service Center GmbH
Europaplatz 3
69115 Heidelberg, Germany

www.ingramcontent.com/pod-product-compliance
Ingram Content Group UK Ltd.
Pitfield, Milton Keynes, MK11 3LW, UK
UKHW051040091026
15624UKWH00011B/605
* 9 7 8 0 3 8 7 9 8 5 3 6 7 *